DEMAND UNIVERSAL HEALTHCARE (DUH!)

Compiled by

Lynn O'Connell

D1400750

DEDICATION

Family, friends and social-media followers of Sue Saltmarsh (26 January 1956 – 18 December 2021) celebrate the joy and passion of her life in advocacy, whether it be her time with Chicago's Hubbard Street Dance Company, the TPAN AIDS community, or the many years she spent as an avid activist for Single Payer healthcare with the founding of DUH (Demand Universal Healthcare) in 2010. In 2013-2015, she and fellow activists drove throughout Illinois and Ohio and the East and West coasts with DUH events in numerous cities – highlighted by DUH's Healthcare Justice March on August 1, 2015 on Washington DC's National Mall. Endorsing candidates became DUH's focus from 2017 thru 2020, and the entire year of 2021 then found Sue transitioning DUH into PEP (https://www.peopleenergizingpolitics.org/) with the goal of dedicating 2022 to endorsing political candidates nationwide who advocate for Universal Health Care and Social Justice. (See Sue and several of her friends in this short video - https://youtu.be/BoiarllLjD4.) Thank you, Sue, for being such an inspiration to so many!

DISCLAIMER

I am not a professional healthcare analyst, simply a passionate advocate for "Medicare for All" wishing to stimulate conversation and advocacy. My intent in publishing this book is to direct students and other readers to the wealth of information written online and in social media by experts.

Articles included in this reference book represent a wide array of subjects and opinions meant to provide the reader with detailed information about our current medical care system in the United States versus "Medicare for All" (aka Universal Health Care).

At the time of publication, the website URLs in this book were active. I make no warranties that their information is free from misstatements or omissions. Multiple efforts have been made to trace all copyright holders but if any have not responded the author will be pleased to include any necessary credits in any subsequent reprint or edition.

FOREWORD

I am not an author or a scholar. I am a rather typical U.S. citizen who graduated from high school in Moorestown, NJ in 1966 and attended The College of Wooster in Ohio for two years before earning a B.A. at The University of Minnesota. My plan was to become a social worker. Hence, in my junior year, I took a class about the fairly new Medicare program that was signed into law in 1965 to provide health coverage for older Americans. At the time, Medicare only included parts A and B. (Compare this to University of Pennsylvania's current "Health Care Innovation" coursework: https://catalog.upenn.edu/courses/hcin/.)

Soon after I was married, I worked in retail management and had to find health insurance on my own since none was provided by my employer. The first time I needed it they paid my claim and then cancelled my policy. After that, I remained uninsured for many years – as was typical for many (invincible) young people. My husband was a veteran and therefore had VA health coverage. It served him very well on two occasions when he found himself in need of medical care at the VA hospital in Minneapolis that was staffed by excellent doctors from the University of Minnesota.

After moving back to New Jersey in 1984 and finding jobs that provided employer-based health insurance, somehow my self-employed husband skipped going through the process of re-registering for VA health insurance, so I maintained a family plan while he traveled internationally several times a year on business. Once I switched from W-2 employment to contract work, the cost of a family plan became untenable and he once again obtained VA coverage.

In 2010, I started becoming curious about "Medicare for All". I searched online and discovered two national organizations: Healthcare-NOW and Health Care for America Now (HCAN). One turned out to advocate for true "Medicare for All" while the other (HCAN) gave private insurance companies a central role to continue to seek to enhance their profit.

Locally, a "Medicare for All" advocacy group in Philadelphia advertised a film event for the showing of "The Healthcare Movie" narrated by Kiefer Sutherland, British-born Canadian actor who is the grandson of the former Premier of Saskatchewan Tommy Douglas (who is widely credited for bringing universal health care to Canada). We viewed the film, continued to attend meetings and rallies, expanded our research, and began to support various organizations advocating for "Medicare for All".

Every year between October and December we are subjected to endless television commercials determined to convince seniors to switch from Medicare B plus a "supplemental" policy to Medicare Advantage ("Medicare C"), whose extra benefits are partially funded by brazenly using taxpayer money. One of the newer ads shows a very resistant "Martha" who refuses to make the phone call – until she is told that the call is FREE. Are (we) seniors that dumb?

And the latest ads are ramping up their focus on having some of your money refunded that is deducted from your monthly Social Security check – but you don't know if you qualify unless you make the call! It is time to demand universal health care and have $0 deducted from our Social Security income. "Medicare for All" would level the playing field and end the advertising pressure from the for-profit insurance companies who provide no useful purpose – they simply bombard us with advertising, take our money and pay our medical bills after first taking their profits and often slowing down the entire system with confusion, obstacles and denials.

The purpose of this book is to act as a reference for others who wish to better understand our current health care system and hopefully "join the choir" to advocate for the comprehensiveness and simplicity of "Medicare for All". It directs the reader (and hopefully the media) to some of the wealth of information on-line and in social media – and to many of the experts who advocate for "Medicare for All".

Personally, I envision a "Medicare for All Smart Card" in your wallet issued once in a lifetime. We are often subjected to endless advertising and required to enroll one year at a time while being told to guess if/when we'll suffer what kind of medical challenges and need which prescriptions. It is time to stop channeling people through traffic lanes: The ACA, Federal Employees, Employer-Based, Medicare B + Supplemental, Medicare Advantage, Indian Health Service, CHIP, Medicaid, VA Health Coverage, World Trade Center Health Program, COBRA, the uninsured, etc. "Medicare for All" would flow with the health challenges you experience at any given time in your life. Your medical issues would be strictly between you and your medical providers.

Will it be abused? I think most people have better ways to spend their time than going to the doctor, and would only use the privilege of "Medicare for All" when appropriate.

Why must many of us select our health insurance plan every year? We are issued a Social Security card and a Medicare card once in our lifetime. E-Z Pass doesn't ask us to tell them every year which bridges and toll roads we will take for the next 12 months. Selecting a health insurance plan and prescription drug plan every year is most likely because it gives the huge for-profit health insurance companies the opportunity every 12 months to convince us to switch to their plans from their competition's. How is this in the interest of simplicity, continuity and cost-effectiveness? Why is our health care system catering to for-profit insurance companies? It should be about US not THEM.

How should it be paid for? By equitable taxation after extremely careful analysis by economists, tax experts and our Congress – taking into consideration the current payments made to the multitude of programs now in existence. Let's identify all current payments: those through tax revenues and those outside tax revenues, such as deductions from social security, paychecks, co-pays, etc. And let's address the hostility by those who feel entitled to comprehensive health care while insisting it should be denied to those they believe to be unentitled to the same.

President Biden and his administration praise the many award-winning economists who support his "Build Back Better" human infrastructure plan. They (and members of Congress) also need to pay attention to the many award-winning economists who explain why "Medicare for All" will be less costly for our country while eliminating frustrating and life-threatening gaps in coverage. There are too many in his administration who have personal interests in seeing the for-profit health insurance industry continue to make huge profits off our current system.

President Biden's White House inadvertently made a strong case recently for the simplicity and cost-effectiveness of "Medicare for All" by outlining a new White House plan, anticipated to take effect in mid-January 2022, which directs Americans to purchase rapid, over-the-counter coronavirus tests and then submit the receipts to their insurance companies so they can be reimbursed.

The plan sparked immediate criticism, given that it will force people to navigate the cumbersome private insurance system to get a refund on tests that remain expensive in the U.S. more than a year and a half into the pandemic.

During a press briefing, NPR reporter Mara Liasson asked White House Press Secretary Jen Psaki why the U.S. continues to lag behind the United Kingdom, Germany, South Korea, and other countries in making rapid Covid-19 tests easily affordable and accessible to all who want or need one – a solution that has long been part of other nations' efforts to combat the pandemic and an objective that has gained importance amid fears of another surge fueled by the Omicron variant.

Psaki's response was viewed as "dismissive" and "out of touch". She rejected the idea of having the federal government mail free Covid-19 tests to households across the United States. "Should we just send one to every American? Then what happens if every American has one test? How much does that cost, and then what happens after that?".

Craig Spencer, the director of global health in emergency medicine at Columbia University Irving Medical tweeted "We spend billions and billions on vaccines that we would never consider charging for. Tests should be no different.". (The solution in this example would be to allow every American to take their valid-for-life "Medicare for All" card to a pharmacy and obtain free tests. Psaki's suggestion that the federal government mail to every household free tests "that might go unused" is yet another irrational attack on a universal healthcare program that is long past due in the U.S.)

In his book "The Case for Medicare for All", Gerald Friedman (University of Massachusetts, Amherst economics professor) closes by saying "Medicare for All will save money and make the United States a richer and happier country. We know that it is the right thing to do; we are only waiting for a political movement and strategy. Let us begin.".

OR – joining up with some of the organizations listed here – let us expand the advocacy and finally make this 100-year-old effort a reality.

AND – Contact your members of Congress in The Senate and The House of Representatives by email on their websites or by phoning the U.S. Capitol switchboard (202.224.3121) where an operator will connect you directly to the office you request.

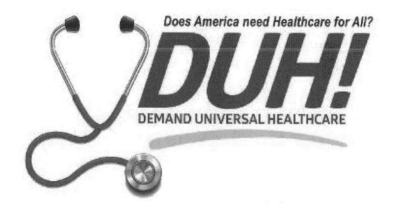

Does America need Healthcare for All?

DUH!

DEMAND UNIVERSAL HEALTHCARE

CHAPTERS

NOW IS THE TIME

For more than 100 years, since 1906 during the administration of Theodore Roosevelt, various proposals have been put forward for Universal Healthcare in The United States of America. And no President, however well-intentioned, has been able to bring the Great Equalizer of Universal Healthcare into law.

Now, with COVID-19 laying bare the weaknesses in our Public Health System, we must press hard for the Biden Administration to take advantage of the Democrat majority in The Senate and The House of Representatives to pass the necessary legislation to put

"a smart-card in every wallet"

An April 2020 Hill-HarrisX survey shows that 69% of registered voters support providing Medicare (we call it Universal Healthcare) to every American (https://pnhp.org/news/two-thirds-of-voters-support-providing-medicare-to-every-american/).

If you read no further than this, please pen a letter without delay to:

President Joseph R. Biden
c/o The White House
1600 Pennsylvania Avenue NW
Washington, DC   20500

and urge President Biden to make Universal Healthcare ("a card in every wallet") a reality. Tell him your personal story about dealing with our current (user-unfriendly) health insurance system.

President Biden rejected Universal Healthcare ("Medicare for All") as too expensive during his campaign and his run against his opponent for the presidency. Yet on January 7, 2022 he stated "Having healthcare is about having peace of mind.". It is time for him to acknowledge that – even with The ACA ("Obamacare") and a Public Option – our healthcare system DOES NOT WORK for millions of Americans. Furthermore, it is time for President Biden to use his knowledge of the workings (obstructionism) of Congress to make Medicare for All a reality.

During the Progressive Era (1901-1909), President Theodore Roosevelt was in power and, although he supported health insurance because he believed that no country could be strong whose people were sick and poor, most of the initiative for reform took place outside of government.

During our COVID crisis of 2020, the weaknesses have been further exacerbated with lay-offs that have caused millions of Americans to lose their health insurance. This impacts not only the employee, but every member of the family.

The FY 2021 defense budget was composed of two parts: a base budget of $671 billion and a warfighting, or Overseas Contingency Operations (OCO), budget of an additional $69 billion. (See: **https://www.defense.gov/Explore/Spotlight/FY2021-Defense-Budget**/) Each year, a massive defense budget is routinely passed by Congress. Yet when the issue of Universal Healthcare is raised, demands are immediately made that its costs be justified. American lives lost to poor healthcare are as surely lost as those lost in military conflicts – and we must value reasonable expenditures to minimize both by honest discussions of the true cost of "Medicare for All".

Think of the children being treated for serious health conditions at hospitals like Shriners and St. Jude's. Does the $19/month donated by so many Americans really need to go for medical treatment when it could instead be utilized for research, family transportation and lodging?

Think of infants born with life-threatening illnesses that require expensive treatment from the moment of their birth. Should their parents, already overwhelmed, be burdened with setting up a "Go Fund Me" page to try to stay financially solvent when that newborn could have been issued a universal healthcare card at birth?

Let President Biden know of your own stories, and of the complexities of shopping for (or renewing) your health insurance every year. Ask him why it needs to be so complicated. Ask why Seniors must have Medicare deducted monthly from their (often modest) Social Security checks.

CEOs and stockholders of for-profit health insurance companies are getting more wealthy every day while millions of Americans experience anxiety or spiral into debt trying to keep up with medical bills (most of which are unknown until the invoice comes in the mail). According to **https://www.fiercehealthcare.com/payer/unitedhealth-s-wichmann-to-earn-2-years-salary-bonuses-post-retirement**, UnitedHealth Group CEO David Wichman's total compensation in 2019 was $18.9 million according to the most recent proxy filing.

This book covers many topics – and many were selected to illustrate just how complex – how absurd – our current healthcare system is. NOW IS THE TIME for "A CARD IN EVERY WALLET" (a hack-proof plastic card the size of a credit card and with an electronic chip tied to one's SS# rather than a quickly-tattered over-sized paper Medicare card).

It is time to simplify the system by having one central billing system, and comprehensive benefits that remove the guessing-game of annually selecting the benefits and prescriptions you individually will need. The profit-motive must be removed from healthcare.

It is time to remove healthcare from union contract negotiations and company payrolls. And it is time to end the plethora of government health programs: Medicare, Medicaid, CHIP, IHS (Indian Health Services), TRICARE, Veterans Administration Health Care, FEHB (Federal Employees Health Benefits Program), etc. – all of which are paid for not by "the government" but by our taxpayer dollars.

Those in power who oppose Universal Healthcare (aka "Medicare For All", aka "Single Payer") do not have the best interests of the majority of Americans at heart. Their objections are nothing more than excuses to maintain power and continue to concentrate wealth in the upper classes. Their excuses are just that – excuses.

- Universal Healthcare is not more costly than our current system – read our chapter on the 22 studies showing that Universal Healthcare is actually cheaper than our current system if ALL costs of our current system are honestly included. **And urge President Biden to read those same studies.**

- Calling Universal Healthcare "socialism" is a tactic that goes back as far as 1917 ("…the US entered WWI and anti-German fever rose. The government-commissioned articles denouncing "German socialist insurance" and opponents of health insurance assailed it as a "Prussian menace" inconsistent with American values."). What is so American about receiving surprise billings for medical care? What is so American about incurring huge medical bills that drive Americans into bankruptcy?

- Scaring Americans into thinking that they cannot keep their own doctor is just that – a scare tactic. Your Universal Healthcare card in your wallet would allow you to go to any doctor and any hospital of your choosing: see S. 1129 ("Medicare for All Act of 2019") and H.R. 1976 ("Medicare for All Act of 2021").

Two chapters of this book address H.R. 1976 – one chapter provides the table of contents of the actual bill as presented in Congress, while another chapter summarizes the bill in plain English. A third chapter provides the table of contents for Senator Bernie Sanders on-hold "Medicare for All" bill introduced in the Senate on 04/10/2019 (S.1129) and needing new attention. These two important bills can be viewed in their entirety at

- S.1129: **https://www.congress.gov/bill/116th-congress/senate-bill/1129/text**

- H.R. 1976: **https://www.congress.gov/bill/117th-congress/house-bill/1976/text**

NOW IS THE TIME for public pressure on President Biden and all of our Senators and Representatives in Congress.

Let's not be complacent and see the "dream" of Universal Healthcare delayed for another 100 years.

<u>True Bipartisanship & Reconciliation</u>

On March 10, 2021 U.S. Representative John Yarmuth (D-KY) said "If the Democrats organized a potluck picnic, Republicans would call it Socialism.".

In the Summer of 2020, Joe Biden pitched himself as a president who could break through Washington's hyperpartisan landscape.

By February of 2021, once the hyperpartisanship of the $1.9T Covid Relief Package seemed almost insurmountable in both Chambers of Congress, the White House began to clarify their definition of "bipartisanship", pointing out that local and state officials - including Republicans and independents, health experts and the majority of Americans - backed Biden's $1.9T Covid Relief Package. More than 400 mayors, including Republicans and independents, and local county officials sent letters to Congress urging lawmakers to pass Biden's package, which includes $350 billion in direct relief to state and local governments.

The package had the support of 75 percent of the American people, including over 50 percent of Republicans," said White House Communications Director Kate Bedingfield in early March 2021. "So we were able to pass this legislation with massive bipartisan support across the country."

(**https://www.washingtonpost.com/opinions/2021/02/10/why-dont-republicans-get-challenged-bipartisanship/**) Jennifer Rubin of The Washington Post wrote: "Biden has attracted considerable support among ordinary Republicans".

This Biden Administration policy of defining bipartisanship as "the support of 75 percent of the American people" is the standard to which HEALTHCARE (not health insurance) coverage for all citizens of the USA must be held – in other words, Medicare For All.

https://www.politifact.com/article/2021/feb/08/what-you-need-know-about-budget-reconciliation-pro/ (See hyperlink for full text and references.)

What You Need to Know about the Budget Reconciliation Process

By Louis Jacobson ; 8 February 2021

PolitiFact.com is an American nonprofit project operated by the Poynter Institute with offices in St. Petersburg, Florida, and in Washington, D.C.

Budget Reconciliation is a process for passing a certain type of fiscal legislation with just a simple majority of 51 Senate votes — rather than the 60 that would be needed if the opposition filibusters. The Democrats have 51 votes if Vice President Kamala Harris is called upon as a tie-breaker. So if Democrats stay united, they can push Biden's agenda through.

The lower vote threshold has made reconciliation the go-to strategy for both parties in recent years. It was used by Republicans during the Trump administration to try — unsuccessfully — to repeal the Affordable Care Act and to enact — successfully — a big tax overhaul bill.

The budget reconciliation process was written into the Congressional Budget Act of 1974 as a tool for lawmakers, but wasn't used until 1980. Since then, it's been used to produce a law 25 times, all but four of which were eventually signed by the president.

"The purpose of the reconciliation process is to enhance Congress's ability to bring existing spending, revenue, and debt limit laws into compliance with current fiscal priorities and goals established in the annual budget resolution," the Congressional Research Service has written.

In the big picture, the idea of budget reconciliation is to use a two-step process for federal budgeting.

The first step is to pass an identical budget resolution through both chambers of Congress that includes "reconciliation instructions" — guidance for committees about how much to reduce the deficit in their areas, or how much to cap spending increases. While reconciliation instructions do not have to be included in a budget resolution, they are required if lawmakers want to use the reconciliation process.

While that resolution does not go to the president for his signature, any subsequent legislation produced through reconciliation does eventually go to the president.

The next step is for lawmakers to hammer out what specific elements go into a reconciliation bill. Individual committees, especially the Budget Committee, play a role in this process, as do party leaders.

Once the legislation is assembled, it is subject to another significant step: challenges under the "Byrd rule."

This is a rule proposed by the late Sen. Robert Byrd, D-W.Va., that was designed to keep budget reconciliation bills focused on topics related to national finances, so that they're not overloaded with extraneous issues.

Applying the rule to a provision in the bill could result in it being removed. One disqualifier would be if the provision doesn't change the level of spending or revenues, or does so only incidentally. Another would be if a provision raises deficits outside of the "budget window" covered by the legislation, typically 10 years. Changes to Social Security are also considered out of bounds.

On the floor, any senator can raise a "point of order" against a provision in the reconciliation bill. Once an objection is raised, the nonpartisan Senate parliamentarian decides whether the provision is OK to stay in the bill. One example from Biden's American Rescue Plan subject to a point of order was raising the minimum wage to $15. The relevant question under the Byrd rule would be whether raising the minimum wage affects federal revenues or spending.

Once debate on a reconciliation bill starts, it is limited to 20 hours, a short time by Senate standards. A simple majority is required to pass the bill. Debate on the final compromise version is limited to 10 hours.

The standard practice is to produce no more than one reconciliation bill per fiscal year. However, it's possible for Democrats to offer two reconciliation bills in the current calendar year: one to cover fiscal year 2021, and another one available this fall for fiscal year 2022, which starts on Oct. 1. That's because the previous Congress did not pass a budget resolution. Historically, reconciliation bills have taken anywhere from a month to a year to finish.

Budget Reconciliation For The People

Congress is widely seen as ineffective by the American people.

According to an April 2021 Rasmussen survey, only 21% of "Likely U.S. Voters" rate the way Congress is doing its job as good or excellent. 54% say it's doing a poor job. **(Reference: https://www.rasmussenreports.com/public_content/politics/mood_of_ameri ca/rate_congress_april13 - See hyperlink for full text).**

The United States spent approximately 18% of its gross domestic product on health care in 2020, and has the highest health spending based on GDP share among developed countries. American families face approximately 530,000 bankruptcies annually due to medical debt – despite the fact that most of them are insured.

Since 1974, Budget Reconciliation has been a process for passing a certain type of fiscal legislation with just a simple majority of 51 Senate votes - rather than the 60 that would be needed if the opposition filibusters.

A frequent argument against Medicare for All as one single comprehensive program to cover all citizens and residents is that it will create a new tax.

It is TAXPAYER money that funds Medicaid, CHIP, the VA, the military and most programs that provide health coverage to U.S. citizens. And it is TAXPAYER money that will someday address the budget deficit created by Budget Reconciliation in 2017 to provide the GOP's huge tax breaks for the wealthy that dropped the effective tax rate on corporations to under 21%.

It is TAXPAYER money to which Congress currently applies its arcane rules for "Budget Reconciliation". Congress needs to redefine "Budget Reconciliation" to address the serious budget needs of American families – especially when it comes to the universal need for health care.

One might say that it is "for the Byrds" not to agree that Medicare For All is one of the most important issues that Congress needs to pass via the process of Budget Reconciliation. Budget Reconciliation for The People is True Bipartisanship.

15

https://www.newsweek.com/69-percent-americans-want-medicare-all-
including-46-percent-republicans-new-poll-says-1500187

69% of Americans Want Medicare for All, Including 46% of Republicans - New Poll
by Daniel Villarreal, 24 April 2020

A newly released poll shows that 69 percent of registered voters support Medicare for All, a plan which would create a national health insurance plan available for all Americans.

The poll also showed 46 percent of Republican voters supporting Medicare for All alongside 88 percent of Democrats and 68 percent of Independents.

While several publications have wondered whether the coronavirus epidemic has bolstered support for a national health insurance plan, the poll found that Democratic support remained steady from a similar poll conducted in 2018, rising only two percentage points since then. Support among Independents remained unchanged, and Republican support actually dropped 6 percentage points from 2018 to 2020. The poll was conducted by the Washington, D.C. newspaper *The Hill* and the market research company HarrisX.

The coronavirus epidemic has raised awareness about flaws in the American health insurance system as many people who lost their jobs due to stay-at-home and social distancing measures also lost their health insurance. Without insurance, many Americans fear getting sick or injured because of the potentially devastating financial impact it could have. Tying insurance to employment also burdens businesses with healthcare and insurance administration costs that can be expensive and time-consuming, according to *The Wall Street Journal*. Employment-based insurance also reduces wages and increases overhead as insurance premiums and deductibles continue to rise, according to the *New York Times*.

However, despite Medicare for All being touted by former Democratic presidential frontrunner Vermont Senator Bernie Sanders, House Speaker Nancy Pelosi and other Senate Democrats focused on healthcare reform have dismissed it.

Many critics of Medicare for All worry also about "rationed" care that discriminates against sicker patients, an overall decline in the quality of care or the taxes that would be required to fund such an overhaul.

The healthcare reform plan touted Joe Biden would leave employer-based health insurance plans intact while also adding a subsidized, Medicare-based public option for small businesses and individuals. However, large employers and their employees wouldn't be able to buy into his public option.

https://www.politico.com/interactives/2019/how-to-fix-politics-in-america/gridlock/   (See hyperlink to read each suggestion.)

GRIDLOCK

Congress is stuck. Here's how we can jolt it into action – or work around it.

Illustration & animation by Ben Fearnley

1
Ditch the Filibuster
HARRY REID

2
Start With Problems, Not Parties
CHARLES KOCH

3
National Ballot Initiatives
TIM WU

4
End the Permanent Campaign
JENNIFER LAWLESS

5
A Permanent Committee to Improve Congress
KEVIN KOSAR

6
Impeachment 2.0
SANFORD V. LEVINSON

7
Return All Legislative Power to Congress
ROBERT P. GEORGE

8
Fix Our Broken Immigration System
MICHAEL ANTON

9
Teach Congress About Science and Technology
M. ANTHONY MILLS

10
A Congressional Pork Barrel Fund
READER SUBMISSION

11
Congressional Bonuses on Merit
READER SUBMISSION

12
Occasional Anonymous Votes
READER SUBMISSION

13
Try Again
READER SUBMISSION

CORRUPTION

What should we do about the influence of money in our campaigns and out

1 Cut Government Salaries BOB WOODSON	2 Give Citizens Vouchers to Hire Lobbyists ARCHON FUNG	3 Shut the Revolving Door Once and For All GARY HART & MICHAEL BENNET
4 Overturn Buckley v. Valeo ELLEN L. WEINTRAUB	5 Disclose Corporate Campaign Spending STEVE BULLOCK	6 Curb Corporate Power FELICIA WONG
7 Public Matching for Small-Dollar Federal Donations BILL DE BLASIO	8 A New Cabinet Position and Federal Agency to Fight Corruption JOE SESTAK	9 Term Limits READER SUBMISSION
10 Make Campaigns Exclusively Public-Funded READER SUBMISSION		

Health Insurance Horror Stories
That Cry Out for Universal Healthcare

We all know others who have had extremely difficult health insurance situations – and many of us have experienced difficult situations of our own. On the emotional side of dealing with illness, we do the best we can. On the financial and bureaucratic side, each would undoubtedly have been a great deal less stressed if our country had had Universal Healthcare (aka "Medicare for All", "Single Payer") – in other words:

"A Card in Your Wallet"

Ideally, our future will provide a "valid-for-life" Medicare For All card that is immediately clipped to the medical chart of every baby born in The United States. When that day arrives, we will no longer have stories like these to tell:

➢ The 911 Responders who, with the help of Jon Stewart, pleaded for years with our U.S. Congress to have their medical costs covered: "Cancers take 20 years to develop … and we might see something different 20 years down the line. (Ultimately, nearly 60 types of cancer were added to the list of illnesses eligible for coverage.) ".

    https://www.cdc.gov/wtc/about.html
    https://nymag.com/intelligencer/2019/06/how-lawmakers-protected-and-failed-9-11-first-responders.html
    https://www.cc.com/video/i58xmo/the-daily-show-with-jon-stewart-worst-responders
    https://abcn.ws/2y1suRx
    https://www.youtube.com/watch?v=zmYiW_xMTKc
    https://www.youtube.com/watch?v=_uYpDC3SRpM
    https://www.youtube.com/watch?v=LdbROxCvEx8
    https://www.youtube.com/watch?v=ICnUJl0t0Xw
    https://en.wikipedia.org/wiki/James_Zadroga_9/11_Health_and_Compensation_Act
    https://fealgoodfoundation.com/

➢The nurses' aide working part-time jobs at two nursing homes in Washington State when COVID hit because, under The Affordable Care Act, an employer does not have to provide health insurance for an employee who works fewer than 30 hours per week. Two PT jobs means this CNA is juggling two schedules and wasting time, energy and transportation expenses instead of having one FT job to focus on. And the elderly residents are deprived of her full energy and focus.

➤The 58 paraprofessionals ("teachers' aides") in a town in southern NJ who each had their part-time hours reduced by 1 hour during the COVID-19 pandemic so they fell below the threshold to qualify for health benefits (per "Obamacare" rules).

➤The very exhausted replacement window sales representative who works long hours for LOWES and tells you he would have retired but he needs the employer health insurance for himself, his wife, and his 2 young adult children who are not yet 26 (a condition of the ACA – which, we guess, is still better than being a 20-year-old orphan!).

➤The woman whose son collides with a parked car on his bicycle and is told that the medical bills must be covered by her auto insurance since the accident involved an automobile.

➤The cost analyst working for an engineering & construction firm that has just announced the closing of their local office. Employees are offered COBRA as a continuation of their employer-based health insurance plan. In speaking with three engineers (all more highly paid than she), she learns that these three men are covered under their wives medical plans. Their wives are all government employees! Hmmmm…she's had premiums deducted from every paycheck – they have not! She will now need (on unemployment insurance) to try to pay the outrageously expensive monthly COBRA premium – they will not! AND, some of her taxes contribute to the health coverage for government employees (as do theirs as well, of course). The playing field certainly would have been more level had they ALL had "a card in our wallet" rather than employer-based health insurance!

➤The retired school teacher who reflects back on how different her life might have been had she arrived on Day 1 with a "valid-for-life" Medicare for All card in her wallet. In addition to rarely getting home before 6pm on school days because of the many things that needed to be done to be prepared for her students the next day, she was also an active member of the teachers' association for her school district and a contract negotiator for her coworkers for a period of time. She recalls the frustration and anger of sitting across the table from School Board members who tried to equate what the teachers did to "glorified babysitting". She remembers sitting in public school board sessions listening to parents asserting that teachers work from 8-3, and "What makes you think you are worth more money?". The lack of respect was hard to accept, especially because of the enormous responsibility of educating her students, a responsibility that weighed heavily on her shoulders daily. During contract negotiations salaries were considered almost hand in hand with the ever rising cost of healthcare. This meant that the teachers were in the position of taking a lower salary settlement in order to maintain their healthcare, while still paying at least 20-25% of their total healthcare premiums in each paycheck. Over the years it was not unusual to meet a former student who was making considerably more money than she, despite the fact that she held two degrees and had far more experience in her career. If Medicare for All had been in place during her 37 year teaching career it would have made a huge difference in the quality of life for her and her family.

➤The 90-year-old woman whose daughter phones AAA for her to ask why mom's auto insurance is $2,000/year when she only drives to church and the grocery store. When cancellation is mentioned, the agent asks the questions: "Does your mother have Medicare?" (at 90? - duh!) & "Does your mother have supplemental health insurance?". Yes to both – on her own and through her deceased husband's Exelon pension! Suddenly, the annual cost of her policy dropped to $1,000/year!

➤In the book CASTE by Elizabeth Wilkerson (Chapter 29), she reminds us: "Leon Lederman was an American physicist who won a Nobel Prize in 1988 for his groundbreaking contributions to our understanding of the particles of nature. Decades afterwards, when he was in his early nineties, he began to suffer memory loss and to require additional care. In 2015, he took the extraordinary step of auctioning off his Nobel Prize medal for $765,000 to cover medical bills that were mounting. In 2018, he died in a nursing home, his Nobel Prize in the hands of someone else."

➤Mary in NJ, in her late 70s, sees the constant ads on TV for "Medicare Advantage". The possible benefits like rides to the doctor, vision, dental, reimbursement of the $170.10/month taken out of your Social Security sure do sound good! "But you don't get these benefits automatically. Call today and see if you qualify." What's the catch? Mary finds the hype so confusing that she decides to stick to her Medicare B +

Supplemental Insurance from United Healthcare (the CEO's total compensation in 2019 was $18.9 million according to the company's proxy filing). Mary is fearful that changing plans might be worse than what she already has – and that she won't know until she needs to use it in a medical emergency.

[Comment from Dr. Margaret Flowers of H.O.P.E. – Health Over Profit for Everyone: "Medicare Advantage plans are private health insurance plans available to people who are eligible for Medicare. While the name sounds positive, Medicare Advantage plans are privatizing Medicare (sending dollars to investors' bank accounts that could be used for care), preventing seniors who need care from getting it and taking us down a wrong path of privatizing Medicare, our public insurance. Due to aggressive marketing of the plans, Medicare Advantage is becoming a bigger share of the Medicare system, now comprising 34% of Medicare enrollees. Medicare Advantage plans receive more money from the government per enrollee than original Medicare and they cover a healthier population than original Medicare. With its high overhead and profits, Medicare Advantage wastes dollars that could be used for health care. Take Action: Spread the word that Medicare Advantage plans are a scam that is hurting seniors and our future Medicare for All healthcare system! Tell your friends and family and write letters to the editor in your local paper about it. Tell your member of Congress that Medicare Advantage plans are ripping off seniors and the federal government."]

https://www.vice.com/en/article/xgq5jw/surprise-medical-bill-stories-and-private-health-care-insurance   (See hyperlink for full text and references.)

Horror Stories about the Cost of Health Care Even When You Have Insurance
By Reina Sultan (Twitter: @SultanReina) ; 4 March 2020

About 27.5 million Americans live without health insurance, leaving them vulnerable to high out-of-pocket costs for medical, dental, and vision care. But having insurance in our current system doesn't mean you'll avoid exorbitant fees — regardless of how high your premiums and copays are. Americans can pay upwards of $4,000 a year just for healthcare coverage, and, still, their insurance plans might not cover mental healthcare, dental, or life-saving surgeries that insurance companies deem "elective." The cost isn't just monetary - **Americans who have private insurance spend an inordinate amount of time collecting documentation, submitting claims, following up on claims, and arguing with their insurance companies.**

I am insured through a PPO plan that most would consider "good insurance," but I've been fighting my insurer for coverage of medically necessary mental healthcare for the past five months. (The issue I'm currently dealing with is *after* they'd refused to cover a registered dietitian to treat my eating disorder, forcing me to pay out of pocket.) This fight has cost me so much time and money. A lot of my debt comes from medical bills.

I'm not alone in that regard. Roughly 137 million Americans have medical debt. This is so common that the leading cause of declaring bankruptcy in the United States is medical bills. Sixty-three percent of people with medical debt had health insurance when treatment began.

Since the number of Americans with medical debt is far higher than the number of uninsured people in this country, we can see that private insurance plans — which we're already paying for — are not protecting us against incurring high costs when we need procedures, prescriptions, or treatments.

Despite this, Joe Biden thinks that Americans want to maintain their private insurance, proposing a plan similar to former candidate Mayor Pete Buttigieg's "Medicare for All who want it," but the private healthcare system remains a barrier to care for many Americans. That's probably why the majority of Americans support Medicare for All.

VICE asked people to tell us about their shocking, infuriating, and straight-up terrible experiences with their insurance companies to see how private coverage often works in the U.S.

Answers edited for length and clarity.

Anna, 30, Washington

My husband and I flew to California to visit my parents and planned to drive their car back up with all my childhood belongings in it. As I was driving through Nevada, the car hit a patch of black ice and flipped over into a ravine. My spine broke on impact. (My husband was OK, aside from breaking his glasses.)

I was taken to a tiny hospital in Ely, where I was immediately pumped full of drugs and sent to get X-rays. Since the doctor couldn't tell whether the break was stable or not from the X-rays, the doctor gave my shaken husband the choice of flying me to Salt Lake City or Las Vegas for an MRI, which would have been a four-hour drive. We flew to Las Vegas within an hour, where I had numerous tests done.

At some point in my morphine haze, a lady came through to explain my insurance while my husband was out getting new glasses. None of this registered because of the medication I was on.

Imagine our surprise when we got back home to a $60,000 bill. Our insurance, Blue Cross Blue Shield, decided that the plane trip was "elective," saying that I could have taken the four-hour ground ambulance ride. We appealed that decision four times, during which the ER doctor clarified that the air ambulance was medically necessary-- which was why they never offered a ground ambulance as a choice. While the appeals were happening, the bill gathered interest and grew to $75,000 for just the air ambulance—including the exams and four days in the hospital, the debt was far over $75,000. All four appeals were denied. We decided declaring bankruptcy was our only option.

Caroline, 26, Massachusetts

I have endometriosis, a chronic reproductive health condition that can cause pain, fatigue, organ damage, and infertility. After an ineffective ablation surgery — where endometriosis lesions are essentially burned off — I found out that excision surgery, where lesions are cut away and removed completely by a specialist, is the gold standard in endometriosis care. There are only a small number of surgeons nationwide skilled enough to perform a successful excision surgery, meaning I would have to locate a qualified surgeon and then travel for care. Most of these surgeons operated out-of-network, due to difficulties in doctors getting fairly reimbursed for complex surgeries. Ablation and excision are coded the same for insurers, meaning a trained specialist is reimbursed the same for excision — which can be an eight-hour surgery — as an unskilled surgeon performing a much quicker and easier procedure. Because of this, most people with endometriosis are looking at tens of thousands in out-of-pocket costs.

I found a surgeon in Maine, about two hours from me. Getting the insurance coverage for the hospital itself was a nightmare. The insurance company was trying not to cover the hospital, which was in-network care. My surgeon was literally on the phone with insurers at the airport while on vacation with his family, fighting to make sure I wouldn't be charged tens of thousands for my hospital care. The company ultimately covered my hospital care, but I still paid thousands out of pocket for my surgeon's care, as well as hundreds for consults and office visits. I have friends who aren't on insurance plans that cover hospital fees, as mine did, and some are out tens of thousands of dollars for surgeries that saved their quality of life.

https://pnhp.org/news/health-care-horror-stories/
From The New York Times. ©April 11, 2008 The New York Times Company. All rights reserved. Used under license.

Health Care Horror Stories
By Paul Krugman, *The New York Times ; 11 April 2008*

Not long ago, a young Ohio woman named Trina Bachtel, who was having health problems while pregnant, tried to get help at a local clinic. Unfortunately, she had previously sought care at the same clinic while uninsured and had a large unpaid balance. The clinic wouldn't see her again unless she paid $100 per visit — which she didn't have.

Eventually, she sought care at a hospital 30 miles away. By then, however, it was too late. Both she and the baby died.

You may think that this was an extreme case, but stories like this are common in America.

Back in 2006, The Wall Street Journal told another such story: that of a young woman named Monique White, who failed to get regular care for lupus because she lacked insurance. Then, one night, "as skin lesions spread over her body and her stomach swelled, she couldn't sleep."

The Journal's report goes on: "Mama, please help me! Please take me to the E.R.," she howled, according to her mother, Gail Deal. "O.K., let's go," Mrs. Deal recalls saying. "No, I can't," the daughter replied. "I don't have insurance."

She was rushed to the hospital the next day after suffering a seizure —

and the hospital spared no expense on her treatment. But it all came too late; she was dead a few months later.

How can such things happen? "I mean, people have access to health care in America," President Bush once declared. "After all, you just go to an emergency room." Not quite.

First of all, visits to the emergency room are no substitute for regular care, which can identify and treat health problems before they become acute. And more than 40 percent of uninsured adults have no regular source of care. Second, uninsured Americans often postpone medical care, even when they know they need it, because of expense.

Finally, while it's true that hospitals will treat anyone who arrives in an emergency room with an acute problem — and it's wonderful that they will — it's also true that hospitals bill patients for emergency-room treatment. And fear of those bills often causes uninsured Americans to hesitate before seeking medical help, even in emergencies, as the Monique White story illustrates.

The end result is that the uninsured receive a lot less care than the insured. And sometimes this lack of care kills them. According to a recent estimate by the Urban Institute, the lack of health insurance leads to 27,000 preventable deaths in America each year.

But are they really preventable? Yes. Stories like those of Trina Bachtel and Monique White are common in America, but don't happen in any other rich country — because every other advanced nation has some form of universal health insurance. We should, too.

If being a progressive means anything, it means believing that we need universal health care, so that terrible stories like those of Monique White, Trina Bachtel and the thousands of other Americans who die each year from lack of insurance become a thing of the past.

http://www.moderntimesbeer.com/blog/medicare-all-yesterday

MEDICARE FOR ALL, YESTERDAY BEER
A message from MTB Founder Jacob McKean

We've publicly and privately supported single payer health care for quite some time now. As a growing business, we've had to deal with privatized health care every step of the way. As an entrepreneur, I had to take the terrifying step of giving up my health insurance when I left my last job in order to start MT (Modern Times Beer). When we opened, I had to navigate the immense difficulty and expense of buying health insurance for a small company. And as we've grown, we've had to cope with the absurd costs and complexities of providing health insurance to hundreds of people across multiple states.

It doesn't have to be this way. It's long been clear to me — as both the CEO of this company and as a human being who needs health care — that privatized health insurance is an on-going disaster for people, for businesses, and for our country. I have not been shy about this stance. A little over a year ago, we hosted a workshop for small business owners to learn about Medicare for All and why they should support it. We have lobbied our elected representatives in meetings, letters, and phone calls. We have joined two different business alliances for Medicare for All and worked in a variety of ways to support their efforts. I have written op-eds and contributed money. But our advocacy does not, and will not, stop there.

In the weeks before the COVID-19 crisis hit, I had set-up a collaboration with a legendary brewery that also strongly supports Medicare for All. It was going to be a benefit for Businesses for Medicare for All, one of the groups we both support. Now, in the throes of this crisis, that plan is obviously on hold: we can't travel, of course, but more importantly, Modern Times is now in a fight for its life. That fight — obscenely, bizarrely, and unnecessarily — is also a fight to prevent our employees from being kicked off their health care in the middle of a pandemic.

Our support for Medicare for All has not changed, and in fact, reality has now loudly endorsed our position. Since we can't release the collaboration beer as we'd originally planned, I decided to name this non-collaborative barrel-aged special release "Medicare for All,

Yesterday," since that is very clearly when we needed it. It is not a benefit beer; frankly, we can't afford it to be. The quantity is also very limited, which makes it suboptimal as an awareness raising thing, but it's the best we could do under the circumstances.

So whether you're able to snag a bottle of this beer or not, we hope you'll consider joining us in the fight for a dignified, coherent, and just health care system. Our lives, and yours, depend on it.

Random Thoughts
That Cry Out for Universal Healthcare

➢ At a Convention of the Medical Committee for Human Rights held in Chicago in March 1966, Martin Luther King Jr. declared: "Of all the forms of inequality, injustice in health care is the most shocking and inhumane."

➢ President Biden remarked (in the Eisenhower Executive Office Briefing Room February 22, 2021) on Helping Small Businesses: "And I want to make it clear: I'm prepared to hear ideas about how to make the American Rescue Plan better and cheaper." - - - Well, Mr. President, "Medicare for All" is the universal opportunity to rescue small businesses by eliminating all obligations of employers to provide health insurance for their employees. It's a "BFD"!

➢ Kamala Harris (10/5/2017 tweet): "A government has three functions: public health, public safety and public education."

➢ Medicare for All would result in job loss or transition for those employed by health insurers (especially highly-paid CEOs). This has happened before and we've adjusted: where are all the telephone operators now? And employees from the telephone booth and typewriter manufacturing industries?

➢ In her book "An American Sickness", Dr. Elisabeth Rosenthal informs us that direct-to-consumer drug advertising rose from $166 million in 1993 to $4.2 billion in 2005 and that, in 2000, Merck spent $160 million advertising Vioxx compared to $146 million spent to advertise Budweiser and $78 million to advertise Nike. She further comments that the Supreme Court has protected drug advertising under the guise of free speech and that "media companies, particularly cable television stations, are ever more dependent on it for survival; healthcare advertising stayed robust even through the Great Recession".

➢ Ad on 12/15/2020 by a private insurer: "The ACA enrollment ends today in several states. Call now." (What is the purpose of enrollment periods? Let's have a card issued at birth that's valid for a lifetime.)

➢ Fidelity Investments (May 6, 2021): According to the Fidelity Retiree Health Care Cost Estimate, an average couple age 65 in 2021 may need approximately $300,000 saved (after tax) to cover health care expenses in retirement.

➢ Independence Blue Cross/Blue Shield advertisement: "We'll never know how many lives we saved by wearing a mask." (Are they buying ads using taxpayer $$$ to falsely imply value for the for-profit premiums and cost-sharing they charge?)

➢ Paycheck.com advertisement ($$$): "Getting healthcare – a big moment for your employee."

➢ Humana advertisement ($$$): "If you have both Medicare and Medicaid, you may get even more benefits with a Medicare Advantage Plan depending on where you live." (Oh, how often that scary word "may" appears in for-profit health insurance advertising!)

➢ Advertising on SilverSneakers.com website (taxpayer $$$): "Enroll in SilverSneakers today. It's all included at no additional cost in many Medicare Advantage plans and select Medicare Supplement plans." (While some Americans get "SilverSneakers" at tax-payer funded "no additional cost", other Americans are uninsured, under-insured or declaring medical bankruptcy.)

➢ Advertising by a "life-settlement" company ($$$): "Paying off medical bills is one of the most common reasons why people are interested in selling their life insurance policies. One client set up a fund to cover medical bills, home renovations, and an income stream for his wife for the rest of her life. People who are terminally ill often consider life settlements to be a means of supporting themselves once they're unable to work. Life settlements help pay for regular expenses such as medical treatment and hospice care. Some people also use them to pay for long-term facilities."

➢ Advertising for Reverse Mortgages ($$$): "There is a vast group that would benefit from home health care though they are unable to afford it on an ongoing basis. On average, a home health aide providing 44 hours of service per week costs $4,576 per month (according to Genworth Financial). Homemaker services, which include services like housekeeping and cooking, run about $4,385 on average. One mechanism to aid this group is home equity. 'Many senior Americans today haven't saved enough for the future, but they may be sitting on an unknown solution: their homes.' Reverse mortgage borrowers can remain in their homes to receive care, and can receive proceeds to pay for it. In comparison, the same borrower could sell the home and use the proceeds to move into a full-time nursing home, spending on average, more than $80,000 per year and exhausting the home equity much sooner. Home health providers and private duty care agencies can benefit from having some knowledge around these loans as a way to pay for their care."

I Am A Republican ...
Can We Talk About A Single Payer System?

By David May, M.D. American College of Cardiology Touch Blog
23 April 2013

I am a Republican. For those who know me that is not a surprise. I live in a red state. I have never voted for a Democratic presidential candidate. I can field strip, clean and reassemble a Remington 12-gauge pump blindfolded. And on top of it, I think we should talk about having a single payer national health care plan. The reason is quite simple. In my view, we already have one; we just don't take advantage of it.

Firstly, Medicare and the Center for Medicare and Medicaid Services (CMS) are de facto setting all of the rules now. They are a single payer system. When we go to lobby the Hill, we lobby Congress and CMS. Talking to Blue Cross, Aetna, Cigna and United Health care is essentially a waste of time. All the third party payers do is play off the Medicare rules to their advantage and profit. They have higher premiums, pay a somewhat higher benefit and have a significantly higher level of regulation which impedes the care of their customers. This is no longer consumer choice but effectively extortion, a less than hidden shake down in which the "choice" for a family of four is company A at $900 per month or company B at $1,100 per month. The payers are simply taking advantage of the system, playing both ends against the middle.

Secondly, in order to move forward with true health care finance we need complete transparency in cost and expense ... and we need it now. As was noted in a recent Time magazine piece on the hidden cost of health care, our current system is a vulgar, less than honorable construct more akin to used car sales than medical care, cloaked under the guise of generally accepted accounting principles and hospital cost shifting.

Thirdly, with a single payer system would potentially come real utilization data, real quality metrics and real accountability. The promise of ICD-10 (https://www.icd10data.com/) with all of its difficulties is that of a much more granular claims-made data. We could use some granularity in health care data and we will never achieve it in big data quantities without a single payer system.

Lastly, I think that the physicians should be in charge of health care and not the insurance companies and hospital systems. With a single price structure, it becomes all about medical decision making, efficiency, the provision of care to our patients, and shared decision making, all of which we do well.

How, you might say, could a Republican come to such a position? The simple answer is I really think it is quite Republican. Oh, I know there will be many raised eyebrows and many critics. I accept that. I understand the fact that no single payer system is perfect, that it is "socialist," that it is "un-American."

I would submit to you, however, that it is un-American to allow many of our citizens to be uninsured, that it is un-American to shunt money away from a strong military in order to support a bloated, inefficient and fraud-laden health care system, that it is un-American not to be open and above board with the cost of what we do, the expense of that service and the profit that we make. Mostly, it is un-American to let this outrageous health care injustice continue.

David May MD, PhD, FACC is a retired interventional cardiologist. From 1990 until 2019 he was the managing partner of Cardiovascular Specialists, PA. Elected to fellowship in the American College of Physicians, the American College of Cardiology and the Society for Cardiovascular Angiography and Intervention, he served as the Chairman of the Board of Governors for the American College of Cardiology from 2013-2014. The author of numerous scientific publications, his current interests include health care disparities, the use of registries to evaluate the quality of care and the impact of electronic health records on the physician-patient relationship.

http://healthoverprofit.org/2020/03/16/453-rural-hospitals-are-failing-medicare-for-all-would-save-them/

453 Rural Hospitals are Failing — Medicare for All would Save Them

By Diane Archer (Founder & President JustCareUSA.org)
for The Hill / 16 March 2020

Our for-profit health care system isn't working for rural Americans. More than 120 rural hospitals have closed since 2010. According to a new report from Chartis Center for Rural Health, another 453 — almost one in four — are at risk of failing. Corporate health insurers can't provide coverage to meet rural patients' needs, and it's endangering the bottom line of rural hospitals. Medicare for All would save them.

In congressional testimony, Dr. Jessica Banthin, Deputy Assistant Director for Health, Retirement, and Long-Term Analysis at the Congressional Budget Office, explains that enacting single-payer Medicare for All could keep rural hospitals afloat. Everyone would have good coverage. And, hospitals would be compensated at Medicare rates, or better, for the care that they deliver.

Other health care reform proposals that allow people the option to buy into Medicare, such as a "public option" or "Medicare buy-in," would not ensure rural residents access to care. A new study published in the Lancet by Yale Professor Alison Galvani et al. finds that these proposals would drive health care costs higher. Health care would continue to be unaffordable for much of rural America. Thousands of rural Americans would continue to die unnecessarily each year.

Right now, our for-profit health care system leaves millions of rural residents uninsured or underinsured and unable to get the care they need. It is not designed to serve rural communities. Mountains of research show that rural Americans with low incomes and chronic conditions often cannot afford needed care or coverage. Not surprisingly, the 46 million rural residents — one in six Americans — have far poorer health outcomes and lower life expectancies than Americans living in urban areas.

Because rural hospitals are not reimbursed for much of the care they deliver, many of them cannot generate the revenue needed to serve their communities. Nearly four in 10 rural hospitals are unprofitable. Low patient numbers contribute to the problem. Hospitals are cutting services and closing. Rural Americans sometimes must travel 30 miles to the nearest hospital.

Public health insurance helps rural hospitals to a limited extent. Rural hospitals are stronger in states that have expanded Medicaid under the Affordable Care Act. The uninsured rate in those states for people with incomes under 138 percent of the federal poverty level has dropped from 35 percent to 16 percent. Medicaid provides necessary revenue to hospitals in those states.

But 14 states have not expanded Medicaid, and the Supreme Court ruled that Congress cannot require states to expand Medicaid. Rural Americans living in the South and in states that have not expanded Medicaid have witnessed the highest number of hospital closures. In states that have not expanded Medicaid, rural hospitals must serve more uninsured patients and deliver a significant amount of uncompensated care. Nearly one in three people with incomes under 138 percent of the federal poverty level are uninsured.

Residents of Texas, Tennessee, Oklahoma and Georgia — none of which expanded Medicaid — are among those at greatest risk of losing access to hospital care. Over the last 10 years, Texas saw 20 rural hospitals close and Tennessee saw 12 hospitals close. Oklahoma and Georgia each saw seven hospitals close.

Beyond struggling to meet their health care needs, rural patients are often burdened with sky-high medical debt. Many are low-wage workers, with little hope of paying off their hospital and medical bills. Rural hospitals and doctors have taken to suing patients for the cost of their care. Thousands of rural Americans are jailed or threatened with jail each year when they don't show up in court for unpaid medical bills.

With Medicare for All, Congress would ensure the viability of rural hospitals. Rural hospitals would be properly compensated for the care they deliver, strengthening their balance sheets.

Medicare for All's guaranteed health care coverage would ensure that rural Americans could get the health care they need, without fear of medical debt. Medicare for All eliminates deductibles and coinsurance, treating rich and poor equally instead of rationing care based on ability to pay.

The cruel and discriminatory logic of the marketplace should not mean that rural Americans go without needed care.

READER ALERT

This book is a reference guide and advocate's tool with the following goals:

1. To encourage President Biden and his administration to embrace MEDICARE FOR ALL ACTS S.1129 (currently on hold) and H.R.1976 as the solution to our current healthcare system's exorbitant costs and complexities. In 2012, then Vice President Biden "evolved" on the issue of same-sex marriage. Now, he needs to listen to people like Senator Sanders and "evolve" on "Medicare for All" aka Universal Health Care.

2. To familiarize readers with the benefits of MEDICARE FOR ALL and encourage curiosity to undertake additional online research – perhaps even joining and donating to one or more MEDICARE FOR ALL organizations – or organizing your own group of advocates in your community or on your campus.

3. To encourage the reader to write to your Representative and your Senators in The U.S Congress, urging them to become co-sponsors of S.1129 or H.R.1976.

4. To write to your favorite TV anchors (MSNBC, CNN, FOX, PBS, etc) and encourage them to interview the many experts highlighted in this book. These amazing Medicare For All experts have been ignored by the media for far too long!

5. To encourage you to donate a copy of this book to your local library, as a copy will be donated by the author to the hundreds of college libraries (including Native American and HBCUs) around the country.

6. To study or skim the following chapters that highlight our COSTLY & COMPLEX CURRENT SYSTEM – if only to know what we now have and ought to replace! And, before MEDICARE FOR ALL becomes a reality, perhaps these chapters will assist you in finding better coverage than you already have.

OUR CURRENT SYSTEM

Our current health insurance ("healthcare") system includes a multitude of complex and costly programs. If we were starting from scratch, no one would design a healthcare system like America's.

If "Medicare For All" (aka Universal Healthcare) were to be enacted by The United States Congress, every BODY would be covered and all or most of these programs would no longer exist, including:

- The Uninsured (treated when necessary in hospital emergency rooms) – including persons without legal residence.

- The Affordable Care Act = ACA ("Obamacare")

- Medicaid

- CHIP (Children's Health Insurance Program)

- Indian Health Service (IHS)

- FEHB Program for Federal Employees

- Veterans' Health Coverage through the Dept. of Veterans' Affairs

- TRICARE

- Employment-based Health Insurance

- Medicare A, B, C & D (plus Medigap "Supplemental")

- Health Savings Accounts & Flexible Savings Accounts

- COBRA

https://www.kff.org/health-reform/issue-brief/no-surprises-act-implementation-what-to-expect-in-2022/
(See hyperlink for full text and references.)

No Surprises Act Implementation: What to Expect in 2022
By Karen Pollitz ; 10 December 2021

The No Surprises Act (NSA) establishes new federal protections against surprise medical bills that take effect in 2022. Surprise medical bills arise when insured consumers inadvertently receive care from out-of-network hospitals, doctors, or other providers they did not choose. Peterson-KFF and other studies find this happens in about 1 in 5 emergency room visits. In addition between 9% and 16% of in-network hospitalizations for non-emergency care include surprise bills from out-of-network providers (such as anesthesiologists) whom the patient did not choose.

Surprise medical bills pose financial burdens on consumers when health plans deny out-of-network claims or apply higher out-of-network cost sharing; consumers also face "balance billing" from out-of-network providers that have not contracted to accept discounted payment rates from the health plan. The federal government estimates the NSA will apply to about 10 million out-of-network surprise medical bills a year.

The NSA will protect consumers from surprise medical bills by:

- requiring private health plans to cover these out-of-network claims and apply in-network cost sharing. The law applies to both job-based and non-group plans, including grandfathered plans

- prohibiting doctors, hospitals, and other covered providers from billing patients more than in-network cost sharing amount for surprise medical bills.

The NSA also establishes a process for determining the payment amount for surprise, out-of-network medical bills, starting with negotiations between plans and providers and, if negotiations don't succeed, an independent dispute resolution (IDR) process.

Protections will apply to most surprise bills for specific types of services provided in certain settings:

- Emergency Services

- Post-emergency stabilization services

- Non-emergency services provided at in-network facilities

For services covered by the NSA, providers are prohibited from billing patients more than the applicable in-network cost sharing amount; a penalty of up to $10,000 for each violation can apply.

How will consumers know if a bill or claim constitutes a surprise medical bill? – It is up to both providers and health plans to identify bills that are protected under the NSA. The regulations also request public comment on whether changes to federal rules governing electronic claims (so-called HIPAA standard claims transactions) are needed to indicate claims for which surprise billing protections apply.

For consumers to be protected, both the health plan and the surprise billing provider will need to comply with the law. If problems arise, consumers might need to seek help from more than one enforcing agency. And, though the NSA is a federal law, states will also have a role in enforcement. The toll free number for the "No Surprises Help Desk" will be 1-800-985-3059.

(The No Surprises Act – NSA – was a 2021 New Year's Eve surprise that became an unplanned last-minute inclusion in this book. Everyone needing health coverage is urged to consider the impact the NSA might have on any one of the potential health insurance programs available to American citizens and residents. The NSA – while well-intentioned – adds further complexity to our current complex health care system. With "Medicare for All", there would be no need for the "No Surprises Act". In general, we need to ask ourselves and each other to define the obligation that we constituents expect of our elected officials. Do we expect them to protect our interests with comprehensive and cost-effective universal health care, or do we find it acceptable for them to protect costly and complex health care programs that ensure huge profits to private insurance companies?)

Currently, there are two "Medicare For All" bills in Congress:

H.R 1976 "Medicare for All Act of 2019" first introduced in the U.S. House of Representatives by Pramila Jayapal on February 27, 2019

S. 1129 "Medicare for All Act of 2019" first introduced in the U.S. Senate by Bernie Sanders on April 10, 2019 (this bill is currently on hold)

For many years prior to these two bills, there was H.R. 676 in the U.S. House of Representatives. H.R. 676 (entitled "The Expanded and Improved Medicare for All Act") deserves attention and gratitude to its author, Representative John Conyers (D-MI). H.R. 676 was first introduced into the U.S. House of Representatives in 2003 with 25 co-sponsors. As of December 2018, it had 124 cosponsors.

Between 2003 and 2018, Representative Conyers' H.R. 676 was the gold standard among organizations and advocates promoting Single Payer Healthcare. Books, articles, films, websites and social media often placed H.R. 676 in a position of prominence. On December 5, 2017, Representative Conyers resigned his seat in the House of Representatives and remained in retirement until his death on October 27, 2019. With Representative Conyers' retirement, Representative Pramila Jayapal revised H.R. 676 and replaced it with H.R.1976.

Special (Inferior?) Treatment of VA Health Programs and Indian Health Service (IHS)

On February 27, 2019 Representative Pramila Jayapal introduced H.R 1976, entitled "Medicare for All Act of 2019". Incorporated into H.R. 1976 is the following provision: "Health insurance exchanges and specified federal health programs terminate upon program implementation. However, the program does not affect coverage provided through the Department of Veterans Affairs or the Indian Health Service.".

This contrasts with the earlier H.R. 676, Section 401, by Representative John Conyers (D-MI) which read as follows:

(a) VA HEALTH PROGRAMS. — This Act provides for health programs of the Department of Veterans' Affairs to initially remain independent for the 10-year period that begins on the date of the establishment of the Medicare For All Program. After such 10-year period, the Congress shall reevaluate whether such programs shall remain independent or be integrated into the Medicare For All Program.

(b) INDIAN HEALTH SERVICE PROGRAMS. — This Act provides for health programs of the Indian Health Service to initially remain independent for the 5-year period that begins on the date of the establishment of the Medicare For All Program, after which such programs shall be integrated into the Medicare For All Program.

When reading the chapters on VA Health Programs and Indian Health Service Programs – with their complexities and high costs – the reader is encouraged to keep this distinction between H.R. 676 and H.R 1976 in mind.

According to Wikipedia: "The proposed 2018 budget proposes to reduce

IHS spending by more than $300 million. This covers the provision of health benefits to 2.5 million Native Americans and Alaskan Natives for a recent average *cost per patient* of less than $3,000, far less than the average cost of health care nationally ($7,700), or for the other major federal health programs Medicaid ($6,200) or Medicare ($12,000)."

Also, keep in mind that the Veterans Health Administration maintains government ownership of its facilities (hospitals, clinics and nursing homes) and employs medical staff (doctors, nurses, etc). This is a very different system than MEDICARE FOR ALL, which simply provides billing services to private medical staff and facilities.

QUESTIONS:

Why don't "Medicare for All" Congressional Bills S. 1129 and H.R. 1976 include members of federally-recognized Native American Tribes and Alaska Native Persons so they would be eligible for all the benefits of universal health care and have a "Medicare for All" card in their possession from birth?

Do federally-recognized Native American Tribes and Alaska Native Persons want the opportunity to be covered under "Medicare For All" with a "card in their wallet" – or are they happy with the health care they currently receive from the Indian Health Service?

Will opponents to "Medicare for All" who falsely label it as "socialism" look at the structure of the Veterans Health Administration (which maintains government ownership of facilities and keeps a full medical staff on government payrolls)? Should veterans have the easy option to have a "Medicare for All Smart Card" in their wallets?

Just asking!

https://www.kff.org/uninsured/report/the-uninsured-and-the-aca-a-primer-key-facts-about-health-insurance-and-the-uninsured-amidst-changes-to-the-affordable-care-act/ (See hyperlink for full text and references.)

The Uninsured and the ACA: A Primer – Key Facts about Health Insurance and the Uninsured amidst Changes to the Affordable Care Act

Rachel Garfield: Follow @RachelLGarfield on Twitter,
Kendal Orgera: Follow @_KendalOrgera on Twitter,
and Anthony Damico ; 25 January 2019

In the past, gaps in the public insurance system and lack of access to affordable private coverage left millions without health insurance, and the number of uninsured Americans grew over time, particularly during economic downturns. By 2013, the year before the major coverage provisions of the Affordable Care Act (ACA) went into effect, more than 44 million nonelderly individuals lacked coverage.

Under the ACA, as of 2014, Medicaid coverage expanded to nearly all adults with incomes at or below 138% of poverty in states that have adopted the expansion, and tax credits are available for people with incomes up to 400% of poverty who purchase coverage through a health insurance marketplace. Millions of people enrolled in ACA coverage, and the uninsured rate dropped to a historic low by 2016. Coverage gains were particularly large among low-income adults in states that expanded Medicaid.

Despite large gains in health coverage, some people continued to lack coverage, and the ACA remained the subject of political debate. Attempts to repeal and replace the ACA stalled in summer 2017, but there have been several changes to implementation of the ACA under the Trump Administration that affect coverage. In 2017, the number of uninsured rose for the first time since implementation of the ACA to 27.4 million. Those most at risk of being uninsured include low-income individuals, adults, and people of color. The cost of coverage continues to be the most commonly cited barrier to coverage.

Health insurance makes a difference in whether and when people get necessary medical care, where they get their care, and ultimately, how healthy they are. Uninsured people are far more likely than those with insurance to postpone health care or forgo it altogether. The consequences can be severe, particularly when preventable conditions or chronic diseases go undetected. While the safety net of public hospitals, community clinics and health centers, and local providers provides a crucial health care source for uninsured people, it does not close the access gap for the uninsured.

For many uninsured people, the costs of health insurance and medical care are weighed against equally essential needs, like housing, food, and transportation to work, and many uninsured adults report financial stress beyond health care. When uninsured people use health care, they may be charged for the full cost of that care (versus insurers, who negotiate discounts) and often face difficulty paying medical bills. Providers absorb some of the cost of care for the uninsured, and while uncompensated care funds cover some of those costs, these funds do not fully offset the cost of care for the uninsured.

Under current law, nearly half (45%) of the remaining uninsured are outside the reach of the ACA either because their state did not expand Medicaid, they are subject to immigrant eligibility restrictions, or their income makes them ineligible for financial assistance. The remainder are eligible for assistance under the law but may still struggle with affordability and knowledge of options. State action to take up the ACA Medicaid expansion could make more people eligible for affordable coverage. The outcome of current debate over health coverage policy in the nation and the states has substantial implications for people's coverage, access, and overall health and well-being.

https://www.kff.org/medicaid/issue-brief/the-coverage-gap-uninsured-poor-adults-in-states-that-do-not-expand-medicaid/
(See hyperlink for full text and references.)

The Coverage Gap: Uninsured Poor Adults in States that Do Not Expand Medicaid
Rachel Garfield: Follow @RachelLGarfield on Twitter,
Kendal Orgera: Follow @_KendalOrgera on Twitter,
and Anthony Damico ; 21 January 2021

The economic downturn and change in Administration are likely to bring renewed attention to gaps in Medicaid coverage in states that have not expanded eligibility under the Affordable Care Act (ACA).

In the 12 states that have not adopted the Medicaid expansion as of January 2021, Medicaid eligibility for adults remains limited. At a time when many are losing income and potentially health coverage during a health crisis, these eligibility gaps leave many without an affordable coverage option and could contribute to growth in the uninsured rate. The Biden Administration is likely to make coverage expansion for low-income populations a priority, including filling in the "coverage gap" that exists for adults in non-expansion states.

Medicaid eligibility for adults in states that did not expand their programs is quite limited: the median income limit for parents in these states is just 41% of poverty, or an annual income of $8,905 for a family of three in 2020, and in nearly all states not expanding, childless adults remain ineligible. Because the ACA envisioned low-income people receiving coverage through Medicaid, it does not provide financial assistance to people below poverty for other coverage. In contrast, in states that have adopted the ACA Medicaid expansion, Medicaid eligibility is extended to nearly all low-income individuals with incomes at or below 138 percent of poverty ($17,609 for an individual in 2020).

Adults left in the coverage gap are spread across the states not expanding their Medicaid programs but are concentrated in states with the largest uninsured populations. More than a third of people in the coverage gap reside in Texas, which has both a large uninsured population and very limited Medicaid eligibility.

Nineteen percent of people in the coverage gap live in Florida, twelve percent in Georgia, and ten percent in North Carolina. There are no uninsured adults in the coverage gap in Wisconsin because the state is providing Medicaid eligibility to adults up to the poverty level under a Medicaid waiver.

The South has relatively higher numbers of poor uninsured adults than in other regions, has higher uninsured rates and more limited Medicaid eligibility than other regions, and accounts for the majority (8 out of 12) of states that opted not to expand Medicaid. As a result, the vast majority of people in the coverage gap in 2019 reside in the South.

If states that are currently not expanding their programs adopt the

Medicaid expansion, all of the nearly 2.2 million adults in the coverage gap would gain Medicaid eligibility.

If all states expanded Medicaid, those in the coverage gap and those who are instead eligible for Marketplace coverage would bring the number of nonelderly uninsured adults eligible for Medicaid to more than 4.3 million people in the twelve current non-expansion states.

The ACA Medicaid expansion was designed to address historically high uninsured rates among low-income adults, providing a coverage option for people with limited access to employer coverage and limited income to purchase coverage on their own. In states that expanded Medicaid, millions of people gained coverage, and the uninsured rate dropped significantly as a result of the expansion. However, with many states opting not to implement the Medicaid expansion, millions of uninsured adults remain outside the reach of the ACA and continue to have limited options for affordable health coverage. In 2019 the uninsured rate in non-expansion states was nearly double that of expansion states (15.5% vs. 8.3%).

By definition, people in the coverage gap have limited family income and live below the poverty level. They are likely in families employed in very low-wage jobs, employed part-time, or with a fragile or unpredictable connection to the workforce. Given the economic downturn and limited offer rates of employer-based coverage for employees with these work characteristics, it is likely that employer-based coverage is not a viable option for them.

It also is unlikely that people who fall into the coverage gap will be able to afford ACA coverage, as they are not eligible for premium subsidies: in 2021, the national average unsubsidized premium for a 40-year-old non-smoking individual purchasing coverage through the Marketplace was $436 per month for the lowest-cost silver plan and $328 per month for a bronze plan.

Most people in the coverage gap live in the South, leading state decisions about Medicaid expansion to exacerbate geographic disparities in health coverage. In addition, because several states that have not expanded Medicaid have large populations of people of color, state decisions not to expand their programs disproportionately affect people of color, particularly Black Americans.

https://www.kff.org/racial-equity-and-health-policy/fact-sheet/health-coverage-of-immigrants/
(See hyperlink for full text, charts and references.)

Health Coverage of Immigrants
Published: July 15, 2021

In 2019, there were 21.3 million noncitizens in the United States, accounting for about 7% of the total U.S. population. Noncitizens include lawfully present and undocumented immigrants. Many individuals live in mixed immigration status families that may include lawfully present immigrants, undocumented immigrants, and/or citizens. One in four children has an immigrant parent, and the majority of these children are citizens.

Noncitizens are significantly more likely than citizens to be uninsured. In 2019, among the nonelderly population, 25% of lawfully present immigrants and more than four in ten (46%) undocumented immigrants were uninsured compared to less than one in ten (9%) citizens. Among citizen children, those with at least one noncitizen parent are more likely to be uninsured compared to those with citizen parents (9% vs. 5%).

Research suggests that the changes to immigration policy enacted by the Trump administration contributed to increased fears among immigrant families about participating in programs and seeking services, including health coverage and care. These include policies focused on curbing immigration, enhancing immigration enforcement, and limiting the use of public assistance among immigrant families.

The pandemic has likely contributed to increased health and financial needs and declines in health coverage among immigrant families. Immigrants' work, living, and transportation situations put them at increased risk for potential exposure to coronavirus. Noncitizen immigrants also face risk of financial difficulties due to the pandemic, as many are working in service industries, such as restaurants and food services that have suffered cutbacks. Initial job losses amid the pandemic were particularly high among immigrants. Given their low incomes, job loss could lead to significant financial pressures and increase the share who are uninsured, as people lose access to employer-sponsored insurance or are no longer able to afford coverage.

Restrictions limit immigrants' access to COVID-relief, and ongoing immigration-related fears are making some reluctant to access assistance, services, and COVID-19 vaccines. Although noncitizen immigrants face increased risks associated with the pandemic, restrictions limit immigrants' eligibility for federal health and financial relief provided in response to COVID-19. Moreover, even though the Biden administration has reversed many immigration policy changes made by the Trump administration that increased fears, recent data suggest that ongoing immigration-related fears are contributing to reluctance to access assistance and services as well as COVID-19 vaccines.

Overview of Immigrants

In 2019, there were 21.3 million noncitizens and 22.9 million naturalized citizens residing in the U.S., who each accounted for about 7% of the total population (Figure 1). About six in ten noncitizens were lawfully present immigrants, while the remaining four in ten were undocumented immigrants (see Text Box 1).[1] Many individuals live in mixed immigration status families that may include lawfully present immigrants, undocumented immigrants, and/or citizens.

A total of 18.6 million or one in four children had an immigrant parent as of 2019, and the majority of these children were citizens. About 9.4 million or 12% were citizen children with a noncitizen parent.

Text Box 1: Overview of Lawfully Present and Undocumented Immigrants

Lawfully present immigrants are noncitizens who are lawfully residing in the U.S. This group includes legal permanent residents (LPRs, i.e. "green card" holders), refugees, asylees, and other individuals who are authorized to live in the U.S. temporarily or permanently.

Undocumented immigrants are foreign-born individuals residing in the U.S. without authorization. This group includes individuals who entered the country without authorization and individuals who entered the country lawfully and stayed after their visa or status expired.

Health Coverage for Nonelderly Noncitizens

In 2019, more than three-quarters of the 28.9 million nonelderly uninsured were U.S.-born and naturalized citizens (Figure 2). The remaining 23% were noncitizens.

However, noncitizens, including lawfully present and undocumented immigrants, were significantly more likely to be uninsured than citizens. Among the nonelderly population, 25% of lawfully present immigrants and more than four in ten (46%) undocumented immigrants were uninsured compared to 9% of citizens (Figure 3).

These differences in coverage also occur among children, with noncitizen children more likely to lack coverage compared to their citizen counterparts. Moreover, among citizen children, those with at least one noncitizen parent were significantly more likely to be uninsured as those with citizen parents (Figure 4).

Barriers to Health Coverage for Noncitizens

The higher uninsured rate among noncitizens reflects limited access to employer-sponsored coverage; eligibility restrictions for Medicaid, CHIP, and ACA Marketplace coverage; and barriers to enrollment among eligible individuals.

Limited Access to Coverage

Although most nonelderly noncitizens live in a family with a full-time worker, they face gaps in access to private coverage. Nonelderly noncitizens are more likely than nonelderly citizens to live in a family with at least one full-time worker, but they also are more likely to be low-income (Figure 5). They have lower incomes because they are often employed in low-wage jobs and industries that are less likely to offer employer-sponsored coverage. Given their lower incomes, noncitizens also face increased challenges affording employer-sponsored coverage when it is available or through the individual market.

Lawfully present immigrants may qualify for Medicaid and CHIP but are subject to certain eligibility restrictions. In general, lawfully present immigrants must have a "qualified" immigration status to be eligible for Medicaid or CHIP, and many, including most lawful permanent residents or "green card" holders, must wait five years after obtaining qualified status before they may enroll. Some immigrants with qualified status, such as refugees and asylees, do not have to wait five years before enrolling. Some immigrants, such as those with temporary protected status, are lawfully present but do not have a qualified status and are not eligible to enroll in Medicaid or CHIP regardless of their length of time in the country (Appendix A). For children and pregnant women, states can eliminate the five-year wait and extend coverage to lawfully present immigrants without a qualified status. As of 2021, 35 states have taken up this option for children and half have elected the option for pregnant women.

In December 2020, Congress restored Medicaid eligibility for citizens of Compact of Free Association (COFA) communities. Compacts of Free Association are agreements between the U.S. government and the Republic of the Marshall Islands, the Federated States of Micronesia, and the Republic of Palau. Certain citizens of these nations can lawfully work, study, and reside in the U.S., but they had been excluded from federally-funded Medicaid since 1996, under the Personal Responsibility and Work Opportunity Reconciliation Act (PRWORA). As part of a COVID-relief package, Congress restored Medicaid eligibility for COFA citizens who meet other eligibility requirements for the program effective December 27, 2020.

Lawfully present immigrants can purchase coverage through the ACA Marketplaces and may receive subsidies for this coverage. These subsidies are available to people with incomes from 100% to 400% FPL who are not eligible for other coverage. In addition, lawfully present immigrants with incomes below 100% FPL may receive subsidies if they are ineligible for Medicaid based on immigration status. This group includes lawfully present immigrants who are not eligible for Medicaid or CHIP because they are in the five-year waiting period or do not have a "qualified" status.

Undocumented immigrants are not eligible to enroll in Medicaid or CHIP or to purchase coverage through the ACA Marketplaces. Medicaid payments for emergency services may be made on behalf of individuals who are otherwise eligible for Medicaid but for their immigration status. These payments cover costs for emergency care for lawfully present immigrants who remain ineligible for Medicaid as well as undocumented immigrants. Since 2002, states have had the option to provide prenatal care to women regardless of immigration status by extending CHIP coverage to the unborn child. In addition, some states have state-funded health programs that provide coverage to some groups of immigrants regardless of immigration status. There are also some locally-funded programs that provide coverage or assistance without regard to immigration status. Under rules issued by the Centers for Medicare and

Medicaid Services, individuals with Deferred Action for Childhood Arrivals (DACA) status are not considered lawfully present and remain ineligible for coverage options.

Enrollment Barriers among Eligible Individuals

Many uninsured lawfully present immigrants are eligible for coverage options under the ACA but remain uninsured, while uninsured undocumented immigrants are ineligible for coverage options. Prior to the pandemic many uninsured lawfully present immigrants were eligible for ACA coverage. The American Rescue Plan Act (ARPA) enacted in 2021 further increased access to health coverage through temporary increases and expansions in eligibility for subsidies to buy health insurance through the health insurance marketplaces. It also includes incentives to states that have not yet adopted the ACA Medicaid expansion to do so and provides a new option for states to extend the length of Medicaid coverage for postpartum women. With the temporary changes under ARPA, nearly eight in ten (79%) uninsured lawfully present immigrants were eligible for ACA coverage, including 27% who were eligible for Medicaid and 52% who were eligible for tax credit subsidies (Figure 6). Many lawfully present immigrants who are eligible for coverage remain uninsured because immigrant families face a range of enrollment barriers, including fear, confusion about eligibility policies, difficulty navigating the enrollment process, and language and literacy challenges. Uninsured undocumented immigrants are ineligible for coverage options due to their immigration status. In the absence of coverage, they remain reliant on safety net clinics and hospitals for care and often go without needed care.

Research suggests that changes to immigration policy made by the Trump administration contributed to growing fears among immigrant families about enrolling themselves and/or their children in Medicaid and CHIP. The Trump administration implemented a range of policies to curb immigration, enhance immigration enforcement, and limit use of public assistance programs among immigrant families. Research shows that, amid this policy climate, some immigrant families avoided enrolling themselves and/or their children in public programs, including Medicaid. In particular, changes to public charge policy that allowed federal officials to consider the use of certain non-cash programs, including Medicaid for non-pregnant adults, when determining whether to provide certain individuals a green card or entry into the U.S., likely contributed to decreases in participation in Medicaid among immigrant families and their primarily U.S.-born children. The Biden administration has since reversed many of these changes, including the changes to public charge policy.

Impact of the Pandemic on Immigrant Health Coverage

The pandemic has likely contributed to increased health and financial needs and declines in health coverage among immigrant families. Immigrants' work, living, and transportation situations put them at increased risk for potential exposure to coronavirus. Noncitizen immigrants also face risk of financial difficulties due to the pandemic, as many are working in service industries, such as restaurants and food services, that have suffered cutbacks. Initial job losses amid the pandemic were particularly high among immigrants. Given their low incomes, job loss could lead to significant financial pressures for them and their families and may increase the share who are uninsured, as people lose access to employer-sponsored insurance or are no longer able to afford coverage.

Restrictions limit immigrants' access to COVID-19 relief, and ongoing immigration-related fears are making some reluctant to access assistance, services, and COVID-19 vaccines. Although noncitizen immigrants face increased risks associated with the pandemic, restrictions limit immigrants' eligibility for federal health and financial relief provided in response to COVID-19. Moreover, even though the Biden administration has reversed many immigration policy changes made by the Trump administration, recent data suggest that ongoing immigration-related fears are contributing to reluctance to access assistance and services as well as COVID-19 vaccines. For example, surveys of Hispanic adults and Asian community health center patients show some are continuing to avoid participating in assistance programs for health, housing, or food due to immigration-related fears. Data also suggest that immigration-related fears are contributing to reluctance to access COVID-19 vaccines among Hispanic adults even though all individuals are eligible for the vaccine regardless of immigration status.

https://www.healthcare.gov/immigrants/lawfully-present-immigrants/
(See hyperlink for full text and references.)

Coverage for Lawfully Present Immigrants

Lawfully present immigrants are eligible for coverage through the Health Insurance Marketplace®.

The term "lawfully present" includes immigrants who have:

- "Qualified non-citizen" immigration status without a waiting period (see details below).

- Humanitarian statuses or circumstances (including Temporary Protected Status, Special Juvenile Status, asylum applicants, Convention Against Torture, victims of trafficking).

- Valid non-immigrant visas.

- Legal status conferred by other laws (temporary resident status, LIFE Act, Family Unity individuals). Here is a list of immigration statuses eligible for Marketplace coverage:
  - Lawful Permanent Resident (LPR/Green Card holder)
  - Asylee
  - Refugee
  - Cuban/Haitian Entrant
  - Paroled into the U.S.
  - Conditional Entrant Granted before 1980
  - Battered Spouse, Child and Parent
  - Victim of Trafficking and his/her Spouse, Child, Sibling or Parent
  - Granted Withholding of Deportation or Withholding of Removal, under the immigration laws or under the Convention against Torture (CAT)
  - Individual with Non-immigrant Status, includes worker visas (such as H1, H-2A, H-2B), student visas, U-visa, T-visa, and other visas, and citizens of Micronesia, the Marshall Islands, and Palau
  - Temporary Protected Status (TPS)
  - Deferred Enforced Departure (DED)
  - Deferred Action Status (Exception: Deferred Action for Childhood Arrivals (DACA) is not an eligible immigration status for applying for health insurance)

> Lawful Temporary Resident
> Administrative order staying removal issued by the Department of Homeland Security
> Member of a federally-recognized Indian tribe or American Indian Born in Canada
> Resident of American Samoa

Lawfully present immigrants and Marketplace savings

If you're a lawfully present immigrant, you can buy private health insurance on the Marketplace. You may be eligible for lower costs on monthly premiums and lower out-of-pocket costs based on your income.

- If your annual income is between 100% and 400% of the federal poverty level (FPL): You may qualify for premium tax credits and other savings on Marketplace insurance.

- If your annual household income is above 400% FPL: You may still qualify for premium tax credits that lower your monthly premium for a 2021 Marketplace health insurance plan.

- If your annual household income is below 100% FPL: If you're not otherwise eligible for Medicaid you'll qualify for premium tax credits and other savings on Marketplace insurance, if you meet all other eligibility requirements.

Immigrants and Medicaid & CHIP

Immigrants who are "qualified non-citizens" are generally eligible for coverage through Medicaid and the Children's Health Insurance Program (CHIP), if they meet their state's income and residency rules.

In order to get Medicaid and CHIP coverage, many qualified non-citizens (such as many LPRs or green card holders) have a 5-year waiting period. This means they must wait 5 years after receiving "qualified" immigration status before they can get Medicaid and CHIP coverage. There are exceptions. For example, refugees, asylees, or LPRs who used to be refugees or asylees don't have to wait 5 years.

The term "qualified non-citizen" includes:

- Lawful Permanent Residents (LPR/Green Card Holder)

- Asylees

- Refugees

- Cuban/Haitian entrants

- Paroled into the U.S. for at least one year

- Conditional entrant granted before 1980

- Battered non-citizens, spouses, children, or parents

- Victims of trafficking and his or her spouse, child, sibling, or parent or individuals with a pending application for a victim of trafficking visa

- Granted withholding of deportation

- Member of a federally recognized Indian tribe or American Indian born in Canada

- Citizens of the Marshall Islands, Micronesia, and Palau who are living in one of the U.S. states or territories (referred to as Compact of Free Association or COFA migrants)

Medicaid & CHIP coverage for lawfully residing children and pregnant women

States have the option to remove the 5-year waiting period and cover lawfully residing children and/or pregnant women in Medicaid or CHIP. A child or pregnant woman is "lawfully residing" if they're "lawfully present" and otherwise eligible for Medicaid or CHIP in the state.

Twenty-nine states, plus the District of Columbia and the Commonwealth of the Northern Mariana Islands, have chosen to provide Medicaid coverage to lawfully residing children and/or pregnant women without a 5-year waiting period. Twenty-one of these states also cover lawfully residing children or pregnant women in CHIP. (See hyperlink to learn if your state has this option in place.)

Getting emergency care

Medicaid provides payment for treatment of an emergency medical condition for people who meet all Medicaid eligibility criteria in the state (such as income and state residency), but don't have an eligible immigration status.

Medicaid, CHIP, & "public charge" status

Applying for or receiving Medicaid or CHIP benefits, or getting savings for health insurance costs in the Marketplace, doesn't make someone a "public charge." This means it won't affect their chances of becoming a Lawful Permanent Resident or U.S. citizen.

There's one exception for people receiving long-term care in an institution at government expense, like in a nursing facility. These people may face barriers getting a green card.

ALSO SEE:

https://www.cbsnews.com/news/does-medicare-for-all-cover-undocumented-immigrants-depends-on-who-you-ask/

The Affordable Care Act of 2010

The Affordable Care Act was a huge step in the right direction, substantially decreasing the number of uninsured - yet only covering 31 million of the US population of 333 million by June 2021. The ACA was layered over many existing programs and depended upon, rather than eliminating, for-profit health insurance with its excessive costs and complexities. Expanded and Improved Medicare for All ("a card in your wallet"), on the other hand, would cover 100% of the US population and eliminate the excessive costs and inequities of the for-profit health insurance industry.

https://en.wikipedia.org/wiki/Affordable_Care_Act
(See hyperlink for full text & references)

The Affordable Care Act
From Wikipedia, the free encyclopedia

The Affordable Care Act (ACA), formally known as the Patient Protection and Affordable Care Act (PPACA), and colloquially known as Obamacare, is a United States federal statute enacted by the 111th United States Congress and signed into law by President Barack Obama on March 23, 2010.

The ACA's major provisions came into force in 2014. By 2016, the uninsured share of the population had roughly halved, with estimates ranging from 20 to 24 million additional people covered. After it went into effect, increases in overall healthcare spending slowed, including premiums for employer-based insurance plans.

The increased coverage was due, roughly equally, to an expansion of Medicaid eligibility and to changes to individual insurance markets. Both received new spending, funded through a combination of new taxes and cuts to Medicare provider rates and Medicare Advantage. Several Congressional Budget Office reports said that overall these provisions reduced the budget deficit, that repealing the ACA would increase the deficit, and that the law reduced income inequality by taxing primarily the top 1% to fund roughly $600 in benefits on average to families in the bottom 40% of the income distribution.

The act largely retained the existing structure of Medicare, Medicaid and the employer market, but individual insurance markets were radically overhauled. Insurers were made to accept all applicants without charging based on preexisting conditions or demographic status (except age). The act mandated that individuals buy insurance (or pay a fine/tax) and that insurers cover a list of "essential health benefits".

Dependents were permitted to remain on their parents' insurance plan until their 26th birthday, including dependents who no longer lived with their parents, are not a dependent on a parent's tax return, are no longer a student, or are married.

The ACA requires members of Congress and their staffs to obtain health insurance either through an exchange or some other program approved by the law (such as Medicare), instead of using the insurance offered to federal employees (the Federal Employees Health Benefits Program).

The ACA explicitly denies insurance subsidies to "unauthorized (illegal) aliens".

The ACA mandated that health insurance exchanges be provided for each state. The exchanges are regulated, largely online marketplaces, administered by either federal or state governments, where individuals, families and small businesses can purchase private insurance plans. Some exchanges also provide access to Medicaid.

By 2019, 12 states and the District of Columbia operated their own own health insurance marketplace. Other states either used the federal exchange, or operated in partnership with or supported by the federal government.

States can apply for a "waiver for state innovation" which allows them to pass legislation setting up an alternative health system that provides insurance at least as comprehensive and as affordable as ACA, covers at least as many residents and does not increase the federal deficit.

PROVISIONS

The individual insurance market was radically overhauled, and many of the law's regulations applied specifically to this market, while the structure of Medicare, Medicaid, and the employer market were largely retained. Some regulations applied to the employer market, and the law also made delivery system changes that affected most of the health care system.

Insurance Regulations: Individual Policies

All new individual major medical health insurance policies sold to individuals and families faced new requirements. The requirements took effect on January 1, 2014. They include:

- Guaranteed issue prohibits insurers from denying coverage to individuals due to preexisting conditions.

- States were required to ensure the availability of insurance for individual children who did not have coverage via their families.

- A partial community rating allows premiums to vary only by age and location, regardless of preexisting conditions.

- Premiums for older applicants can be no more than three times those for the youngest.

- Essential health benefits must be provided.

- Preventive care and screenings for women. "All FDA-approved contraceptive methods, sterilization procedures, and patient education and counseling for all women with reproductive capacity." This mandate applies to all employers and educational institutions except for religious organizations.

- Annual and lifetime coverage caps on essential benefits were banned.

- Insurers are forbidden from dropping policyholders when they become ill.

- All policies must provide an annual maximum out of pocket (MOOP) payment cap for an individual's or family's medical expenses (excluding premiums).

- Preventive care, vaccinations and medical screenings cannot be subject to co-payments, co-insurance or deductibles.

- The law established four tiers of coverage: bronze, silver, gold and platinum. The categories vary in their division of premiums and out-of-pocket costs.

- Insurers are required to implement an appeals process for coverage determination and claims on all new plans.

- Insurers must spend at least 80–85% of premium dollars on health costs; rebates must be issued if this is violated.

Individual Mandate

The individual mandate required everyone to have insurance or pay a penalty. The mandate was intended to increase the size and diversity of the insured population, including more young and healthy participants to broaden the risk pool, spreading costs.

The Individual mandate tax was $695 per individual or $2,085 per family at a minimum, reaching as high as 2.5% of household income (whichever was higher).

The Tax Cuts and Jobs Act of 2017 reduced to $0 the fine/tax for violating the individual mandate, starting in 2019. (The requirement itself is still in effect.)

Among the groups who were not subject to the individual mandate are:

- Illegal immigrants, estimated at around 8 million, are ineligible for insurance subsidies and Medicaid. They remain eligible for emergency services.

- Medicaid-eligible citizens not enrolled in Medicaid.

- Citizens whose insurance coverage would cost more than 8% of household income.

- Citizens who live in states that opt out of Medicaid expansion and who qualify for neither existing Medicaid coverage nor subsidized coverage.

Employer Mandate (and Part-Time Work)

Businesses that employ fifty or more people but do not offer health insurance to their full-time employees are assessed additional tax ($4,060 per full-time employee in 2021) if the government has subsidized a full-time employee's healthcare through tax deductions or other means. This is commonly known as the employer mandate. This provision was included to encourage employers to continue providing insurance once the exchanges began operating.

Most policy analysts (both right and left) were critical of the employer mandate provision. They argued that the perverse incentives regarding part-time hours were real and harmful; that the raised marginal cost of the 50th worker for businesses could limit companies' growth; that the costs of reporting and administration were not worth the costs of maintaining employer plans; and noted that the employer mandate was not essential to maintain adequate risk pools. The provision generated vocal opposition from business interests and some unions who were not granted exemptions.

In 2015 the progressive Center for Economic and Policy Research found no evidence that companies were reducing worker hours to avoid ACA requirements for employees working more than 30 hours per week.

Premium Subsidies

Individuals whose household incomes are between 100% and 400% of the federal poverty level (FPL) are eligible to receive federal subsidies applied towards premiums for policies purchased via an ACA exchange, provided they are not eligible for Medicare, Medicaid, the Children's Health Insurance Program, or other forms of public assistance health coverage, and provided they do not have access to affordable coverage through their own or a family member's employer. Households below the federal poverty level are not eligible to receive these subsidies. Enrollees must have U.S. citizenship or proof of legal residency to obtain a subsidy.

The subsidies for an ACA plan purchased on an exchange stop at 400% of the federal poverty level (FPL). According to the Kaiser Foundation, this results in a sharp "discontinuity of treatment" at 400% FPL, which is sometimes called the "subsidy cliff".

The amount of subsidy is sufficient to reduce the premium for the second-lowest-cost silver plan (SCLSP) from 2-10%. The subsidy can be used towards any plan available on the exchange, but not catastrophic plans. The subsidy may not exceed the premium for the purchased plan.

Small businesses are eligible for a tax credit provided they enroll in the Small Business Health Option Program (SHOP) Marketplace.

In March 2018, the CBO reported that ACA had reduced income inequality measured after taxes (due to the income tax surcharges and subsidies) in 2014, saying the law led the bottom 40% to receive an average of an additional $560-$690 while causing households in the top 1% to pay an additional $21,000 due mostly to the net investment income tax and the additional Medicare tax. The law placed relatively little burden on households in the top 20% outside of the top 1%.

CBO estimated that subsidies paid under the law in 2016 averaged $4,240 per person for 10 million individuals receiving them, roughly $42 billion. The tax subsidy for the employer market was approximately $1,700 per person (for approximately 156.5 million) in 2016, or $266 billion total.

Cost-sharing Reduction Subsidies

As written, the ACA mandated that insurers reduce copayments and deductibles for ACA exchange enrollees earning less than 250% of the FPL. Medicaid recipients were not eligible for the reductions.

So-called cost-sharing reduction (CSR) subsidies were to be paid to insurance companies to fund the reductions. During 2017, approximately $7 billion in CSR subsidies were to be paid, versus $34 billion for premium tax credits.

The latter were defined as mandatory spending that does not require an annual Congressional appropriation. CSR payments were not explicitly defined as mandatory. This led to litigation and disruption later.

Risk Management for Private Insurers

The ACA implemented multiple approaches to helping mitigate the disruptions to insurers that came with its many changes: Risk Corridors (temporary through 2016), Reinsurance (temporary through 2016), and Risk Adjustment.

Risk adjustment involves transferring funds from plans with lower-risk enrollees to plans with higher-risk enrollees, intended to encourage insurers to compete based on value and efficiency rather than by attracting healthier enrollees.

Medicaid Expansion

The ACA revised and expanded Medicaid eligibility starting in 2014. All U.S. citizens and legal residents with income up to 133% of the poverty line, including adults without dependent children, would qualify for coverage in any state that participated in the Medicaid program.

As of December 2019, 37 states (including Washington DC) had adopted the Medicaid extension. States that expanded Medicaid had a 7.3% uninsured rate on average in the first quarter of 2016, while the others had a 14.1% uninsured rate, among adults aged 18 to 64. Over half the national uninsured population lived in those states.

The Centers for Medicare and Medicaid Services (CMS) estimated that the cost of Medicaid expansion was $6,366 per person for 2015, about 49 percent above previous estimates. An estimated 9 to 10 million people had gained Medicaid coverage, mostly low-income adults. The Kaiser Family Foundation estimated in October 2015 that 3.1 million additional people were not covered because of states that rejected the Medicaid expansion.

Many states did not make Medicaid available to childless adults at any income level. Because subsidies on exchange insurance plans were not available to those below the poverty line, such individuals had no new options.

A 2016 study found that residents of Kentucky and Arkansas, which both expanded Medicaid, were more likely to receive health care services and less likely to incur emergency room costs or have trouble paying their medical bills. Residents of Texas, which did not accept the Medicaid expansion, did not see a similar improvement during the same period.

Importantly, issues with cost-related unmet medical needs, skipped medications, paying medical bills, and annual out-of-pocket spending have been significantly reduced among low-income adults in Medicaid expansion states compared to non-expansion states.

Expanded Medicaid has led to a 6.6% increase in physician visits by low-income adults, as well as increased usage of preventative care such as dental visits and cancer screenings among childless, low-income adults. Other notable health outcomes associated with Medicaid expansion include improved glucose monitoring rates for patients with diabetes, better hypertension control, and reduced rates of major post-operative morbidity.

ACA Taxes and Excise Taxes

Annual excise taxes totaling $3 billion were levied on importers and manufacturers of prescription drugs.

An excise tax of 2.3% on medical devices and a 10% excise tax on indoor tanning services were applied as well.

Excise taxes from the Affordable Care Act raised $16.3 billion in fiscal year 2015. $11.3 billion came from an excise tax placed directly on health insurers based on their market share.

In fiscal year 2018, the individual and employer mandates yielded $4 billion each. Excise taxes on insurers and drug makers added $18 billion.

Income tax surcharges produced $437 billion.

The Health Insurance Tax (repealed beginning 2021) was applied to all insurers that offered fully-insured health insurance in the group market, the marketplaces, or public programs (such as Medicare or Medicaid).

The ACA includes an excise tax of 40% on total employer premium spending in excess of specified dollar amounts (initially $10,200 for single coverage and $27,500 for family coverage) indexed to inflation. This "Cadillac" tax was originally scheduled to take effect in 2018, but was delayed until 2020 by the Consolidated Appropriations Act, 2016.

In 2019 Congress repealed the so-called "Cadillac" tax on health insurance benefits, an excise tax on medical devices, and the Health Insurance Tax.

Delivery System Reforms

The ACA includes delivery system reforms intended to constrain costs and improve quality.

Medicare switched from fee-for-service to bundled payments. A single payment was to be paid to a hospital and a physician group for a defined episode of care (such as a hip replacement) rather than separate payments to individual service providers.

Health care cost/quality initiatives included incentives to reduce hospital infections, adopt electronic medical records, and to coordinate care and prioritize quality over quantity.

The ACA allowed the creation of Accountable Care Organizations (ACOs), which are groups of doctors, hospitals and other providers that commit to give coordinated care to Medicare patients. ACOs were allowed to continue using fee-for-service billing. They receive bonus payments from the government for minimizing costs while achieving quality benchmarks that emphasize prevention and mitigation of chronic disease. Missing cost or quality benchmarks subjected them to penalties.

THE HEALTHCARE DEBATE, 2008–2010

In February 2009, President Obama announced to a joint session of Congress his intent to work with Congress to construct a plan for healthcare reform. On November 7, the House of Representatives passed the Affordable Health Care for America Act on a 220–215 vote and forwarded it to the Senate for passage.

On December 23, the Senate voted 60–39 to end debate on the bill: a cloture vote to end the filibuster. The bill then passed, also 60–39, on December 24, 2009, with all Democrats and two independents voting for it and all Republicans against, except one who did not vote. The bill was endorsed by the American Medical Association and AARP.

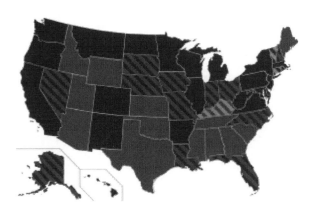

Senate vote by state:

▌Democratic yes (58)

▌Independent yes (2)

▌Republican no (39)

▌Republican not voting (1)

House vote by congressional district:

▌Democratic yes (219)

▌ Democratic no (34)

▌ Republican no (178)

▐ No representative seated (4)

Obama held a meeting with both parties' leaders on February 25, 2010. The Democrats decided the House would pass the Senate's bill, so as to avoid another Senate vote.

The House passed the Senate bill with a 219–212 vote on March 21, 2010, with 34 Democrats and all 178 Republicans voting against it. The next day, Republicans introduced legislation to repeal the bill. Obama signed The ACA into law on March 23, 2010.

House Democrats then drafted the Health Care and Education Reconciliation Act (HCERA), which could be passed by the reconciliation process. Per the Congressional Budget Act of 1974, reconciliation cannot be subject to a filibuster, but is limited to budget changes. Most of House Democrats' demands were budgetary: "these changes - higher subsidy levels, different kinds of taxes to pay for them, nixing the Nebraska Medicaid deal - mainly involve taxes and spending. In other words, they're exactly the kinds of policies that are well-suited for reconciliation." Obama signed HCERA into law on March 30, 2010.

Since passage, Republicans have voted to repeal all or parts of the Affordable Care Act more than sixty times; none have been successful.

IMPLEMENTATION OF THE ACA

At the beginning of the 2015, 11.7 million had signed up (ex-Medicaid). By the end of the year about 8.8 million consumers had stayed in the program (2016 US population of 323 million).

An estimated 9 to 10 million people had gained Medicaid coverage in 2016, mostly low-income adults. The ACA reduced the percent of Americans between 18 and 64 who were uninsured from 22.3 percent in 2010 to 12.4 percent in 2016.

The five major national insurers expected to lose money on ACA policies in 2016, in part because the enrollees were lower income, older and sicker than expected.

In response to Trump's executive order on January 20, 2017, the IRS announced that it would not require that tax returns indicate a person has health insurance, reducing the effectiveness of the individual mandate. Starting in 2019, the individual mandate was repealed via the Tax Cuts and Jobs Act.

More than 9.2 million people (3.0 million new customers and 6.2 million returning) enrolled on the national exchange in 2017, down some 400,000 from 2016. The eleven states that run their own exchanges signed up about 3 million more.

By 2019, 35 states and the District of Columbia had either expanded coverage via traditional Medicaid or via an alternative program. The CBO estimated that the repeal of the individual mandate would cause 13 million fewer people to have health insurance in 2027.

EMPLOYER VS. NON-EMPLOYER INSURANCE COSTS

For the group market (employer insurance), a 2016 survey found that:

- Deductibles grew 63% from 2011 to 2016, while premiums increased 19% and worker earnings grew by 11%.

- In 2016, 4 in 5 workers had an insurance deductible, which averaged $1,478. For firms with less than 200 employees, the deductible averaged $2,069.

- The percentage of workers with a deductible of at least $1,000 grew from 10% in 2006 to 51% in 2016. The 2016 figure dropped to 38% after taking employer contributions into account.

For the non-group market, of which two-thirds are covered by ACA exchanges, a survey of 2015 data found that:

- 49% had individual deductibles of at least $1,500 ($3,000 for family), up from 36% in 2014.

- Many exchange enrollees qualify for cost-sharing subsidies that reduce their net deductible.

- While about 75% of enrollees were "very satisfied" or "somewhat satisfied" with their choice of doctors and hospitals, only 50% had such satisfaction with their annual deductible.

- While 52% of those covered by The ACA exchanges felt "well protected" by their insurance, in the group market 63% felt that way.

HEALTH OUTCOMES: ACA & MEDICAID EXPANSION

According to a 2014 study, The ACA likely prevented an estimated 50,000 preventable patient deaths from 2010 to 2013. Himmelstein and Woolhandler wrote in January 2017 that a rollback of The ACA's Medicaid expansion alone would cause an estimated 43,956 deaths annually.

A July 2019 study by the National Bureau of Economic Research (NBER) indicated that states enacting Medicaid expansion exhibited statistically significant reductions in mortality rates. "The lifesaving impacts of Medicaid expansion are large: an estimated 39 to 64 percent reduction in annual mortality rates for older adults gaining coverage."

Dependent Coverage Expansion (DCE) under the ACA has had a demonstrable effect on various health metrics of young adults, a group with a historically low level of insurance coverage and utilization of care. Studies have also found that DCE was associated with improvements in cancer prevention, detection, and treatment among young adult patients.

A 2019 *JAMA* study found that ACA decreased emergency department and hospital use by uninsured individuals. A 2020 *JAMA* study found that Medicaid expansion under the ACA was associated with reduced incidence of advanced-stage breast cancer, indicating that Medicaid accessibility led to early detection of breast cancer and higher survival rates.

From the start of 2010 to November 2014, 43 hospitals in rural areas closed. Between January 2010 and 2015, a quarter of ER doctors said they had seen a major surge in patients, while nearly half had seen a smaller increase. Seven in ten ER doctors claimed they lacked the resources to deal with large increases in the number of patients. The biggest factor in the increased number of ER patients was insufficient primary care providers to handle the larger number of insured.

FEDERAL DEFICIT as ASSESSED by CBO

The CBO (Congressional Budget Office) reported in multiple studies that The ACA would reduce the deficit, and repealing it would increase the deficit, primarily because of the elimination of Medicare reimbursement cuts. The 2011 comprehensive CBO estimate projected a net deficit reduction of more than $200 billion during the 2012–2021 period. The

CBO claimed the bill would "substantially reduce the growth of Medicare's payment rates for most services; impose an excise tax on insurance plans with relatively high premiums; and make various other changes to the federal tax code, Medicare, Medicaid, and other programs" - ultimately extending the solvency of the Medicare trust fund by eight years.

This estimate was made prior to the Supreme Court's ruling that enabled states to opt out of the Medicaid expansion, thereby forgoing the related federal funding.

Health economist Uwe Reinhardt, wrote, "The rigid, artificial rules under which the Congressional Budget Office must score proposed legislation unfortunately cannot produce the best unbiased forecasts of the likely fiscal impact of any legislation."

Noam Scheiber and Jonathan Cohn noted that the CBO had a track record of overestimating costs and underestimating savings of health legislation; stating, "innovations in the delivery of medical care, like greater use of electronic medical records and financial incentives for more coordination of care among doctors, would produce substantial savings while also slowing the relentless climb of medical expenses. But the CBO would not consider such savings in its calculations, because the innovations hadn't really been tried on such large scale or in concert with one another - and that meant there wasn't much hard data to prove the savings would materialize."

PUBLIC OPINION

In 2015, a poll reported that 47% of Americans approved the health care law. This was the first time a major poll indicated that more respondents approved than disapproved.

Separate polls from Fox News and NBC/*WSJ*, both taken during January 2017, indicated more people viewed the law favorably than did not for the first time. Another January 2017 poll reported that 35% of respondents believed "Obamacare" and the "Affordable Care Act" were different or did not know. (About 45% were unsure whether "repeal of Obamacare" also meant "repeal of the Affordable Care Act".) 39% did not know that "many people would lose coverage through Medicaid or subsidies for private health insurance if the ACA were repealed and no replacement enacted," with Democrats far more likely (79%) to know that fact than Republicans (47%).

LEGAL CHALLENGES TO THE ACA

Medicaid Expansion

In *National Federation of Independent Business v. Sebelius* (June 2012), the Supreme Court ruled that states could choose not to participate in the law's Medicaid expansion, but upheld the law as a whole.

Contraception mandate

In *Burwell v. Hobby Lobby* (June 2014) the Supreme Court exempted closely held corporations with religious convictions from the contraception rule.

In *Little Sisters of the Poor Saints Peter and Paul Home v. Pennsylvania*, the Supreme Court ruled 7–2 on July 8, 2020, that employers with religious or moral objections to contraceptives can exclude such coverage from an employee's insurance plan.

California v. Texas

Texas and nineteen other states filed a civil suit in the United States District Court for the Northern District of Texas in February 2018, arguing that with the passage of the Tax Cuts and Jobs Act of 2017, which eliminated the tax for not having health insurance, the individual mandate no longer had a constitutional basis and thus the entire ACA was no longer constitutional.

In December 2019, the Fifth Circuit agreed the individual mandate was unconstitutional. It did not, however, agree that the entire law should be voided. Instead, it remanded the case to the District Court for reconsideration of that question. The Supreme Court accepted the case in March 2020, but to be heard in the 2020–2021 term, with the ruling likely falling after the 2020 elections.

Democrats pointed out that the effect of invalidating the entire law would be to remove popular provisions such as the protection for preexisting conditions, and that the Republicans had still not offered any replacement plan.

REPEAL EFFORTS

The ACA was the subject of many unsuccessful repeal efforts

by Republicans in the 111th, 112th, and 113th Congresses (January 2009 – December 2014). On February 3, 2015, the House of Representatives added its 67th repeal vote to the record (239 to 186). This attempt also failed, as did other attempts in 2017.

ACTIONS TO HINDER IMPLEMENTATION

The American Health Care Act (AHCA aka "Trumpcare") was written by Republicans in the House of Representatives as a replacement for The ACA. It was voted on and passed in the House on May 4, 2017. Senate Republican Leadership released a draft of the legislation – called the Better Care Reconciliation Act of 2017 – on June 22, 2017 and was rejected by a 49-51 vote on July 28, 2017 (thanks to Senator John McCain's famous "thumbs down" vote).

Under both the ACA and the AHCA, CBO reported that the health exchange marketplaces would remain stable. However, Republican politicians took a variety of steps to undermine it, creating uncertainty that adversely impacted enrollment and insurer participation while increasing premiums. Past and ongoing Republican attempts to weaken the law have included:

- President Trump ended the payment of cost-sharing reduction subsidies to insurers on October 12, 2017. Premium increases expected to be 10% or less in 2018 became 28 - 40% instead. Since most premiums are subsidized, the federal government would cover most of the increases.
- Trump weakened the individual mandate with his first executive order, which limited enforcement of the tax. For example, tax returns without indications of health insurance ("silent returns") will still be processed, overriding Obama's instructions to reject them.
- Trump reduced funding for advertising for exchange enrollment by up to 90%, with other reductions to support resources used to answer questions and help people sign-up for coverage. CBO said the reductions would reduce ACA enrollment.
- Trump reduced the enrollment period for 2018 by half, to 45 days.
- Trump made public statements that the exchanges were unstable or in a death spiral.

- President Donald Trump rescinded the federal tax penalty for violating the individual mandate through the Tax Cuts and Jobs Act of 2017, starting in 2019.
- Many economically conservative opponents called the ACA "socialist" or "socialized medicine", pointing to the government redistribution of wealth via subsidies for low-income purchasers, expansion of the government-run Medicaid insurance, government requirements as to what products can be sold on the exchanges, and the individual mandate, which reduces freedom of consumer choice to be uninsured.

https://xpostfactoid.blogspot.com/2016/05/
(See hyperlink for full text and references.)

98% of Americans with Health Insurance are Subsidized. How 'bout the other 2%?
By Andrew Sprung, Healthcare Writer, 25 May 2016

While the ACA has reduced the ranks of the U.S. uninsured by some 17 million, and currently subsidizes private health insurance plans for about 9.4 million people, it has also raised the price of health insurance for most of those who have to buy their own insurance, and don't qualify for ACA premium subsidies.

Those who buy their insurance in the individual market and get no subsidy at all are the only insured Americans whose insurance is unsubsidized, and they are a tiny minority of the insured population. 147 million people who get their insurance through an employer are subsidized via the tax exclusion for employer-sponsored health insurance. 72.4 million Medicaid enrollees and 55.5 million Medicare enrollees are subsidized, as are about 9 million VA-enrolled veterans and, again, 9.4 million ACA marketplace enrollees.

In fact, one substantial group of those who are shut out of marketplace subsidies does have access to a tax credit. That is the self-employed health insurance tax deduction, which can be claimed by any self-employed person with a positive net income. If that income exceeds the cost of insurance purchased in the individual market, the whole premium paid for insurance is deductible.

If 36% of individual market enrollees who don't get ACA credits are self-employed, approximately 3 million of them should be eligible for the self-employment health insurance deduction, the value of which varies according to income. That leaves about 5.3 million current enrollees without access to any subsidy at all. Some enrollees at any income level may also benefit from the medical expenses deduction, allowing a taxpayer to deduct medical expenses that exceed 10% of income.

One relatively simple way to help the currently unsubsidized would be to simply extend the self-employed health insurance deduction to anyone who buys insurance in the individual market and does not qualify for the ACA premium tax credit. If the deduction were capped at 20% -- so that someone in, say, a 39% bracket could only deduct 20% of the cost of insurance from their tax bill -- that would help pay for the eligibility expansion, since some self-employed are presumably taking the deduction at top tax rates.

To hazard a guess, perhaps a quarter of the country's 28 million uninsured have incomes outside of subsidy range. Extending the health insurance deduction to those among them who are not self-employed might entice more into the market, improving the risk pool.

Andrew Sprung is also the author of (and recommends) "A post-ACA subsidy that already exists: Is deductibility of health premiums a promising 'repeal' component? See how it works for over 4 million who already take the deduction." (https://www.healthinsurance.org/blog/a-post-aca-subsidy-that-already-exists/).

OBAMACARE WILL SOON HELP MORE MIDDLE-CLASS FAMILIES

Rick Newman / 10 March 2021

Most of the headlines regarding the American Rescue Plan Congress passed on March 10 focus on $1,400 stimulus checks and a 4-month extension of federal unemployment benefits. Less noticed are a set of changes to Obamacare, aka the Affordable Care Act, that are the biggest revamp of health care policy in more than a decade.

The American Rescue Plan, as it's known, will address one of the main flaws in the ACA by expanding health care subsidies to several million middle-income families that haven't been eligible for assistance up till now. Originally, the ACA offered subsidies that covered some or all of the cost of health insurance for lower-income Americans. The benefit declined as income rose, and phased out completely for incomes at 400% of the poverty line. For a family of four, that would be $106,000 in income, which meant above that level they'd get no help purchasing insurance.

Many people above that income level get coverage through an employer, which is generally affordable. But those who have to buy it on their own can easily spend $20,000 or more on insurance premiums alone. Costs are highest for those in their 50s or early 60s who aren't yet eligible for Medicare. Some people stuck in this category simply forego insurance because it's too expensive.

The new law eliminates the income cap and limits the amount any family pays for health insurance to 8.5% of household income. That means families that previously earned too much for subsidies can now enroll through an ACA marketplace, and the government will reimburse any amount paid for insurance above 8.5% of annual income.

The change covers calendar years 2021 and 2022, but the catch for 2021 is that it only covers plans offered through an ACA exchange. Families on a non-exchange plan can't ask for a rebate - but they can switch plans. The Biden administration has opened a special ACA enrollment period that lasts until May 15, which would allow people to cancel an unsubsidized plan and get a cheaper plan through an exchange.

The savings could make it well worth the hassle. A family earning $150,000 got no ACA subsidies up till now. But the change in the law means if that family joins an ACA plan, the most it will have to pay for premiums is 8.5% of its income, or $12,750. Some families now pay considerably more than that. They still have to pay other costs, such as deductibles and co-pays. But more affordable insurance could also allow families to buy more comprehensive plans with better coverage than they've been used to.

There's no upper income limit on the benefit because the cost of insurance available through an exchange has a ceiling. Somebody earning a million dollars couldn't pay $100,000 in premiums for an ACA plan, with the government covering $15,000 of the cost. Such lavish health coverage might exist in the private market, but not in any ACA plan.

A key issue in 2022 midterm elections

The ACA changes would only last for two years, because new federal spending that's not offset by new revenues must be temporary. Democrats have already said, however, they'd like to make the changes permanent. That will make it a potent issue in the 2022 midterm elections, with Democrats saying they must retain control of Congress in order to lock in a treasured new middle-class benefit. Republicans have opposed any expansion of the ACA, but they've been surprisingly quiet about the latest move. There's no GOP alternative to the ACA so it's not clear how they'll battle the Democrats.

About 23 million Americans get coverage through the ACA, and eliminating the income cap for subsidies could bring a few million more into the program. It would also mark an important redo, dating to President Obama's mistaken claim that anybody who liked their insurance would be able to keep it under Obamacare. That wasn't true, because the law essentially banned inexpensive plans with limited coverage. Some people found they suddenly had to buy more expensive coverage. Over time, the biggest hikes in premiums came in the so-called individual market, where people who didn't get coverage through the ACA or an employer had to pay whatever insurers demanded, or go without.

Expanding the benefit will cost about $24 billion for both years, according to the Congressional Budget Office. Additional cost has been a barrier to expansion in the past, but Congress has authorized $6 trillion in economic relief during the last 12 months, an unprecedented spending blowout. Voters don't seem to mind. Approval of the Biden rescue is well above 60% in several polls, which suggests voters would be fine with a few billion per year to keep the ACA expansion in place after 2022.

There's disappointment among some progressives that this may be the extent of health care reform during Biden's first two years, and perhaps during his entire term. Biden has proposed a "public option," similar to Medicare, that would be available to people who can't get affordable coverage any other way. But opening ACA subsidies to many of those same people will accomplish at least part of the goal, and perhaps do it without the angry opposition that threatened the ACA for nearly a decade after Congress first passed it. American health care is becoming slightly more rational.

Rick Newman is the author of four books, including **"Rebounders: How Winners Pivot from Setback to Success."** *Follow him on Twitter: @rickjnewman.*

https://www.macpac.gov/medicaid-101/
(See hyperlink for full text and references.)

MEDICAID 101

Medicaid is a joint federal-state program that provided health care coverage to an estimated 74.6 million people in fiscal year (FY) 2018. As a major payer in the U.S. health care system, it accounted for about 16.4 percent of national health care spending in calendar year 2018.

Medicaid's role among payers is unique. It provides coverage for health and other related services for the nation's most economically disadvantaged populations, including low-income children and their families, low-income seniors, and low-income people with disabilities. These populations are distinguished by the breadth and intensity of their health needs; the impact of poverty, unemployment, and other socioeconomic factors on their ability to obtain health care services; and the degree to which they require assistance in paying for care.

Medicaid provides benefits not typically covered (or covered to a lesser extent) by other insurers, including long-term services and supports. It also pays for Medicare premiums and cost sharing for more than 12 million people who are enrolled in both programs. It is also a major source of financing for care delivered by certain providers, particularly safety net institutions that serve both low-income and uninsured individuals.

The Medicaid program was enacted as part of the Social Security Amendments of 1965 (P.L. 89-97), the same legislation that created Medicare. Like Medicare, Medicaid is an entitlement program. Eligible individuals have rights to payment for medically necessary health care services defined in statute; the federal government is obligated to fund a share of the outlays for those services.

Variability in Medicaid is the rule rather than the exception. States establish their own eligibility standards, benefit packages, provider payment policies, and administrative structures under broad federal guidelines, effectively creating 56 different Medicaid programs — one for each state, territory, and the District of Columbia. States also differ in Medicaid financing.

Note: MACPAC (The Medicaid and CHIP Payment and Access Commission) is a non-partisan legislative branch agency that provides policy and data analysis and makes recommendations to Congress, the Secretary of the U.S. Department of Health and Human Services, and the states on a wide array of issues affecting Medicaid and the State Children's Health Insurance Program (CHIP). The U.S. Comptroller General appoints MACPAC's 17 commissioners, who come from diverse regions across the United States and bring broad expertise and a wide range of perspectives in Medicaid and CHIP.

Medicare v. Medicaid

MEDICARE is an insurance program. Medical bills are paid from trust funds which those covered have paid into. It primarily serves people over 65, whatever their income, and serves younger disabled people and dialysis patients and ALS patients. Patients pay part of costs through deductibles for hospital and other costs.

MEDICAID is a combination federal-state medical and long-term care assistance program that helps low-income people of every age. The Centers for Medicare and Medicaid Services (CMS) is the federal agency that monitors Medicaid programs offered by each state. It is run within federal guidelines but varies from state to state. Patients usually pay no part of costs for covered medical expenses, but a small co-payment is sometimes required. If a family earns too much to qualify for Medicaid but their children need low-cost care, the children may be covered through CHIP (Children's Health Insurance Program) under that program's rules and requirements. (To see if you qualify for your state's Medicaid or CHIP program, see https://www.healthcare.gov/medicaid-chip/eligibility/ or http://www.medicaid.gov)

In 2010, the Affordable Care Act (ACA) attempted to expand healthcare coverage to more Americans. As a result, all legal residents and citizens of the United States with incomes of up to 138% of the poverty line qualify for coverage in Medicaid participating states. However, states are not required to participate in the expansion, and many states have chosen not to expand eligibility requirements. Those states, due to a Supreme Court ruling, maintained their already-established levels of Medicaid funding.

Medicaid has strict income and eligibility requirements that vary by state. Because the program is designed to help the poor, many states require that Medicaid recipients have no more than a few thousand dollars in liquid assets to qualify. Upon reaching age 65, Medicaid recipients become eligible for Medicare, triggering revisions in the assistance they receive through Medicaid going forward based upon their individual circumstances.

While Medicaid benefits vary by state, the Federal government mandates coverage for many services including hospitalization, laboratory services, x-rays, doctors' services, nursing and nursing facility services, family planning, midwife services and home healthcare for those eligible for nursing facility services.

Additional (optional) benefits by state include prescription drug coverage, vision and dental services, physical therapy, prosthetic devices and medical transportation.

Medicaid is the nation's largest source of long-term care funding – a benefit not covered by Medicare and usually not covered by private health insurance.

https://www.kff.org/medicaid/issue-brief/status-of-state-medicaid-expansion-decisions-interactive-map/
(See hyperlink for full text and references.)

STATUS OF STATE ACTION
on the MEDICAID EXPANSION DECISION
9 July 2021

To date, 39 states (including DC) have adopted the Medicaid expansion and 12 states have not adopted the expansion. Current status for each state is based on KFF tracking and analysis of state expansion activity.

Coverage under the Medicaid expansion became effective January 1, 2014 in all states that have adopted the Medicaid expansion except for the following: Michigan (4/1/2014), New Hampshire (8/15/2014), Pennsylvania (1/1/2015), Indiana (2/1/2015), Alaska (9/1/2015), Montana (1/1/2016), Louisiana (7/1/2016), Virginia (1/1/2019), Maine (1/10/2019 with coverage retroactive to 7/2/2018), Idaho (1/1/2020), Utah (1/1/2020), Nebraska (10/1/2020), Oklahoma (planned for 7/1/2021), and Missouri (adopted but not implemented as of 7/1/2021).

Arizona, Arkansas, Indiana, Iowa, Michigan, Montana, Nebraska, New Hampshire, New Mexico, Ohio, and Utah have approved Section 1115 waivers to operate their Medicaid expansion programs in ways not otherwise allowed under federal law. Some of these Section 1115 waivers include work requirements, which the Biden Administration has recently begun the process of withdrawing.

https://www.nj.com/coronavirus/2020/05/this-troubled-nursing-home-has-most-deaths-in-nj-but-there-were-problems-long-before-deadly-outbreak.html   (See hyperlink for full text)

This Troubled Nursing Home has Most Deaths in New Jersey. But there were Problems Long Before Deadly Outbreak.

Published: 1 May 2020

See hyperlink for full text – note this excerpt re: Medicaid billings

In 2017, then under the management of another company, Andover agreed to pay $888,000 to resolve allegations it provided substandard or worthless nursing services to some patients, federal authorities said. The nursing home allegedly billed Medicaid "for materially substandard or worthless nursing services provided to certain patients that failed to meet federal standards of care and federal statutory and regulatory requirements" between July 1, 2010, and Dec. 31, 2012, according to the U.S. Attorney's Office in New Jersey.

Andover did not admit to any liability, but agreed to settle the case by paying $395,508 to the United States and $492,492 to the state, and entered into a five-year corporate integrity agreement that included a mandate that a committee shall assess the nursing and mental health staffing provided at Andover and make recommendations regarding how to improve such staffing.

Children's Health Insurance Program

The Children's Health Insurance Program (CHIP) is a federal healthcare program administered by the United States Department of Health and Human Services. It provides matching funds to states for low-cost health insurance for children under 19 whose parents earn too much to qualify for Medicaid. Often, these parents are unable to obtain health insurance coverage for their children through an employer or can't afford private insurance.

There is a lot of confusion as to whether Medicare, CHIP, or the Affordable Care Act should be used for children in low-income families. In 2009, Congress allocated federal funds to help raise visibility and also help more children enroll.

Parents must apply for CHIP and many are unaware of the program's existence. Sometimes children will qualify for children's Medicaid rather than CHIP. An adult who lives more than half the time with the child may apply for the child. CHIP coverage can begin at any time throughout the year with benefits becoming available immediately.

Responsibility for managing CHIP programs falls under each state's Medicaid administration and is therefore administered differently by each state. States are allowed to use Medicaid and CHIP funds for premium assistance programs that help eligible individuals purchase private health insurance.

CHIP typically covers routine check-ups, immunizations, doctor visits, inpatient and outpatient hospital care, dental and vision care, prescriptions, laboratory and X-ray services, and emergency services. Some states have received authority to use CHIP funds to cover certain adults, including pregnant women and parents of children receiving benefits from both CHIP and Medicaid.

A family of four earning up to $45,000 a year will usually qualify for CHIP, but the limits vary on a state-by-state basis. Some states require a monthly premium that cannot exceed 5 percent of annual income. Benefits and co-payments are not consistent among the various programs. Many services covered by CHIP are free but some require a co-payment.

CHIP is also named differently by each state: "All Kids" in Alabama, "Denali Kidcare" in Alaska, "KidsCare" in Arizona, "ARKids First" in Arkansas . . . "CHIP" in Mississippi and Pennsylvania and Texas and Utah and West Virginia . . . "BadgerCare Plus" in Wisconsin. (See https://www.kff.org/other/state-indicator/chip-program-name-and-type/?currentTimeframe=0&sortModel=%7B%22colId%22:%22Locatio n%22,%22sort%22:%22asc%22%7D for complete list.)

CHIP grew out of years of work in the U.S. Congress to improve Americans' health coverage. Quickly after his election in 1992, President Bill Clinton assembled a task force to write a comprehensive health reform bill, and he worked with Congress to introduce the Health Security Act (HSA) in November 1993. It included provisions such as universal coverage and a basic benefit package, health insurance reform, and consumer choice of health plans.

After the HSA failed in the fall of 1994, congressional leaders and the administration recognized the need for an incremental, bipartisan approach to health care reform.

CHIP (as SCHIP) was formulated in the aftermath of the failure of President Bill Clinton's comprehensive health care reform proposal. In December 1996 First Lady Hillary Rodham Clinton examined several possible initiatives and decided expanding health care insurance to children who had none was the one to advance, especially as its focus on children would be politically popular.

The new initiative was proposed at Bill Clinton's January 1997 State of the Union address, with the stated goal of coverage of up to five million children. Organizations from the Children's Defense Fund to the Girl Scouts of the USA lobbied for its passage, putting public pressure on Congress.

SCHIP was then passed and signed into law by Bill Clinton on August 5, 1997 as part of the Balanced Budget Act of 1997, to take effect the following month.

At the time of its creation, SCHIP represented the largest expansion of taxpayer-funded health insurance coverage for children in the U.S. since the establishment of Medicaid in 1965.

CHIP was designed as a federal-state partnership similar to Medicaid;

programs are run by the individual states according to requirements set by the federal Centers for Medicare and Medicaid Services. States are given flexibility in designing their CHIP policies within broad federal guidelines, resulting in variations regarding eligibility, benefits, and administration across different states.

Many states contract with private companies to administer some portions of their CHIP benefits. These programs, typically referred to as Medicaid managed care, allow private insurance companies or health maintenance organizations to contract directly with a state Medicaid department at a fixed price per enrollee. The health plans then enroll eligible individuals into their programs and become responsible for assuring CHIP benefits are delivered to eligible beneficiaries.

States may design their CHIP programs as an independent program separate from Medicaid (separate child health programs), use CHIP funds to expand their Medicaid program (CHIP Medicaid expansion programs), or combine these approaches (CHIP combination programs). States receive enhanced federal funds for their CHIP programs at a rate above the regular Medicaid match.

By February 1999, 47 states had set up CHIP programs. By April 1999, some 1 million children had been enrolled.

CHIP covered 7.6 million children during federal fiscal year 2010, and every state has an approved plan. Nonetheless, the number of uninsured children continued to rise after 1997, particularly among families that did not qualify for CHIP.

Children from birth through age 18 who live in families with incomes above the Medicaid thresholds in 1996 and up to 200% of the federal poverty level are eligible for the CHIP Medicaid expansion program (with some states being more generous or restrictive in the number of children they allow into the program).

In 2007, researchers from Brigham Young University and Arizona State found that children who drop out of CHIP cost states more money because they shift away from routine care to more frequent emergency care situations. The conclusion of the study is that an attempt to cut the costs of a state healthcare program could create a false savings because other government organizations pick up the tab for the children who lose insurance coverage and later need care.

Reauthorization

➢ On December 21, 2007 President Bush signed into law an extension of CHIP funding through March 31, 2009.

➢ On January 14, 2009, the House passed H.R. 2 on a vote of 290-138. The bill authorized spending and added $32.8 billion to expand the health coverage program to include about 4 million more children, including coverage of legal immigrants with no waiting period for the first time.

➢ The 2010 passage and signing of the Patient Protection and Affordable Care Act included funding for CHIP through 2015.

➢ In 2015, Congress passed the Medicare Access and CHIP Reauthorization Act of 2015 (MACRA), and it was signed by President Obama.

➢ CHIP expired on September 30, 2017. At the time, most states had sufficient funds to keep the program running for a period of months. On November 3, 2017, the House of Representatives passed the CHAMPION Act, which would fund CHIP until 2022.

➢ On January 22, 2018, President Trump signed legislation that reauthorized CHIP for six years.

➢ On February 9, 2018, Congress passed the Bipartisan Budget Act of 2018, which reauthorized CHIP for an additional four years. The bill was passed by vote of 71-28 in the Senate and by a vote of 240-186 in the House of Representatives. President Trump signed the bill into law that same day, allowing for CHIP's extension through 2027.

See hyperlinks for full text and references:

https://en.wikipedia.org/wiki/Children%27s_Health_Insurance_Program

https://www.healthcare.gov/medicaid-chip/childrens-health-insurance-program/

Indian Health Service
From Wikipedia, the free encyclopedia

The **Indian Health Service (IHS)** is an operating division (OPDIV) within the U.S. Department of Health and Human Services (HHS). IHS is responsible for providing direct medical and public health services to members of federally-recognized Native American Tribes and Alaska Native people. IHS is the principal federal health care provider and health advocate for Indian people.

The IHS provides health care in 36 states to approximately 2.2 million out of 3.7 million American Indians and Alaska Natives (AI/AN). As of April 2017, the IHS consisted of 26 hospitals, 59 health centers, and 32 health stations. Thirty-three urban Indian health projects supplement these facilities with a variety of health and referral services. Several tribes are actively involved in IHS program implementation. Many tribes also operate their own health systems independent of IHS.

Formation and Mission of IHS

The provision of health services to members of federally recognized tribes grew out of the special government-to-government relationship between the federal government and Indian tribes. This relationship, established in 1787, is based on Article I, Section 8 of the Constitution, and has been given form and substance by numerous treaties, laws, Supreme Court decisions, and Executive Orders.

Health services for the needs of American Indian and Alaska Natives in the United States were first provided through the Department of War from the early 19th century until the Office of Indian Affairs came into creation and took over the mission. After the mission again changed departmental authority to the Department of Health, Education, and Welfare's Public Health Service in 1955, the IHS was established.

The original priorities were stated to be:

1. Assemble a competent health staff

2. Institute extensive curative treatment for the seriously ill

3. Develop a full-scale prevention program that would reduce the excessive amount of illness and early deaths, especially for preventable diseases

Employment by IHS

IHS employs approximately 2,650 nurses, 700 physicians, 700 pharmacists, 100 physician assistants and 300 dentists, as well as a variety of other health professionals such as nutritionists, registered medical-record administrators, therapists, community health representative aides, child health specialists, and environmental sanitarians. It is one of two federal agencies mandated to use Indian Preference in hiring. This law requires the agency to give preference to qualified Indian applicants before considering non-Indian candidates for employment, although exceptions apply.

IHS draws a large number of its professional employees from the U.S. Public Health Service Commissioned Corps. This is a non-armed service branch of the uniformed services of the United States. Professional categories of IHS Commissioned corps officers include physicians, physician assistants, nurses, dentists, pharmacists, engineers, environmental health officers, and dietitians.

Many IHS positions are in remote areas as well as its headquarters outside of Rockville, Maryland, and at Phoenix Indian Medical Center in Phoenix, Arizona. In 2007, most IHS job openings were on the Navajo reservation. 71% of IHS employees are American Indian/Alaska Native.

The IHS also hires Native/non-Native American interns, who are referred to as "externs". Participants are paid based on industry standards, according to their experience levels and academic training, but are instead reimbursed for tuition and fees if the externship is used for an academic practical experience requirement.

Legislation

The Snyder Act of 1921 (23 U.S.C. 13) was the first formal legislative authority allowing health services to be provided to Native Americans. In 1957, the Indian Facilities Act authorized funding for community hospital construction. This authority was expanded in 1959 with the Indian Sanitation and Facilities Act, which also authorized construction and maintenance of sanitation facilities for Native American homes, communities, and lands.

Indian Self-Determination Act of 1975 (Public Law 93-638)

ExpectMore.gov lists four rated areas of IHS: federally administered activities (moderately effective), healthcare-facilities construction (effective), resource-and patient-management systems (effective), and sanitation-facilities construction (moderately effective). All federally recognized Native American and Alaska Natives are entitled to health care. This health care is provided by the Indian Health Service, either through IHS-run hospitals and clinics or tribal contracts to provide healthcare services.

Indian Health Care Improvement Act of 1976

The passing of the Indian Health Care Improvement Act of 1976 (Public Law 94-437) expanded the budget of the IHS to expand health services. The IHS was able to build and renovate medical facilities and focus on the construction of safe drinking water and sanitary disposal facilities. The law also developed programs designed to increase the number of Native American professionals and improve urban Natives' health care access.

Other Legislation

Title V of the Indian Health Care Improvement Act of 1976 and Title V of the Indian Health Care Amendment of 1980 have increased the access to healthcare that Native Americans living in urban areas receive. The IHS now contracts with urban Indian health organizations in various U.S. cities in order to expand outreach, referral services, and comprehensive healthcare services.

Administration

The Indian Health Service is headed by a director. As of mid-2017 the agency had seen five different directors since the beginning of 2015.

Reporting to the director are a chief medical officer, deputy directors (Operations, Government Affairs, Management, and Quality), and Offices for Tribal Liaison, Urban Health, and Contracting. Twelve regional area offices each coordinate infrastructure and programs in a section of the United States.

A 2010 report by Senate Committee on Indian Affairs Chairman Byron

Dorgan, D-N.D., found that the Aberdeen Area of the IHS was in a "chronic state of crisis". "Serious management problems and a lack of oversight of this region have adversely affected the access and quality of health care provided to Native Americans in the Aberdeen Area, which serves 18 tribes in the states of North Dakota, South Dakota, Nebraska and Iowa," according to the report.

Areas

A network of twelve regional offices oversees clinical operations for individual facilities and funds. As of 2010, the federally operated sites included twenty-eight hospitals and eighty-nine outpatient facilities.

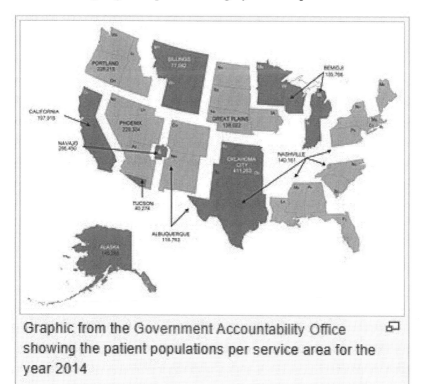

Graphic from the Government Accountability Office showing the patient populations per service area for the year 2014

- Alaska Area (Aleut Community of St. Paul, Alaska)

- Albuquerque Area (Navajo)

- Bemidji Area (Chippewa)

- Billings Area

- California Area (Cherokee)

- Great Plains Area (Rosebud Sioux): The name of this area was changed in 2014 from the Aberdeen Area.

- Nashville Area (Mississippi Choctaw)

- Navajo Area

- Oklahoma Area

- Phoenix Area (Three Affiliated Sioux Tribes)

- Portland Area (Confederated Tribes of Warm Springs)

- Tucson Area (Three Affiliated Sioux Tribes)

Services and benefits

The IHS provides a variety of health services in outpatient and inpatient settings, with benefits including pharmacy, dental, behavioral health, immunizations, pediatrics, physical rehabilitation, and optometry. A more extensive list can be found at the official IHS website, and it is recommended for patients to contact their particular IHS facility to confirm services provided since benefits may differ by location.

Eligibility

To qualify for health benefits from the IHS, individuals must be of American Indian and/or Alaska Native descent and be a part of an Indian community serviced by IHS. Individuals must be able to provide evidence such as membership in a federally-recognized tribe, residence on tax-exempt land, or active participation in tribal affairs. Federally-recognized tribes are annually defined by the Bureau of Indian Affairs (BIA). Non-Indians can also receive care if they are the child of an eligible Indian, the spouse (including same-sex spouses) of an eligible Indian, or a non-Indian woman pregnant with an eligible Indian's child. The exact policy can be found in the IHS Indian Health Manual (IHM).

To apply for benefits through the IHS, individuals can enroll through the patient registration office of their local IHS facility. Individuals should be prepared to show proof of enrollment in a federally recognized tribe.

Direct Care versus Purchased/Referred Care (PRC)

"Direct Care" refers to medical and dental care that American Indians and Alaska Natives receive at an IHS or tribal medical facility. If patients are referred to a non-IHS/tribal medical facility, there is the option to request for coverage via the IHS "Purchased/Referred Care (PRC) Program". Due to limited funds from U.S. Congress, referrals through PRC are not guaranteed coverage. Authorization of these payments is determined through several factors, including confirmation of AI/AN tribal affiliation, medical priority, and funding availability.

IHS National Core Formulary

The IHS National Pharmacy and Therapeutics Committee (NPTC) is composed of administrative leaders and clinical professionals, including pharmacists and physicians, who regulate the IHS National Core Formulary (NCF) to reflect current clinical practices and literature. The NCF is reviewed every quarter and revised as needed based on arising health needs within the Native American communities, pharmacoeconomic analyses, recent guidelines, national contracts, and clinician advice. Fibric acid derivatives and niacin extended release were removed from the formulary in February 2017, but there were no changes made to the NCF during the May 2017 meeting. The complete National Core Formulary can be found on the IHS website.

Necessity for Hepatitis C Coverage

The National Health and Nutrition Examination Survey provides national prevalence data for hepatitis C but excludes several high risk populations including federal prisoners, homeless individuals and over one million Native Americans residing on reservations. To address this concern, in 2012 IHS implemented a nationwide hepatitis C virus (HCV) antibody testing program for persons born between 1945 and 1965. This resulted in a fourfold increase in the number of patients screened. IHS facilities of the Southwest reported the largest gains in number of patients tested and the percentage of eligible patients that received testing. Currently, the incidence rate of acute hepatitis C in Native Americans is higher in comparison to any other racial/ethnic group (1.32 cases per 100,000). Additionally, Native Americans have the highest rate of hepatitis C related deaths (12.95% in 2015) in comparison to any other racial/ethnic group.

Despite this prevalent need, IHS currently does not include any new direct acting anti-retroviral (DAA) hepatitis C medications on its

National Core Formulary. New DAA drugs provide a cure to hepatitis C in most cases but are costly. Due to their lack in funding and quality of care, the IHS has not been able to effectively combat the Native American HCV issue, unlike the Veterans Affairs system, which was able to eradicate much of the disease through adequate resources from the federal government.

TRIBAL SELF-DETERMINATION

Notable Self-determination Legislation

In 1954, the Indian Health Transfer Act included language that recognized tribal sovereignty, and the Act additionally "afforded a degree of tribal self-determination in health policy decision-making." The Indian Self Determination and Education Assistance Act (ISDEAA) allows for tribes to request self-determination contracts with the Secretaries of Interior and Health and Human Services. The tribes take over IHS activities and services through an avenue called '638 contracts' through which tribes receive the IHS funds that would have been used for IHS health services and instead manage and use this money for the administration of health services outside of the IHS.

Self-determination Successes and Concerns

The benefits and drawbacks of Tribal Self Determination have been widely debated. Many tribes have successfully implemented elements of health-related Self Determination. An example is the Cherokee Indian Hospital in North Carolina. This community-based hospital, funded in part by the tribe's casino revenues, is guided by four core principles:

- "The one who helps you from the heart,"

- "A state of peace and balance,"

- "it belongs to you" and

- "Like family to me" "He, she, they, are like my own family".

The hospital is based on the adoption of an Alaska Native model of healthcare called the "Nuka System of Care," a framework that focuses on patient-centered, self-determined health service delivery that heavily relies on Patient participation.

The Nuka System of Care was developed by the Southcentral

Foundation in 1982, a non-profit healthcare organization that is owned and composed of Alaska Natives. The Nuka System's vision is "A Native community that enjoys physical, mental, emotional and spiritual wellness". Every Alaska Native in the health system is a "customer-owner" of the system and participates as a self-determined individual who has a say in the decision-making processes and access to an intimate, integrated, long-term care team. When a customer-owner seeks care, their primary care doctors' foremost responsibility is to build a strong and lasting relationship with the beneficiary, and customer-owners have various options through which they can give input and participate in decisions about their health. These options include surveys, focus groups, special events and committees. The board is made up entirely of Alaska Natives who helped design the system and actively participate in running it effectively.

Following the implementation of the Nuka System of Care in Alaska Native health, successes in improved standards of care have been achieved, such as increases in the number of Alaska Natives with a primary care provider, in childhood immunization rates, and customers satisfaction in regard to respect of culture and traditions. In addition, decreases in wait times for appointments, wait lists, emergency department and urgent care visits, and staff turnover have been reported. The North Carolina Cherokee Indian Hospital in 2012 as well as other tribes have implemented the Nuka System approach when planning their new or revamped health centers and systems.

Some tribes are less optimistic about the role of Self Determination in Indian healthcare or may face barriers to success. Tribes have expressed concern that the 638 contracting and compacting could lead to "termination by appropriation," the fear that if tribes take over the responsibility of managing healthcare programs and leave the federal government with only the job of funding these programs, then the federal government could easily "deny any further responsibility for the tribes, and cut funding". The fear of potential termination has led some tribes to refuse to participate in Self Determination contracting without a clear resolution of this issue.

Some tribes also renounce Self Determination and contracting because of the chronic underfunding of IHS programs. They do not see any benefit in being handed the responsibility of a "sinking ship" due to the lack of a satisfactory budget for IHS services.

Other tribes face various barriers to successful Self Determination. Small tribes lacking in administrative capabilities, geographically-isolated tribes with transportation and recruitment issues, and tribes with funding issues may find it much harder to contract with the IHS and begin self-determination. Poverty and a lack of resources can thus make Self Determination difficult.

Budget

The IHS receives funding as allocated by the United States Congress and is not an entitlement program, insurance program, or established benefit program.

The 2017 United States federal budget includes $5.1 billion for the IHS to support and expand the provision of health care services and public health programs for American Indians and Alaska Natives. The proposed 2018 budget proposed to reduce IHS spending by more than $300 million.

This covers the provision of health benefits to 2.5 million Native Americans and Alaskan Natives for a recent average *cost per patient* of less than $3,000, far less than the average cost of health care nationally ($7,700), or for the other major federal health programs Medicaid ($6,200) or Medicare ($12,000).

Current Issues

In 2013, the IHS experienced funding cuts of $800 million, representing a substantial percentage of its budget. Over the past twenty years, the gap between spending on federally recognized American Indian/Alaska Natives and spending on Medicare beneficiaries has grown eightfold. This inequity has a large impact on service rationing, health disparities and life expectancy, and can lead to preventive services being neglected. Other issues that have been highlighted as challenges to improving health outcomes are social inequities such as poverty and unemployment, cross-cultural communication barriers, and limited access to care.

Data from the 2014 National Emergency Department Inventory survey showed that only 85% of the 34 IHS respondents had continuous physician coverage. Of these 34 sites only 4 sites utilized telemedicine while a median of just 13% of physicians were board certified in emergency medicine. The majority of IHS emergency department from the survey reported operating at or over capacity.

Since its beginnings in 1955, the IHS has been criticized by those it serves in medical deserts and by public officials.

Native Americans who are not of a federally-recognized tribe or who live in urban areas have trouble accessing the services of the IHS.

Note: See Wikipedia link for full text and references:
https://en.wikipedia.org/wiki/Indian_Health_Service

QUESTIONS:

Why don't "Medicare for All" Congressional Bills S. 1129 (on hold) and H.R. 1976 include members of federally-recognized Native American Tribes and Alaska Native Persons so they would be eligible for all the benefits of universal health care and have a "Medicare for All" card in their possession from birth?

Do federally-recognized Native American Tribes and Alaska Native Persons want that opportunity – or are they happy with the health care they currently receive from the Indian Health Service?

Just asking!

https://www.cdc.gov/wtc/about.html
(See hyperlink for full text and references.)

World Trade Center Health Program

Monitoring and Treatment

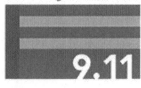

WTC Health Program

The World Trade Center (WTC) Health Program is a limited federal health program administered by the National Institute for Occupational Safety and Health, part of the Centers for Disease Control and Prevention in the U.S. Department of Health and Human Services and is authorized through 2090. The Program provides no-cost medical monitoring and treatment for certified WTC-related health conditions to those directly affected by the 9/11 attacks in New York, the Pentagon, and in Shanksville, Pennsylvania.

The Program also funds medical research into physical and mental health conditions related to 9/11 exposures.

The WTC Health Program is dedicated to helping those who were there during and after the attacks of September 11, 2001. The Program provides services to the following categories of individuals when the individual meets activity, location, time period, and minimum hour requirements.

- WTC Responders: Workers or volunteers who provided rescue, recovery, debris cleanup, and related support services on or in the aftermath of the September 11, 2001, attacks for certain amounts of time during the period between September 11, 2001, and July 31, 2002. There are three types of responders: FDNY Responders, WTC General Responders (including NYPD), and Pentagon and Shanksville, PA, Responders.

- WTC Survivors: Individuals who were present in the New York City (NYC) Disaster Area in the dust or dust cloud on September 11, 2001; who worked, resided, or attended school, childcare, or adult

94

daycare in the NYC Disaster Area from September 11, 2001, to July 31, 2002; who were eligible for certain residential grants or whose place of employment was eligible for certain grants following the September 11, 2001, attacks.

The WTC Health Program pays for medically necessary treatment of certified conditions, as well any certified medically associated health condition(s), as long as the treatment is provided by a WTC Health Program affiliated provider or pharmacy. The member MUST have a certified or medically associated health condition(s) in order to be covered. To learn more about covered conditions, visit "Covered Conditions". (**Please Note:** This list is not exhaustive. Contact your Clinical Center of Excellence (CCE) or call the WTC Health Program if you have any questions about whether your condition may be covered by the program.)

Acute and Traumatic Injuries

Acute traumatic injuries are characterized by physical damage to your body caused by hazards or adverse conditions. Examples include:

- Burn
- Complex sprain
- Eye injury
- Fracture
- Head trauma
- Tendon tear

Airway and Digestive Disorders

Airway and digestive disorders, also known as Aerodigestive Disorders, are a group of disorders that affect breathing airways, such as your sinuses or lungs, or upper digestive tract, such as your esophagus. Examples include:

- Asthma
- Chronic cough syndrome
- Chronic laryngitis
- Chronic nasopharyngitis
- Chronic respiratory disorder- fumes and vapors
- Chronic rhinosinusitis
- Gastroesophageal reflux disorder (GERD)
- Interstitial lung disease

- New-onset, and WTC-exacerbated chronic obstructive pulmonary disease (COPD)
- Reactive airway dysfunction syndrome (RADS)
- Sleep apnea (medically associated to another airway or digestive disorder)
- Upper airways hyperreactivity

Cancers

Cancer may be defined as the uncontrolled growth and spread of cells. It may occur at any place in the body, and it makes it difficult for the body to function normally. Examples include:

- Blood and lymphoid tissue (including lymphoma, myeloma, and leukemia)
- Breast
- Childhood cancers
- Digestive system (including colon and rectum)
- Eye and orbit
- Ovary
- Head and neck (oropharynx and tonsil)
- Prostate
- Mesothelioma
- Rare cancers (read a statement from the Administrator about Rare Cancers for more information)
- Respiratory system (including lung and bronchus)
- Skin (melanoma, non-melanoma and carcinoma in situ)
- Soft and connective tissue
- Thyroid
- Urinary system (including kidney and bladder)

Mental Health Conditions

Mental health conditions include a wide range of conditions that affect your mood, thinking, and behavior. Examples include:

- Acute stress disorder
- Adjustment disorder
- Anxiety disorders
- Depression
- Dysthymic disorder
- Generalized anxiety disorder
- Major depressive disorder
- Panic disorder

- Post-traumatic stress disorder (PTSD)
- Substance use disorder

Musculoskeletal Disorders (applies to WTC Responders only)

Musculoskeletal disorders are chronic or recurring disorder of the musculoskeletal system caused by heavy lifting or repetitive strain on the joints. Examples include:

- Carpal tunnel syndrome (CTS)
- Low back pain
- Other musculoskeletal disorders

Maximum Time Interval and Cancer Latency Period

To be certified for some airway and digestive health conditions, your condition must meet an additional requirement known as maximum time interval. Maximum time intervals are the maximum amount of time that could have gone by between the date of your last 9/11 exposure and the onset of symptoms of your airway and digestive health condition. Specific requirements are included in the Member Handbook in the Maximum Time Intervals for Aerodigestive Disorders section.

To be certified for cancer, minimum cancer latency requirements must be met. Latency is the amount of time that has passed between your initial 9/11 exposures and the date you were first diagnosed with cancer. Specific requirements are included in the Member Handbook in the Cancer Latency section.

Members can access services without having to pay any co-payments, deductibles, or other out-of-pocket expenses for medically necessary treatment of certified WTC-related health conditions.

The WTC Health Program provides care through multiple Clinical Centers of Excellence (CCE) and the Nationwide Provider Network (NPN).

CCEs treat members in the NY metropolitan area. Responders, survivors, and FDNY have specific clinics.

Care is provided in all US states and territories through the Nationwide Provider Network (NPN). The NPN is a network of health care providers across the country under contract with the Program to provide care for members who live outside the NY metropolitan area.

Members of the WTC Health Center Health Program have important health needs and powerful stories of hope and healing. Visit our Program Videos page to see members share their stories of where they were and how they've been helped through the WTC Health Program. (https://www.cdc.gov/wtc/programvideos.html)

For Health Care Providers - 9/11 Health Information: **Could your patient be sick due to 9/11 exposures?** Learn how best to help an exposed patient in the factsheet (see hyperlink): 9/11 Health Information for Health Care Providers [PDF, 212 KB, 2 pages, May 2021]

NOTE: The National Institute for Occupational Safety and Health, the government agency that houses the World Trade Center Health Program, awarded Logistics Health Inc. (LHI), then headed by Tommy Thompson, former governor of Wisconsin and former U.S. Secretary of Health and Human Services (2001-2004), its first $11 million federal contract in 2008. LHI, founded in 1999 to address military medical readiness concerns, is a subsidiary of OptumServe, the federal health services business of Optum and UnitedHealth Group. LHI operates as a middleman between the 9/11 community and the health benefits they're promised. There are many complaints about the program's bureaucracy and lost paperwork. Yet John Feal, a key 9/11 Survivor Advocate with the FealGood Foundation (https://fealgoodfoundation.com/updates/), believes in the program and at one point in 2018 simply said it needs to increase its staff to keep up with the growing demand. "I'm not going to say anything mean about them. But they need to do a better job." said Feal.

References:

- https://fealgoodfoundation.com/

- www.fox6now.com/news/there-needs-to-be-a-better-system-in-place-wisconsin-9-11-responder-left-waiting-for-treatment

- https://wisconsintechnologycouncil.com/logistics-health-story-is-bright-spot-for-wisconsin/

- **"No Responders Left Behind"**: This documentary follows the work of the men and women including first responder and 9/11 social activist, John Feal, FDNY hero Ray Pfeifer, and 22-time Primetime Emmy award-winner and former host of The Daily Show, Jon Stewart in their fight to get health benefits and compensation for 9/11 first responders. This is a model of advocacy that should be emulated by the entire "Medicare for All" movement.

NOTE: It took years of advocacy, pain, suffering and many deaths for Congress to finally enact the "World Trade Center (WTC) Health Program". Yet it took no time at all for the program to find its way into the control of the for-profit health system.

Federal Employees Health Benefits Program
From Wikipedia, the free encyclopedia

The **Federal Employees Health Benefits (FEHB) Program** is a system of "managed competition" through which employee health benefits are provided to civilian government employees and annuitants of the United States government. The program was created in 1960.

The FEHB program allows some insurance companies, employee associations, and labor unions to market health insurance plans to governmental employees. The program is administered by the United States Office of Personnel Management (OPM).

(In 2010, about 250 plans participated in the program. About 20 plans were nationwide or almost nationwide, such as the ones offered by some employee unions such as the National Association of Letter Carriers, by some employee associations, and by national insurance companies such as Aetna and the Blue Cross and Blue Shield Association on behalf of its member companies. There were about 230 locally available plans, almost all HMOs.)

Premiums vary from plan to plan and are paid in part by the employer (the U. S. government agency that the employee works for or, for annuitants, OPM) and the remainder by the employee.

The government contributes 72% of the weighted average premium of all plans, not to exceed 75% of the premium for any one plan (calculated separately for individual and family coverage). This dollar amount is recalculated each year as health care costs and plans' premiums increase.

The FEHB program is open to most federal employees. For example, as of 2014, members of the United States Congress and their staff are excluded from the FEHB and required to purchase health insurance through the health care exchange due to the Affordable Care Act. However, the federal government provides a premium contribution for the purchase of this health insurance.

Certain employees (such as postal workers) have a higher portion of their premiums paid as the result of collective bargaining agreements.

Enrollees pay the entire cost of their costly choices, but reap rewards if they make frugal choices. This creates constant pressure on the plans, since to attract enrollees the plans must hold down costs, while balancing this incentive against benefit offerings and customer service, to reach a position that will maximize their enrollment revenues and profits.

This feature of the program is arguably its greatest strength and the primary reason that one expert summarized it as having "outperformed Medicare every which way — in containment of costs both to consumers and to the government (taxpayer!), in benefit and product innovation and modernization, and in consumer satisfaction," decade after decade.

The FEHBP's cost was about $40 billion in 2010, including both premiums and out-of-pocket costs. It enrolls about four million employees and annuitants (with their dependents, eight million persons in total). While its enrollment is about one-fifth that of the nation's largest health insurance program, Medicare, it spends less than one-tenth as much because most enrollees are below age 65 and cost far less on average than the elderly and disabled who constitute Medicare's enrollees.

Premiums can vary substantially, and in 2010 the lowest cost plan option had a self-only premium cost of about $2,800 and the highest cost plan option for self-only enrollment was about $7,200. As an example of benefit variation, a cap of about $5,000 a year on potential out-of-pocket costs for self-only enrollment is found in a number of plans, but in some plans the cap may reach $15,000 or more.

Choices among health plans are available to employees during an "open enrollment" period, or "open season," after which the employee will be covered fully in any plan he or she chooses without limitations regarding pre-existing conditions. After the annual enrollment, changes can be made only upon a "qualifying life event" such as marriage, divorce, adoption or birth of a child, or change in employment status of a spouse, until the next annual open season, during which employees can enroll, disenroll, or change from one plan to another. In practice, there is a great deal of inertia in enrollment, and only about 5 percent of employees change plans in most open seasons.

The FEHB program relies on consumer choices among competing private plans to determine costs, premiums, benefits, and service. This model is in sharp contrast to that used by original Medicare. In Medicare, premiums, benefits, and payment rates are all centrally determined by law or regulation (there is no bargaining and no reliance on volume discounts in original Medicare; these parameters are set by fiat).

Some have criticized the FEHB model because neither the "monopsony" power ("*market situation in which there is only one buyer*") nor purchasing power of the federal government is utilized to control costs. This controversy is similar to that which surrounded legislation for the Medicare Prescription Drug Coverage passed during the George W. Bush administration. Over time, however, the FEHB program has outperformed original Medicare not only in cost control, but also in benefit improvement, enrollee service, fraud prevention, and avoidance of "pork barrel" spending and earmarks.

One of the most prominent features of the FEHB program is the choices it allows. There are three broad types of plans: fee-for-service and preferred provider organization (PPO), usually offered in combination; HMOs; and high-deductible health plans and other consumer-driven plans.

In the FEHB program, the federal government sets minimal standards that, if met by an insurance company, allow it to participate in the program. The result is numerous competing insurance plans that are available to federal employees.

In the Washington, D.C., metropolitan area, plans open to all federal employees and annuitants include 10 fee-for-service and PPO plans, seven HMOs, and eight high-deductible and consumer-driven plans. A similar number of choices is offered in almost all large metropolitan areas, and in many smaller cities and rural areas.

The program is sometimes criticized for offering this broad array of choices, but there are many ways enrollees can obtain advice and assistance, including advice from office colleagues and friends, newspaper and magazine articles in both the general press and publications that specialize in federal employees or retirees, OPM publications and Web site, and several online tools that compare plans' costs, benefits, and services. **(REALLY????)**

As a noticeably consumer-friendly service, OPM requires that all plans publish brochures that describe benefits in plain English and in a standardized format that facilitates plan comparison and that can easily be downloaded in PDF format. Almost all plans provide Web sites that provide detailed information not only on their benefits, but also on their provider panels and their drug formularies.

The underlying legislation for the FEHB program is minimal and remarkably stable, particularly in comparison to Medicare. The FEHB statute is only a few dozen pages long, and only a few paragraphs are devoted to the structure and functioning of the program. Regulations are minimal; only another few dozen pages. In contrast, the Medicare statute found in title 18 of the Social Security Act is about 400 pages long and the accompanying regulations consume thousands of pages in the U.S. Code of Federal Regulations.

The FEHB program has often been proposed as a model for national health insurance and sometimes as a program that could directly enroll the uninsured. In the 2004 presidential campaign, Senator John Kerry proposed opening enrollment in this plan to all Americans.

In enacting the Medicare Modernization Act in 2003, the Congress explicitly modeled the reformed Medicare Advantage program and the new Medicare Part D Prescription Drug program after the FEHB program.

One of the prominent proposals for health reform in the United States, the proposed bipartisan Wyden-Bennett Act is largely modeled after the FEHB program, as have recent "Republican Alternative" proposals by Representative Paul Ryan.

NOTE: This article serves as a strong argument that we need to replace our complicated current system with IMPROVED MEDICARE FOR ALL – aka "A card in your wallet". How amazing that the OPM (United States Office of Personnel Management) needs to protect Federal employees by requiring that "all plans publish brochures that describe benefits in plain English and in a standardized format that facilitates plan comparison and that can easily be downloaded in PDF format.". And that the way to get the best health insurance is "advice from office colleagues and friends, newspaper and magazine articles in both the general press and publications that specialize in federal employees or retirees, OPM

publications and Web site, and several online tools that compare plans' costs, benefits, and services". Like President Biden often says: "Give me a break".

https://www.health.mil/About-MHS
(See hyperlink for full text, references and video.)

MILITARY HEALTH SYSTEM

The Military Health System (MHS) is one of America's largest and most complex health care institutions, and the world's preeminent military health care delivery operation. Our MHS saves lives on the battlefield, combats infectious disease around the world, and is responsible for providing health services through both direct care and Private Sector Care to approximately 9.6 million beneficiaries, composed of uniformed service members, military retirees, and family members.

The MHS enables the National Defense Strategy by providing a Medically Ready Force, a Ready Medical Force, and improving the health of all those entrusted to its care.

Our Mission

The missions of the MHS are complex and interrelated:

- To ensure America's 1.4 million active duty and 331,000 reserve-component personnel are healthy so they can complete their national security missions.
- To ensure that all active and reserve medical personnel in uniform are trained and ready to provide medical care in support of operational forces around the world.
- To provide a medical benefit commensurate with the service and sacrifice of more than 9.6 million active duty personnel, military retirees and their families.

The Elements of the MHS

The MHS is a federated system of uniformed, civilian and contract personnel and additional civilian partners at all levels of the Department of Defense and beyond – from senior officials in the Office of the Secretary of Defense to doctors and other health care providers in nearly every community across the nation.

MHS Initiatives and Areas of Impact

In order to provide quality care in wartime and peacetime, the MHS is among the nation's leading health systems, not just in size or complexity, but in several areas of healthcare. Those include:

- Trauma Care
- Research and Development
- Civilian Partnerships
- Global Health Engagement

We are more than combat medicine. The MHS is a complex system that weaves together:

- Health care delivery
- Medical education
- Public health
- Private sector partnerships
- Cutting edge medical research and development

Exemplified by personal courage and a drive for excellence, the MHS is changing how health care is delivered throughout the United States and the world.

The MHS is led by office of the Assistant Secretary of Defense for Health Affairs under the Office of the Undersecretary of Defense for Personnel and Readiness.

https://www.health.mil/About-MHS

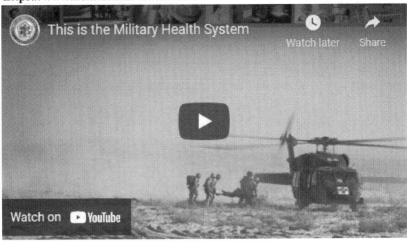

See LHI (https://logisticshealth.com/our-company.aspx) – a subsidiary of OptumServe ("the federal health services business of Optum and UnitedHealth Group").

TRICARE
From Wikipedia, the free encyclopedia

TRICARE, formerly known as the Civilian Health and Medical Program of the Uniformed Services (CHAMPUS), is a health care program of the United States Department of Defense Military Health System. TRICARE provides civilian health benefits for U.S Armed Forces military personnel, military retirees, and their dependents, including some members of the Reserve Component. TRICARE is the civilian care component of the Military Health System, although historically it also included health care delivered in military medical treatment facilities. The TRICARE program is managed by the Defense Health Agency (DHA).

The Department of Defense operates a health care delivery system that served approximately 9.4 million beneficiaries in 2018. The Department of Defense's unified medical program represents $50.6 billion or 8% of total FY2019 U.S. military spending.

With the exception of active duty service members (who are assigned to the TRICARE PRIME option and pay no out-of-pocket costs for TRICARE coverage), Military Health System beneficiaries may have a choice of TRICARE plan options depending upon their status (e.g., active duty family member, retiree, reservist, child under age 26 ineligible for family coverage, Medicare-eligible, etc.) and geographic location.

TRICARE'S OPTIONS

TRICARE SELECT

TRICARE SELECT is available to retirees from the Active Component, retirees from the Reserve Component age 60 or older, and their eligible family members. TRICARE SELECT is also available to Reservist and their family under the TRICARE RESERVE SELECT COMPONENT.

Under TRICARE SELECT, beneficiaries can use any civilian health care provider that is payable under TRICARE regulations. The beneficiary is responsible for payment of an annual deductible and coinsurance, and may be responsible for certain other out-of-pocket expenses. As of

January 1, 2021 the fees are $12.50 per month or $150 a year for individuals and $25 per month or $300 per year for families.

TRICARE PRIME

TRICARE PRIME is a health maintenance organization (HMO) style plan available to active duty personnel, retirees from the Active Component, retirees from the Reserve Component age 60 or older, and their eligible family members. Under TRICARE PRIME, beneficiaries must choose a primary care physician and obtain referrals and authorizations for specialty care. In return for these restrictions, beneficiaries are responsible only for small copayments for each visit (retirees and their families only). There is an annual enrollment fee for TRICARE PRIME for military retirees and their family members. There is no enrollment fee for active duty military and their family members. The majority of TRICARE PRIME enrollees must exclusively use the MTF (Military Treatment Facility) to receive their care, as long as the MTF has capacity. If the MTF does not have capacity, the commander of the MTF notifies the region's contractor and the contractor's provider network is used to supplement the MTF's capacity. If the MTF regains capacity, the MTF reserves the right to move the beneficiaries back to receiving their care at the MTF in a process known as "recapture."

TRICARE RESERVE SELECT (TRS)

TRICARE RESERVE SELECT is a premium-based health plan that active status qualified National Guard and Reserve members may purchase. The classification is sometimes referred to as TRICARE RESERVE COMPONENT (RC). It requires a monthly premium and offers coverage similar to TRICARE STANDARD and TRICARE EXTRA for the military member and eligible family members. It has a partial premium cost sharing arrangement with DOD similar to civilian private or public sector employer plans, although typically at a lower cost than civilian plans. The program coverage is available worldwide to SELECT RESERVE (SELRES) members of both the Title 10 USC Federal Reserve Components (Army Reserve, Navy Reserve, Air Force Reserve, Marine Corps Reserve), Title 14 USC Federal Reserve Component (Coast Guard Reserve) and the Title 32 National Guard (Army National Guard and Air National Guard) in a drill pay (also known as "paid") status. Retired RESERVE COMPONENT personnel under the age of 60, actively drilling Individual Ready Reserve (IRR) personnel in a non-paid status, or actively drilling Volunteer Training Unit (VTU) personnel in a non-paid status do not qualify for TRICARE RESERVE SELECT. IRR and VTU members are eligible for reinstatement under TRS if they return to a SELRES status. Reserve Component personnel who are also Federal civil servants (to include Army Reserve Technicians and Air Reserve Technicians (ART) in the Army Reserve, Army National Guard, Air Force Reserve and Air National Guard) and eligible for the Federal Employee Health Benefit Program (FEHBP) are also excluded from TRS. Retired Reserve Component personnel and eligible dependent family members become eligible TRICARE STANDARD, TRICARE EXTRA or TRICARE PRIME on the service member's 60th birthday in the same manner as Active Component retirees and their eligible dependents are eligible immediately upon retirement from active service.

TRICARE RESERVE RETIRED (TRR)

TRICARE RESERVE RETIRED is a premium-based health plan that qualified retired members of the National Guard and Reserve under the age of 60 may purchase for themselves and eligible family members. It is similar to TRICARE RESERVE SELECT (TRS), but differs in that there is no premium cost-sharing with DOD as there is with TRS. As such, retired Reserve Component members who elect to purchase TRR must pay the full cost (100%) of the calculated premium plus an additional administrative fee. Payments could range as high as $900.00 a month. Although open to all eligible retired Reserve Component personnel under the age of 60, the program's principal focus is often perceived as being focused on recent Reserve Component retirees who are self-employed or otherwise ineligible for civilian employer provided/subsidized health insurance, especially those who were mobilized for full-time active duty service subsequent to 11 September 2001 in support of Operations Enduring Freedom, Iraqi Freedom, New Dawn and/or Noble Eagle. Retired Reserve Component personnel who elect to participate in TRR will exit TRR when the service member reaches age 60 and he/she and their eligible dependent family members become eligible for the same TRICARE STANDARD, TRICARE EXTRA or TRICARE PRIME options as Active Component retirees and, in the case of TRICARE PRIME, at the same cost as Active Component retirees.

TRICARE FOR LIFE (TFL)

TRICARE FOR LIFE was enacted by Congress in response to growing complaints from beneficiaries that as Medicare out of pocket costs increased a benefit was needed to pay these costs in lieu of TRICARE retirees being required to purchase Medicare Supplemental Coverage to pay for prescriptions, physician and hospital dispensed drugs, cost shares and deductibles. Before TRICARE FOR LIFE, TRICARE beneficiaries immediately lost TRICARE coverage upon attaining Medicare eligibility at age 65, placing them at the same level of coverage as U.S. citizens who had never served full 20 to 30-plus year careers in the armed forces. This included becoming Medicare eligible due to disability. TRICARE FOR LIFE is designed to pay patient liability after Medicare payments. In some instances TRICARE FOR LIFE is the primary payer when the services are normally a TRICARE benefit but not covered by Medicare. This includes drug charges, when Medicare benefit limits are attained and services performed outside the United States or in a Veterans Affairs facility where Medicare does not pay. TFL does not pay patient liability for services that are not a TRICARE benefit even though they may be paid by Medicare, such as chiropractic benefits. The policy limitations applying to TRICARE also apply to TFL and must therefore be deemed medically necessary and skilled care. Medical claims are processed by the national TRICARE DUAL ELIGIBLE FISCAL INTERMEDIARY CONTRACTOR (TDEFIC-Wisconsin Physicians Service Insurance Corporation). Pharmacy claims are processed by the TRICARE PHARMACY CONTRACTOR (Express Scripts) and Overseas TFL claims are processed by the TRICARE INTERNATIONAL SOS using Wisconsin Physicians Service as their Fiscal Intermediary partner.

TRICARE YOUNG ADULT (TYA)

The signing of the National Defense Authorization Act in January 2011 aligned TRICARE with the provisions of the 2010 Patient Protection and Affordable Care Act, and led to the creation of TYA.

TRICARE YOUNG ADULT (TYA) is a premium-based health care plan available for purchase by qualified dependents who have aged out of TRICARE at age 21, or age 23 for full-time college students (and not yet 26). Dependents are eligible if they are unmarried, not eligible for either TRICARE coverage or their own employer-sponsored health care coverage, and their sponsor is TRICARE eligible. Eligible dependents have the option to purchase TRICARE STANDARD/EXTRA health coverage on a month-to-month basis. Purchased coverage includes medical and pharmacy benefits but does not include dental.

TRICARE SUPPLEMENT

In addition to the TRICARE options listed above, military retirees can opt for a TRICARE SUPPLEMENT plan. TRICARE SUPPLEMENT was designed to help military retirees and their families save money on unexpected out of pocket expenses that are not covered by TRICARE. Out of pocket costs that may be alleviated by TRICARE SUPPLEMENT can include specialists, surgeries, and hospital stays. The TRICARE SUPPLEMENT plan can be beneficial for TRICARE STANDARD beneficiaries who are covered under a 75/25 plan that does not cover all expenses in the event of an unexpected illness or accident.

https://www.va.gov/health-care/family-caregiver-benefits/champva/
(See hyperlink for full text and references.)

Am I eligible for health care through CHAMPVA?

You may only be eligible for health care through CHAMPVA if you don't qualify for TRICARE and at least one of these descriptions is true for you.

At least one of these must be true:

- You're the spouse or child of a Veteran who's been rated permanently and totally disabled for a service-connected disability by a VA regional office, **or**

- You're the surviving spouse or child of a Veteran who died from a VA-rated service-connected disability, **or**

- You're the surviving spouse or child of a Veteran who was at the time of death rated permanently and totally disabled from a service-connected disability, **or**

- You're the surviving spouse or child of a service member who died in the line of duty, not due to misconduct (in most of these cases, family members qualify for TRICARE, not CHAMPVA).

A service-connected disability is a disability that we've concluded was caused—or made worse—by the Veteran's active-duty service. A permanent disability is one that's not expected to improve.

Note: A Veteran who's the qualifying CHAMPVA sponsor for their family may also qualify for the VA health care program based on their own Veteran status. If 2 spouses are both Veterans who qualify as CHAMPVA sponsors for their family, they both may now qualify for CHAMPVA benefits. Each time they need medical care, they may choose to get care through the VA health care program or using their CHAMPVA coverage.

VETERANS HEALTH ADMINISTRATION
From Wikipedia, the free encyclopedia

The **Veterans Health Administration** (VHA) is the component of the United States Department of Veterans Affairs (VA) led by the Under Secretary of Veterans Affairs for Health that implements the healthcare program of the VA through the administration and operation of numerous VA Medical Centers (VAMC), Outpatient Clinics (OPC), Community Based Outpatient Clinics (CBOC), and VA Community Living Centers (VA Nursing Home) Programs.

The VHA is distinct from the U.S. Department of Defense Military Health System of which it is not a part.

The VHA division has more employees than all other elements of the VA combined.

The Veterans Health Administration is a form of nationalized healthcare service in the United States that provides healthcare to veterans.

What makes this type of healthcare different from other forms in the United States is that everything is owned by and operated by the Department of Veterans Affairs as opposed to private companies which is what we see in other parts of the health care market. This means that all the medical facilities that are part of the VHA are owned by the US Government and all the doctors and workers at the facilities are paid by the government.

Since the VHA is nationalized they receive funding from the Department of Veterans Affairs, which is allocated (taxpayer) funds by the federal government. Because of this, Veterans that qualify for VHA healthcare do not pay premiums or deductibles for their healthcare, but may have to make copayments depending on what procedure they are having.

The funding the VA receives is split into mandatory, which is an amount of spending dictated by law, and discretionary spending, which is spending that can be adjusted year to year. In 2020 the budget given to the VA was $220.2 billion, of which 56% was mandatory spending and 44% was discretionary. From the discretionary funding, 87.6% was allocated to medical programs which came to a total VHA budget of $85 billion.

The 1994 VA Primary Care Directive required all VA facilities to have primary care teams by year 1996. As a result, the percentage of patients receiving primary care at the VA increased from 38 percent to 95 percent from 1993 to 1999.

In 2014, Congress passed the Veterans Access, Choice, and Accountability Act. VA Secretary Robert Wilkie assured veterans that the VA wouldn't be privatized and that veterans would still be able to get the same quality of care they had been receiving.

Research revealed that three out of four veterans would leave the VA network if a national healthcare system were adopted. They also found that there was a high demand for primary care throughout the VA system. Studies show that 66.9 percent of women who do not use the VA for women's services consider private practice physicians more convenient. Also, 48.5 percent of women do not use women's services at the VA due to a lack of knowledge of VA eligibility and services.

VHA is especially praised for its efforts in developing a low cost open source electronic medical records system VistA which can be accessed remotely with secure passwords by health care providers. The system, which has been adopted by all veterans' hospitals and clinics and continuously improved by users, has cut the number of dispensing errors in half at some facilities and saved thousands of lives. Technology has helped the VHA achieve cost controls and care quality that the majority of private providers cannot achieve.

Eligibility for VA Health Care Benefits

To be eligible for VA health care benefit programs one must have served in the active military, naval or air service and separated under any condition other than dishonorable. Current and former members of the Reserves or National Guard who were called to active duty (other than for training only) by a federal order and completed the full period for which they were called or ordered to active duty also may be eligible for VA health care.

General care includes health evaluation and counseling, disease prevention, nutrition counseling, weight control, smoking cessation, and substance abuse counseling and treatment as well as gender-specific primary care.

Mental health includes evaluation and assistance for issues such as depression, mood, and anxiety disorders; intimate partner and domestic violence; elder abuse or neglect; parenting and anger management; marital, caregiver, or family-related stress; and post-deployment adjustment or post-traumatic stress disorder (PTSD). The percentage of patients with a mental illness was 15 percent in 2007. The percentage of veterans with mental illnesses has trended up. The VHA allocated an extra $1.4 billion per year to mental health program between 2005 and 2008.

Management and screening of chronic conditions includes heart disease, diabetes, cancer, glandular disorders, osteoporosis and fibromyalgia as well as sexually transmitted diseases such as HIV/AIDS and hepatitis.

Reproductive health care includes maternity care, infertility evaluation and limited treatment; sexual problems, tubal ligation, urinary incontinence, and others. VHA is prohibited from providing either in-vitro fertilization or abortion services.

Rehabilitation, home care, and long-term care referrals are given to those in need of rehabilitation therapies such as physical therapy, occupational therapy, speech-language therapy, exercise therapy, recreational therapy, and vocational therapy.

Doctors who work in the VHA system are typically paid less in core compensation than their counterparts in private practice. However, VHA compensation includes benefits not generally available to doctors in private practice, such as lesser threat of malpractice lawsuits, freedom from billing and insurance company payment administration, and the availability of the government's open source electronic records system VistA.

Covered Services/Acute Care Standard Benefits

Preventive Care Services
- Counseling on inheritance of genetically determined disease
- Immunization
- Nutrition Education
- Physical Examinations (including eye and hearing)

- Health Care Assessments
- Screening Test
- Health Education Programs

Ambulatory (Outpatient) and Hospital (Inpatient), Diagnostic and Treatment Services

- Medical
- Surgical (Including reconstructive/plastic surgery as a result of disease or trauma)
- Mental Health
- Dialysis
- Substance Abuse
- Prescription Drugs (when prescribed by a VA Physician)

Covered Services/Acute Care Limited Benefits

The following care services have limitations and may have special eligibility criteria:

- Ambulance Services
- Chiropractic Care (at 47 VA hospitals)
- Dental Care
- Durable Medical Equipment (walkers, crutches, canes, etc)
- Eyeglasses
- Hearing Aids
- Home Health Care
- Maternity and Parturition (Childbirth) Services usually provided in non-VA contracted hospitals at VA expense; care is usually limited to a mother. (VA may furnish health care services to a newborn child of a woman Veteran who is receiving maternity care furnished by VA for not more than seven days after the birth if the Veteran delivered the child in (1) a VA facility, or (2) another facility pursuant to a VA contract for services relating to such delivery)
- Non-VA Health Care Services

Long Term Standard Benefits

- Geriatric Evaluation. Geriatric evaluation is the comprehensive assessment of a Veteran's ability to care for him/herself physical health and social environment, which leads to a plan of care.

- Adult Day Health Care. The adult day health care (ADHC) program is a therapeutic day care program, providing medical and rehabilitation services to disabled Veterans in a combined setting.

- Respite Care. Respite care provides supportive care to Veterans on a short-term basis to give the caregiver planned relief from the physical and emotional demands associated with providing care. Respite care can be provided in the home or other institutional settings.

- Home Care. Skilled home care is provided by VA and contract agencies to Veterans that are home bound with chronic diseases and includes nursing, physical/occupational therapy and social services.

- Hospice/Palliative Care. Hospice/Palliative care programs offers pain management, symptom control and other medical services to terminally ill Veterans or Veterans in the late stages of the chronic disease process. Services also include respite care as well as bereavement counseling to family members.

Long Term Limited Benefits

- Nursing Home Care. VA provides nursing home services to Veterans through three national programs: VA owned and operated Community Living Centers (CLC), State Veterans' Homes owned and operated by the states, and the community nursing home program.

- Domiciliary Care. Domiciliary care provides rehabilitative and long-term, health maintenance care for Veterans who require some care, but who do not require all services provided in nursing homes. Domiciliary care emphasizes rehabilitation and return to the community.

Home Health Care

- Skilled Home Health Care Services (SHHC): SHHC services are in-home services provided by specially trained personnel, including nurses, physical therapists, occupational therapists and social workers.

- Homemakers/Home Health Aide Services (H/HHA): H/HHA Services are personal care and related support services that enable frail or disabled Veterans to live at home.

- Family Caregivers Program: VA's Family Caregivers Program provides support and assistance to caregivers of post 9/11 Veterans and Service members being medically discharged. Eligible primary Family Caregivers can receive a stipend, training, mental health services, travel and lodging reimbursement, and access to health insurance if they are not already under a health plan care. Each state has their own criteria and Board Members for approval, denial, and appeal.

Vet Centers

All community based Vet Centers provide readjustment counseling, outreach services and referral services to help veterans make a satisfying post-war readjustment to civilian life. Services are also available for their family members for military related issues.

OEF/OIF/OND Care Management Team

The Operation Enduring Freedom / Operation Iraqi Freedom / Operation New Dawn (OEF/OIF/OND) Care Management Team helps returning service members achieve a smooth transition of health care services. A specialized OEF/OIF/OND care management team provides case management and care coordination for all severely ill, injured and impaired combat veterans.

Domiciliary Care Program

The Domiciliary Care Program of the Department of Veterans Affairs provides residential rehabilitative and clinical care to veterans who have a wide range of problems, illnesses, or rehabilitative care needs which can be medical, psychiatric, substance use, homelessness, vocational, educational, or social.

VA Travel Reimbursement

Veterans may be eligible for mileage reimbursement or special mode transport in association with obtaining VA health care services.

Medical Programs

• The Civilian Health and Medical Program of the Department of Veterans Affairs (CHAMPVA) is a health benefit program in which the Department of Veterans Affairs (VA) shares the cost of certain health care services and supplies with eligible beneficiaries. The program is available to spouses and children of veterans with permanent and total service-connected disability ineligible for the DoD TRICARE, and also to the surviving spouse or child of a veteran who died from a VA service-connected disability or who at the time of death was rated permanently and total disabled.

- The Spina Bifida Program (SB) is a comprehensive health care benefits program administered by the Department of Veterans Affairs for birth children of certain Vietnam and Korea War veterans who have been diagnosed with spina bifida (except spina bifida occulta).

- The Children of Women Vietnam Veterans (CWVV) Health Care Program is a federal health benefits program administered by the Department of Veterans Affairs for children of women Vietnam War veterans born with certain birth defects.

- Patient Aligned Care Team (PACT): The Department of Veterans Affairs' Office of Patient Care Services has a Primary Care Program Office that has implemented a new patient-centered medical home (PCMH) model at VHA primary care sites. PAC Teams provide accessible, patient-centered care and are managed by primary care providers with the active involvement of other clinical and non-clinical staff.

- Transplant Service: If the need arises, veterans are eligible for transplant service.

- VA Dental Care: For VA dental care a veteran must have a service-connected compensable dental disability or condition. Those who were prisoners of war (POWs) and those whose service-connected disabilities have been rated at 100 percent or who are receiving the 100 percent rate by reason of individual unemployability (IU) are eligible for any needed dental care, as are those veterans actively engaged in a 38 USC Chapter 31 vocational rehabilitation program and veterans enrolled who may be homeless and receiving care under VHA Directive 2007-039.

https://kim.house.gov/media/press-releases/reps-kim-and-kelly-introduce-bill-expand-no-fee-healthcare-reserve-and-national
(See hyperlink for full text and references.)

Reps. Kim and Kelly Introduce Bill to Expand No-Fee Healthcare for Reserve and National Guard

On 25 May 2021, Congressman Kim and Congressman Trent Kelly (MS-01) introduced the Healthcare for our Troops Act, a bill that would make no-fee healthcare available to the over 800,000 Americans serving our nation in the Reserve and National Guard. The bipartisan bill is co-sponsored by the two co-chairs of the National Guard and Reserve Caucus, Congressman Tim Ryan (OH-13) and Congressman Steven Palazzo (MS-04), as well as Congressman Scott DesJarlais (TN-04), Congresswoman Elise Stefanik (NY-21), Congressman Marc Veasey (TX-33) Congressman Kai Kahele (HI-01), Congresswoman Marie Newman (IL-03), Congresswoman Marilyn Strickland (WA-10), and Congressman Jim Cooper (TN-05). The bill would ensure that every member of the Reserves and National Guard, including the roughly 130,000 members who don't have private health insurance, can access TRICARE Reserve Select at no cost.

May 25, 2021 PRESS RELEASE
Reps. Kim and Kelly Introduce Bill to Expand No-Fee Healthcare for Reserve and National Guard

WASHINGTON, DC – Today, Congressman Andy Kim (NJ-03) and Congressman Trent Kelly (MS-01) introduced the Healthcare for our Troops Act, a bill that would make no-fee healthcare available to the over 800,000 Americans serving our nation in the Reserve and National Guard. The bipartisan bill is co-sponsored by the two co-chairs of the National Guard and Reserve Caucus, Congressman Tim Ryan (OH-13) and Congressman Steven Palazzo (MS-04), as well as Congressman Scott DesJarlais (TN-04), Congresswoman Elise Stefanik (NY-21) and Congressman Marc Veasey (TX-33).

"Americans who wear the uniform and protect our nation should not be without healthcare. It's that simple," said Congressman Kim. "We owe our Reservists and National Guard so much, and this bill fulfills a basic bipartisan promise: that we will be there for them as they are there for us every day to keep our country safe. I want to thank Congressman Kelly for his partnership on this mission to make sure that every one of our Reservists and National Guard members has the health care they deserve. I look forward to working with our colleagues across the aisle to get this across the finish line and deliver for those who serve."

The bill would ensure that every member of the Reserves and National Guard, including the roughly 130,000 members who don't have private health insurance, can access TRICARE Reserve Select at no cost. The bill also addresses a recent call by the head of the National Guard Bureau, Army General Daniel Hokanson, for no-cost healthcare for every member of the National Guard. General Hokanson called the issue, "one of my most pressing concerns."

"From being deployed nonstop, protecting our nation's capital, and handling pandemic relief efforts, we witnessed an unprecedented use of our military," said Congressman Kelly. "Current bureaucratic policies prevent some of our service members from having the same healthcare benefits as their counterparts on active-duty. Providing health care for all service members is a readiness issue that is easily fixed. Our Guardsmen and Reservists deserve to have access to preventive and routine healthcare. The Healthcare for our Troops Act ensures that no military member will have to worry about paying for medical bills."

Specifically, if enacted, the Healthcare for our Troops Act would:

- Ensure Reservists and National Guard members have no-fee healthcare through TRICARE Reserve Select that covers medical and dental coverage

- Increases military readiness by ensuring service members can access physicals needed to be ready for no-notice deployments which have increased over the past year

- Provide an incentive for small businesses to hire Reserve and National Guard members by ensuring their healthcare costs are covered

- Require a study on eliminating annual physicals during drill and replacing them with forms to be completed by civilian providers to assess medical readiness--giving commanders back valuable training days and saving over $162 Million annually in contracted medical assessments

- Eliminate the statutory language that excludes Federal Employees Health Benefits Program eligible service members from TRICARE Reserve Select eligibility.

- Fix the parity gap for Reserve Component retirees receiving early retirement pay due to deployment credits making them eligible for TRICARE upon receipt of retirement pay

"As a Cochair of the National Guard and Reserve Caucus, I could not be more proud of the work that these service members have done for our country – especially over this last year," said Congressman Ryan. "But back-to-back deployments, whether overseas or here at home, take their toll. This legislation represents a huge step forward in making sure our citizen Soldiers, Airmen, Sailors, and Marines not only have access to the health care they need to take care of themselves, but also to do their jobs. I'm honored to support this bill,"

"I am proud to support the Tricare Reserve Select expansion bill, to ensure that our National Guard and Reserve members are not over-paying for the healthcare they deserve. As a Mississippi National Guardsman and Co-chair of the National Guard and Reserve Caucus, I can attest to how this legislation improves Tricare by increasing affordability and retention rates," said Congressman Palazzo. "This year, we saw our National Guardsmen and Reservists drop everything to serve this country. They have had our backs, this bill helps us have theirs."

This bill has the support of: National Guard Association of the U.S. (NGAUS), Military Officers Association of America (MOAA), Enlisted Association of the National Guard of the U.S. (EANGUS), Association of the United States Army (AUSA), Chief Warrant Officers Association of the U.S. Coast Guard, Naval Enlisted Reserve Association, Reserve Organization of America (formerly Reserve Officers Association), Air Force Sergeants Association, VoteVets, and the Wounded Warrior Project.

https://stanmed.stanford.edu/2017spring/how-health-insurance-changed-from-protecting-patients-to-seeking-profit.html
(See hyperlink for full text and references.)

Insurance Policy: How an Industry Shifted from Protecting Patients to Seeking Profit

By Elisabeth Rosenthal, Spring 2017

Jeffrey Kivi, PhD, was receiving monthly infusions of Remicade to treat psoriatic arthritis, an autoimmune disease he'd had since childhood. The drug enabled the high school science teacher to stand all day in his classroom and to walk down the school's hallways. Each monthly infusion cost $19,000, which his insurance covered. Then his doctor switched hospitals.

The cost of Kivi's infusions ballooned, soon surpassing $132,000 a month. He still wasn't responsible for any of the cost, but he was stunned. What could account for this disparity in price?

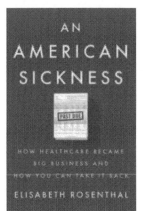

Plenty of factors, writes Elisabeth Rosenthal, MD, in her new book *An American Sickness*. The new hospital spent more on amenities and marketing. It held the patent on Remicade, and stood to benefit from its administration if profits were high enough. And Kivi's insurer didn't push back against the higher price — instead, it paid three-quarters of it. Kivi was so appalled he switched to a medication he could take at home.

The United States spends almost 20 percent of its gross domestic product on health care, and if we want to reduce that, Rosenthal argues, we're all going to have to be more like Jeffrey Kivi. Rosenthal, editor-in-chief of *Kaiser Health News*, itemizes the ills that have befallen health care, including opaque and inequitable pricing, perverse financial incentives and an ethos of putting profits before patients. She then writes a prescription for reform, including short-term strategies to reduce costs and long-term policy goals.

In this excerpt, Rosenthal explains how the transformation of the United States' health care economy began: with the creation of insurance companies and their evolution into for-profit entities.

The very idea of health insurance is in some ways the original sin that catalyzed the evolution of today's medical-industrial complex.

The people who founded the Blue Cross Association in Texas nearly a century ago had no idea how their innovation would spin out of control. They intended it to help the sick. And, in the beginning, it did.

A hundred years ago medical treatments were basic, cheap and not terribly effective. Often run by religious charities, hospitals were places where people mostly went to die. "Care," such as it was, was delivered at dispensaries by doctors or quacks for minimal fees.

Disease was very time-consuming. Without antibiotics and nonsteroidal medicines, or anesthetics and minimally invasive surgery, sickness and injury took much longer to heal. The earliest health insurance policies were designed primarily to compensate for income lost while workers were ill. Long absences were a big problem for companies that depended on manual labor, so they often hired doctors to tend to workers. In the 1890s, lumber companies in Tacoma, Washington, paid two enterprising doctors 50 cents a month to care for employees. It was perhaps one of the earliest predecessors to the type of employer-based insurance found in the United States today.

As medical treatments and knowledge improved in the early 20th century, the concept of insurance evolved. The archetype for today's insurance plans was developed at Baylor University Medical Center in Dallas, Texas (now part of Baylor Scott & White Health, since it merged with another health system in 2013, forming a giant health care conglomerate), which was founded in 1903 in a 14-room mansion by the Baptist Church. A devout cattleman provided the initial $50,000 in funding to open what was then called the Texas Baptist Memorial Sanitarium, "a great humanitarian hospital." By the 1920s, more and more Texans were coming for treatment. When Justin Ford Kimball, a lawyer who was Baylor's vice president, found out that the hospital was carrying a huge number of unpaid bills, he offered the local teachers' union a deal. For $6 a year, or 50 cents a month, teachers who subscribed were entitled to a 21-day stay in the hospital, all costs included. But there was a deductible. The "insurance" took effect after a week and covered the full costs of hospitalization, $5 a day, which is about $105 in 2016 dollars.

Soon, employees for the *Dallas Morning News* and local radio stations were also signing up for what we today would call catastrophic care insurance. It was a good deal. The cost of a 21-day hospitalization, $525, would have bankrupted many at the time. In that era, given the treatments available, within 21 days you were likely dead or cured.

Within a decade, the model spread across the country. Three million people had signed up by 1939 and the concept had been given a name: Blue Cross Plans. The goal was not to make money, but to protect patient savings and keep hospitals — and the charitable religious groups that funded them — afloat. Blue Cross Plans were then not-for-profit.

Despite this, before World War II, when most treatments were still relatively unsophisticated and cheap, few Americans had health insurance. The invention of effective ventilators, breathing machines that moved air in and out of the lungs, enabled a vast expansion of surgery suites and intensive care units. That meant more people could be saved, including soldiers injured during the war and victims of polio outbreaks.

Transformative technologies rapidly spread across the developed world. Abbott Laboratories made and patented the first intravenous anesthetic, thiopental, in the 1930s. Massachusetts General Hospital started the first anesthesia department in the United States in 1936. The first intensive care unit armed with ventilators opened during a polio epidemic in Copenhagen in the early 1940s.

Five dollars a day and a 21-day maximum stay were no longer enough. Insurance with a capital "I" was increasingly needed. A private industry selling direct to customers could have filled the need — as it has for auto and life insurance. But a quirk of history and some well-meaning policy helped etch in place employer-based health insurance in the United States. When the National War Labor Board froze salaries during and after World War II, companies facing severe labor shortages discovered that they could attract workers by offering health insurance instead. To encourage the trend, the federal government ruled that money paid for employees' health benefits would not be taxed. This strategy was a win-

win in the short term, but in the long term has had some very losing implications.

The policies offered were termed major medical, meaning they paid for extensive care but not routine doctor visits and the like. The original purpose of health insurance was to mitigate financial disasters brought about by a serious illness, such as losing your home or your job, but it was never intended to make health care cheap or serve as a tool for cost control. Our expectations about what insurance should do have grown.

Blue Cross and its partner, Blue Shield, were more or less the only major insurers at the time and both stood ever ready to enroll new members. The former covered hospital care and the latter doctors' visits. Between 1940 and 1955, the number of Americans with health insurance skyrocketed from 10 percent to over 60 percent. That was before the advent of government programs like Medicare and Medicaid. The Blue Cross/Blue Shield logo became ubiquitous as a force for good across America. According to their charter, the Blues were nonprofit and accepted everyone who sought to sign up; all members were charged the same rates, no matter how old or how sick. Boy Scouts handed out brochures and preachers urged their congregants to join. By some accounts, Blue Cross Blue Shield became, like Walter Cronkite, one of the most trusted brands in postwar America.

But the new demand for health insurance presented a business opportunity and spawned an emerging market with other motivations. Suddenly, at a time when medicine had more of value to offer, tens of millions of people were interested in gaining access and expected their employers to provide insurance so they could do so. For-profit insurance companies moved in, unencumbered by the Blues' charitable mission. They accepted only younger, healthier patients on whom they could make a profit. They charged different rates, depending on factors like age, as they had long done with life insurance. And they produced different types of policies, for different amounts of money, which provided different levels of protection.

Aetna and Cigna were both offering major medical coverage by 1951. With aggressive marketing and closer ties to business than to health care, these for-profit plans slowly gained market share through the 1970s and 1980s. It was difficult for the Blues to compete. From a market perspective, the poor Blues still had to worry about their mission of "providing high-quality, affordable health care for all."

By the 1990s, the Blues, which offered insurance in all 50 states, were hemorrhaging money, having been left to cover the sickest patients. In 1994, after state directors rebelled, the Blues' board relented and allowed member plans to become for-profit insurers. Their primary motivation was not to charge patients more, but to gain access to the stock market to raise some quick cash to erase deficits. This was the final nail in the coffin of old-fashioned noble-minded health insurance.

Many of the long-suffering Blue plans seized the business opportunity. Blue Cross and Blue Shield of California was particularly aggressive, gobbling up its fellow Blues in a dozen other states. Renamed WellPoint, it is the biggest of the for-profit companies descended from the original nonprofit Blue Cross Blue Shield Association; today it is the second-largest insurer in the United States. Most of its plans still operate under the name Anthem BlueCross BlueShield, but in New York the plans operate under the Emblem brand. The insurer for New York City teachers, which reimbursed about $100,000 for each of Jeffrey Kivi's outpatient infusions, has evolved a long way from its not-for-profit mission and $5-a-day hospital payments.

WellPoint's first priority appears no longer to be its patient/members or even the companies and unions that choose it as an insurer, but instead its shareholders and investors. As in any for-profit enterprise, executives are compensated for how well they perform that financial function and are compensated well. In 2010 WellPoint had intended to hike premiums in California by 39 percent, before an attorney general effectively nixed the plan. CEO Angela Braly received total annual compensation of more than $20 million in 2012, despite the fact that she resigned under pressure that year because the company revenues were down. Joe Swedish, the new CEO appointed in 2013, is a longtime health care executive who served at the for-profit Hospital Corporation of America. His starting salary and bonus totaled about $5 million, not including stock options.

Then, in August 2014, WellPoint announced that it planned to change its name to Anthem Blue Cross (pending approval by shareholders), presumably to take advantage of whatever nostalgic good feelings patients had retained toward the Blues, before raising premiums on some of its California ACA policies by 25 percent in 2015. Dave Jones, California's vocal insurance commissioner, accused Anthem of "once again imposing an unjustified and unreasonable rate increase on its individual members." Using his bully pulpit to publicly voice his objections was Jones' only recourse, since he, like many state insurance commissioners, can make only nonbinding determinations and has no legal authority to deny rates. To express their collective frustration, members gathered signatures for a MoveOn.org petition: "Anthem Blue Cross: Stop Playing Politics with Our Premiums." They urged their insurer "to stop spending corporate funds on political campaigns, disclose everything it has spent directly or indirectly on political campaigns, and use the money to lower rates for Anthem policy-holders and California taxpayers."

In 1993, before the Blues went for-profit, insurers spent 95 cents out of every dollar of premiums on medical care, which is called their "medical loss ratio." To increase profits, all insurers, regardless of their tax status, have been spending less on care in recent years and more on activities like marketing, lobbying, administration and the paying out of dividends. The average medical loss ratio is now closer to 80 percent. Some of the Blues were spending far less than that a decade into the new century. The medical loss ratio at the Texas Blues, where the whole concept of health insurance started, was just 64.4 percent in 2010.

The framers of the Affordable Care Act tried to curb insurers' profits and their executives' salaries, which were some of the highest in the U.S. health care industry, by requiring them to spend 80 to 85 percent of every premium dollar on patient care. Insurers fought bitterly against this provision. Its inclusion in the ACA was hailed as a victory for consumers. But even that apparent "demand" was actually quite a generous gift when you consider that Medicare uses 98 percent of its funding for health care and only 2 percent for administration.

Why did EmblemHealth agree to pay nearly $100,000 for each of Jeffrey Kivi's infusions, even though they cost only $19,000 at another hospital just down the street? First, it's less trouble for insurers to pay it than not. NYU is a big client that insurers don't want to lose, and an insurer can compensate for the high price in various ways — by raising premiums, co-payments, or deductibles. Second, now that they suddenly have to use 80 to 85 percent rather than, say, 75 percent of premiums on patient care, insurers have a new perverse motivation to tolerate such big payouts. In order to make sure their 15 percent take is still sufficient to maintain salaries and investor dividends, insurance executives have to increase the size of the pie. To cover shortfalls, premiums are increased the next year, passing costs on to the consumers. And 15 percent of a big sum is more than 15 percent of a smaller one. No wonder 2017 premiums for the most common type of ACA plan are slated to rise by double digits in many cities, despite economists' assurances that the growth of health care spending is slowing.

To some extent insurers do better if they negotiate better rates for your care. But that is true only under certain circumstances and in a limited way. "They are methodical money takers, who take in premiums and pay claims according to contracts — that's their job," said Barry Cohen, who owns an Ohio-based employee benefits company. "They don't care whether the claims go up or down 20 percent as long as they get their piece. They're too big to care about you."

Excerpt from *AN AMERICAN SICKNESS: HOW HEALTHCARE BECAME BIG BUSINESS AND HOW YOU CAN TAKE IT BACK* by Elisabeth Rosenthal, Copyright © 2017 by Elisabeth Rosenthal. Used by permission of Penguin Press, an imprint of Penguin Publishing Group, a division of Penguin Random House LLC. All rights reserved. Elisabeth Rosenthal, MD, is the editor-in-chief of Kaiser Health News.

https://www.commonwealthfund.org/publications/newsletter-article/us-workers-employment-based-health-insurance-continues-decline
(See hyperlink for full text and references.)

For U.S. Workers, Employment-Based Health Insurance Continues to Decline, Report Says
By Jane Norman, CQ HealthBeat Associate Editor

September 27, 2012 -- When it comes to health insurance coverage for those under 65 in the United States, research released last week shows the trends are like two trains rushing past one another: Coverage in public programs is growing, while traditional private insurance through employers is contracting.

That will continue, predicts a report written by Paul Fronstin, of the nonpartisan Employee Benefits Research Institute (EBRI), who dove deep into recently released census numbers. "Until the economy gains enough strength to have a substantial impact on the labor market, a rebound in employment-based coverage is unlikely," the report said.

EBRI also found that those Americans who still have employer-based insurance are far more likely to earn more than $75,000 a year, work in a managerial or professional occupation, be employed by a big firm - and be white. Where a person or his or her spouse works is the most important factor in determining whether he or she is insured.

The report by the organization gives a glimpse into the makeup of the working-age uninsured population likely to be enrolling in Medicaid or buying policies in the state-based or federal health insurance exchanges once they are up and running in 2014 under the health care law (PL 111-148, PL 111-152). Many are in the South. For example, in 13 states, uninsured people made up 20 percent or more of the population between 2009 and 2011, said the report. Those states are Arkansas, Arizona, California, Florida, Georgia, Louisiana, Mississippi, Montana, Nevada, New Mexico, Oklahoma, South Carolina and Texas.

The report also says that in general, employers want to provide health insurance because it makes for a better workforce - but may reconsider if the economy continues to be sour or the health care law "changes the value proposition" of offering insurance, thus speeding up the trend toward less employer-based insurance.

Health insurance is the benefit most valued by employees and provides them with a hedge against devastating losses from sickness, notes Fronstin. Employers offer it to increase productivity and raise esteem. But that may shift, the report cautions, because "the recent enactment and ongoing implementation of federal health reform legislation may change that equation." Employers are penalized under the law for not offering affordable health insurance, but opponents of the overhaul have warned that many businesses may decide to pay the penalty rather than sustain the costs of adding coverage. Studies have been mixed on whether that will happen.

The institute, a private group based in Washington that studies issues such as health, retirement and savings, based its study on the latest 2011 numbers from the census on the uninsured, focusing on the non-elderly population, those under 65. It found that employer-based health insurance for this group shrank again in 2011, to 58.4 percent, compared to 69.3 percent in 2000.

At the same time, EBRI said, 22.5 percent of the non-elderly in 2011, or more than a fifth of the population, were enrolled in a public program. That's compared to 14.1 percent in 1999. Sources of coverage for this group include Medicaid, the Children's Health Insurance Program, Medicare for people with disabilities, Tricare and veterans' health benefits.

And 7.1 percent of Americans bought their insurance in the individual market, a target for major overhaul in the health care law.

Fronstin noted that overall, the percentage of people under 65 with some kind of insurance coverage actually increased between 2010 and 2011, the first time that's happened since 2007, even if it's a slight rise. Now 82 percent of these Americans have health insurance, up from 81.5 percent in 2010. But 18 percent still lack insurance, though that, again, was slightly better than the 18.5 percent in 2010, the highest share of people without insurance between 1994 and 2010, the report said.

Who has employer-based health insurance, and who has the best health insurance? The report says 71.8 percent of people in families headed by a full-time, full-year worker had employer-provided insurance, compared to 34.2 percent of those in families whose head works part of the time and just part of the year.

The size of the employer matters, too. Nearly two-thirds of the uninsured - 61 percent - either were self-employed or worked at companies with fewer than 100 employees, the report said.

Race is a stark divider. The report said 66.9 percent of whites had employer-based coverage in 2011, compared to 46.7 percent of blacks and 38.8 percent of Hispanics.

As for profession, 33.3 percent of people who work in agriculture, forestry, fishing, mining and construction in 2011 were uninsured, which was even worse than people employed in the service industry — 23.4 percent of them were uninsured. Among those in wholesale and retail trade, 19.5 percent were uninsured, and 15.7 percent of those in manufacturing lacked insurance.

It's about money, too. A third of people without insurance were in families with annual incomes of less than $20,000. That compared with 6.7 percent of those in families with annual incomes of $75,000 or more, the report said.

https://thehill.com/opinion/healthcare/499907-its-time-to-say-goodbye-to-employment-based-health-insurance (See hyperlink for full text and references.)

It's Time to Say Goodbye
to Employment-Based Health Insurance

By Deborah Gordon and Akshaya Kannan, Opinion Contributors
28 May 2020, The views expressed by Contributors are their own and not the view of The Hill.

America's employment-based health insurance system was problematic before the pandemic. Now, with millions of Americans both unemployed and uninsured, it seems absurd.

In May 2020, the jobless rate hit nearly 15 percent and more than 36 million Americans filed for unemployment. Many of these jobs may never come back. An estimated 12.7 million Americans have lost their job-based health insurance; this number could grow to 43 million Americans. Although a recent study estimates that millions of newly unemployed Americans will be eligible for Medicaid or marketplace subsidies, at least 5.7 million will remain uninsured.

COVID-19 re-opening and recovery plans must include a new way to ensure people that don't tie health insurance to employment status.

Even before the pandemic, employment-based insurance wasn't working for many Americans. First offered as an employee incentive to offset wage freezes during World War II's tightly constrained labor market, health insurance benefits became table stakes for attracting and retaining talent. However, as insurance expanded to cover more services and medical inflation grew, employers have shifted rising costs onto employees.

The resulting value erosion defeats the original purpose, and worse leaves employers open to blame from employees feeling financially squeezed. Still, many assume it's the best they can get. For many, it is.

The employment-based system traps many Americans in jobs they would otherwise leave. In our research at the Harvard Kennedy School, we saw firsthand the cost to consumers who felt stuck in their jobs due to health benefits.

We heard from one woman who stayed in a job she did not love because she wanted to have a second child; she didn't trust she'd be able to replace her "amazing health insurance." Economists call this phenomenon "job-lock," where stagnation and workforce immobility hamper employee engagement and block self-employment and entrepreneurship, which rise with access to health insurance outside of a job.

Job-lock now seems almost quaint luxury from another era. COVID-19 lays bare the problem with an insurance system that leaves people economically vulnerable when they are least able to absorb the costs and more likely to need the care. Untethered from stable employment, millions of Americans are desperate for a new way to access insurance. Many businesses have nothing to offer.

COVID-19 reveals urgency for a new approach, yet consumers fear losing what they have. Time and again, voters have favored incrementalism, craving familiarity. But now, the pandemic has shaken the foundation to which many Americans have clung. Instead of timidly repairing that foundation when the dust settles, we should boldly sever those ties once and for all.

We must then forge a new path that offers affordability, access, portability, and choice. Such a path runs through the health insurance marketplaces - often called exchanges - created by the ACA. Already a viable option for millions of Americans without employer-sponsored insurance, these marketplaces need not be simply health insurance of last resort.

Rather, marketplaces present the opportunity to improve choice, optimize benefits, and create insurance portability for consumers. These platforms enable comparisons and create transparency into insurance pricing, spurring competition with the potential to drive down prices and expand the assortment. They empower consumers to select their own plan where their employer plan was chosen for them based on aggregate corporate needs.

The federal government could also offer a subsidized public option or extend current subsidies to protect lower-income consumers. A recent Gallup poll estimates that while 54 percent of Americans support a private health care system, 42 percent support a government-run system. In an open marketplace, consumers are free to choose private or public options that work with their budgets and their families' needs.

Employers will also benefit from an open marketplace. Absolved of the burden of choosing health insurance plans for their employees, businesses can focus on what they need to most - getting back on their feet in the wake of COVID-19. Small businesses, struggling greatly during this pandemic, could compete for talent on a more level playing field without having to fight to attract employees drawn to corporate benefits.

Employers heavily subsidize employee health insurance costs and might welcome the chance to drop these financial obligations. These contributions are vital to financing health care. If businesses get out of the business of buying health insurance for their employees, they will have to pay a price. Taxes equivalent to employer contributions must be levied in order to offer affordable marketplace options.

Opponents might argue that employers have negotiating power to reduce the cost of insurance; without employers in the mix, this leverage could be lost. However, medical inflation and cost-sharing trends suggest employers are not using that power to reduce health costs nor to protect employees from the increases.

2020 is the year for a health care overhaul. COVID-19 has destabilized employment-based insurance. Facing a pandemic and a recession, Americans have the opportunity to break the link entirely and empower consumers to shop on open insurance marketplaces. Now, more than ever, Americans need affordable access to health insurance and the economic security that would come with controlling their own health insurance destiny.

Deborah Gordon is a former health insurance executive and author of The Health Care Consumer's Manifesto; follow her on Twitter @gordondeb. Akshaya Kannan, M.D., MPP, is a graduate of Emory University School of Medicine and Harvard Kennedy School. She is currently a resident physician in Obstetrics and Gynecology at the University of California, San Francisco.

A Majority of Americans with Employer-based Health Insurance Don't Mind if it Changes to Medicare for All — as Long as They Can Keep Their Current Coverage

By Joseph Zeballos-Roig and Walt Hickey, 8 August 2019

Over 59% of respondents who receive health insurance through their employer said in a new INSIDER poll they would be fine if that plan changed, as long as it meant no change in coverage. ... Mainly people just like being covered in general, bearing little loyalty to a specific insurer.

And the respondents' attitude toward "Medicare for All" reflects a dynamic that candidates who champion it — like Sen. Bernie Sanders — are counting on: If the system provides equal or more comprehensive benefits, then broad swaths of Americans are likely to support it. ...

Under Medicare for All, there would be a national health insurance system that would be funded by tax revenue and cover everyone who lives in the US. It would also pay for every medically-needed service, ranging from doctor visits to mental healthcare to prescription drugs.

...(T)he plan would ... replace employer-based health insurance, which is the most important source of health coverage for non-elderly Americans. ...

The results showed that, among all respondents ... 59% said they would support switching their employer-based health insurance to a government plan under Medicare for All. ...

Joe Biden said Americans should be able to keep their plans if they like them. He's criticized Sanders' plan since it would virtually do away with private health insurance. ...

INSIDER's polling ... indicates that even if people think their employer plan is great, that doesn't necessarily mean that they're opposed to changing it. For Democrats, it means the final policy should carry out a clean reform of the healthcare system that doesn't disrupt it in a way that Americans can feel, lest they face a political backlash.

# # #

AND, per the Bartleby Column "Managing the Great Resignation" in the 11/27/2021 issue of The Economist: "Salaries matter to everyone but, for lower-wage workers in particular, benefits like health care have also become central. A recent survey by Jeffries, an investment bank, found that health concerns were the prime reason why people with only a high-school education had quit their jobs." - - - - A strong argument for providing Medicare For All ("a card in your wallet") to everyone seeking employment.

Original Medicare Part A & Part B

It used to be that young adults lamented the approach of age 30. Now we often hear "I can't wait until I turn 65 and qualify for Medicare". That alone should make it clear that "Medicare For All" is long past due in our country!

Medicare is the federal health insurance program created in 1965 to provide health coverage for Americans aged 65 and older. The program – administered by the Centers for Medicare and Medicaid Services – was expanded in 1972 to cover people younger than 65 who have permanent disabilities, including those diagnosed with end-stage renal disease (ESRD). And in 2001, Congress added ALS (Amyotrophic Lateral Sclerosis aka "Lou Gehrig's disease") as a diagnosis that makes a person eligible for Medicare prior to age 65.

The program is currently comprised of Original Medicare (Parts A & B), Medicare Advantage (Part C), Part D prescription drug coverage and Medigap.

In 2019, according to the 2020 Medicare Trustees Report, Medicare provided health insurance for approximately 61.2 million individuals: 52.6 million people aged 65 and older, and 8.7 million disabled younger people. Total expenditures in 2019 were $796.2 billion and total income was $794.8 billion, with assets of $303.3 billion held in special issue U.S. Treasury securities.

According to annual Medicare Trustees reports and research by the government's MedPAC group, Medicare A and Medicare B cover about half of healthcare expenses of those enrolled. Enrollees almost always cover most of the remaining costs of Medicare A & B by taking additional private insurance (known as "MEDIGAP" or "Supplemental Insurance") and/or by joining a Part C (Medicare Advantage) or Part D Medicare health plan.

Beneficiaries also have other healthcare-related costs. These additional so-called out of pocket (OOP) costs can include deductibles and co-pays; the costs of uncovered services such as for long-term custodial, dental, hearing, and vision care; the cost of annual physical exams (for those not on Part C health plans that include physicals); and the costs related to basic Medicare's lifetime and per-incident limits.

Some people are automatically enrolled in Medicare Part A (Hospital Insurance) and Medicare Part B (Medical Insurance), while other people have to sign up for it. Generally speaking, you are eligible for Medicare if one of the following applies:

- you are 65 years old, and have been a legal permanent US resident for at least five continuous years.

- you will be getting benefits from Social Security or the Railroad Retirement Board (RRB) at least 4 months before turning 65.

- you are 65 and have paid into Medicare for at least 10 years even if you plan to delay collecting Social Security until a later age.

- you are under 65 and have amyotrophic lateral sclerosis (ALS – also known as Lou Gehrig's Disease) – or end-stage renal disease (ERSD); or

- you are not yet 65, but have been entitled to Social Security Disability benefits for at least 24 months.

MEDICARE PART A

Medicare Part A – often called "hospital insurance" – is devoted to inpatient care, covering the costs of inpatient hospital stays (of at least one night), skilled nursing facility stays (if they meet specific criteria), home health care and hospice care.

In order to get premium-free Medicare Part A, you need to have paid into the Medicare system. This means that you or your spouse (or a parent, if you're enrolling a disabled child) must have worked for at least ten years prior to enrolling in Medicare. If not, you're still eligible, but will have to pay a premium for Medicare Part A.

You can get premium-free Part A at 65 if:

- You already get retirement benefits from Social Security or the Railroad Retirement Board.

- You're eligible to get Social Security or Railroad benefits but haven't filed for them yet.

- You or your spouse had Medicare-covered government employment.

If you're under 65, you can get premium-free Part A if:

- You got Social Security or Railroad Retirement Board disability benefits for 24 months.

- You have End-Stage Renal Disease (ESRD) or Amyotrophic Lateral Sclerosis (ALS) and meet certain requirements.

If you don't qualify for premium-free Part A, you can buy Part A. People who buy Part A will pay a premium of either $259 or $471 each month in 2021 depending on how long they or their spouse worked and paid Medicare taxes. In most cases, if you choose to buy Part A, you must also have Medicare Part B (Medical Insurance).

If you choose NOT to buy Part A, you can still buy Part B.

Part A Deductible & Copays & Coinsurance

You must first meet an insurance deductible before Part A helps with your medical costs. The Part A deductible for 2021 was $1,484.

A copayment or cost sharing may apply to specific services, such as extended stays in a hospital or skilled nursing facility.

Part A has coinsurance for:

- Inpatient hospital care lasting between 61 and 90 days total per benefit period.

- Inpatient mental health care lasting between 61 and 90 days total per benefit period.

- Skilled nursing care lasting between 21 and 100 days total per benefit period.

- Coinsurance is also available for a limited number of additional days.

The following coverage restrictions apply to Medicare Part A:

- Inpatient hospital care is limited to 90 days total per benefit period.

- Inpatient mental care is limited to 90 days total per benefit period.

- Skilled nursing care is limited to 100 days total per benefit period.

For each type of care, you can receive coverage for 60 additional days throughout your lifetime. These are known as "lifetime reserve days."

MEDICARE PART B

Medicare Part B – often called "medical insurance" – covers certain doctors' and preventive services, outpatient care, medical supplies and durable medical equipment as well as some providers' services while inpatient at a hospital, outpatient hospital charges, most provider office visits even if the office is "in a hospital", and most professionally administered prescription drugs.

Complex rules control Part B benefits, and periodically-issued advisories describe coverage criteria.

Most Medicare Part B enrollees pay an insurance premium based on when you enroll and your annual household income. The standard Part B premium for 2021 was $148.50 a month. It is separate from the health insurance premiums you will pay if you choose Medigap, Medicare Advantage (Part C) or Prescription Drug Coverage (Part D).

Your Part B premium will be automatically deducted from your benefit payment if you get benefits from Social Security, the Railroad Retirement Board or the Office of Personnel Management. If you don't get these benefit payments, you'll get a bill.

If an individual does not sign up for Part B when they are first eligible, they may have to pay a late enrollment penalty for as long as they have Medicare. Their monthly premium for Part B may go up 10% for each full 12-month period that they could have had Part B, but did not sign up for it.

If your modified adjusted gross income as reported on your IRS tax return from 2 years ago is above a certain amount, you'll pay the standard premium amount and an Income Related Monthly Adjustment Amount (IRMAA). This is your most recent tax return information provided to Social Security by the IRS. IRMAA is an extra charge added to your premium.

See the following chart to view your (2021) monthly Medicare Part B premium based upon your (2019) yearly income:

CHART: What you pay in 2021 based upon your 2019 yearly income

➢ You pay in 2021: $148.50/month

- File individual tax return: $88,000 or less

- File joint tax return: $176,000 or less

- File married & separate tax return: $88,000 or less

➤ You pay in 2021: $207.90/month

- File individual tax return: Above $88,000 up to $111,000

- File joint tax return: Above $176,000 up to $222,000

- File married & separate tax return: Not applicable

➤ You pay in 2021: $297.00/month

- File individual tax return: Above $111,000 up to $138,000

- File joint tax return: Above $222,000 up to $276,000

- File married & separate tax return: Not applicable

➤ You pay each month (in 2021): $386.10

- File individual tax return: Above $138,000 up to $165,000

- File joint tax return: Above $276,000 up to $330,000

- File married & separate tax return: Not applicable

➤ You pay each month (in 2021): $475.20

- File individual tax return: Above $165,000 & less than $500,000

- File joint tax return: Above $330,000 & less than $750,000

- File married & separate tax return: Above $88,000 & less than $412,000

➤ You pay each month (in 2021): $504.90

- File individual tax return: $500,000 or above

- File joint tax return: $750,000 and above

- File married & separate tax return: $412,000 and above

Part B Deductible & Copays & Coinsurance

You must first meet an insurance deductible before Part B helps with your medical costs. In 2021, you pay $203 for your Part B deductible.

After you meet your deductible for the year, you typically pay 20% coinsurance of the Medicare-approved amount for some medical services, such as doctor services (including most doctor services while you're a hospital inpatient), outpatient therapy and durable medical equipment.

A copayment or cost sharing may apply to specific services, such as those received in an outpatient hospital setting.

No deductibles, copays or coinsurance are required for Medicare-covered preventive care services, such as annual wellness visits and mammograms for women.

Under Medicare Part B, there are annual limits on services for physical therapy, occupational therapy and speech language pathology.

MEDICARE PART C (for clarification)

Medicare Part C is an alternative called Managed Medicare or Medicare Advantage which allows patients to choose health plans with at least the same service coverage as Parts A and B (and most often more), often the benefits of Part D, and always an annual out-of-pocket spend limit which A and B lack. A beneficiary must enroll in Parts A and B first before signing up for a Part C Medicare Advantage plan.

COSTS & GUIDELINES FOR ORIGINAL MEDICARE

Generally, there's a cost for each Medicare A and Medicare B service. Here are some general guidelines:

- In Original Medicare you don't need to choose a primary care doctor. You can select any doctor, health care provider, hospital, or facility in the United States that is enrolled in Medicare and accepting new Medicare patients.

- In Original Medicare, you don't need a referral to see a specialist, but the specialist must be enrolled in Medicare.

- Most hospitals in the U.S. participate in Medicare.

- With a few exceptions, most prescriptions aren't covered in Original Medicare. You can add drug coverage by joining a Medicare Part D drug plan.

- You may already have employer or union coverage that may pay costs that Original Medicare doesn't. If not, you may want to buy a Medicare Supplement Insurance (Medigap) policy.

- You generally pay a deductible for your Medicare Parts A and B health care before Medicare pays its share.

- You usually pay a monthly premium for Part B. Part B premiums and standard deductibles and cost sharing amounts generally change annually on January 1st.

- You pay your share (coinsurance / copayment) for covered services and supplies. There's no yearly limit for what you pay out-of-pocket.

- You generally don't need to file Medicare claims. The law requires providers and suppliers to file your claims for the covered services and supplies you get. Providers include doctors, hospitals, skilled nursing facilities, and home health agencies.

- If you're in a Medicare Advantage Plan or other Medicare plan, your plan may have different rules. But your plan must give you at least the same coverage as Original Medicare. Some services may only be covered in certain settings or for patients with certain conditions.

Two ways to find out if Medicare Parts A/B cover what you need:

- Talk to your doctor or other health care provider about why you need certain services or supplies. Ask if Medicare will cover them. You may need something that's usually covered but your provider thinks that Medicare won't cover it in your situation. If so, you'll have to read and sign a notice. The notice says that you may have to pay for the item, service, or supply.

- Find out if Medicare covers your item, service, or supply at https://www.medicare.gov/coverage.

Information in the above portion of this chapter is extracted from the following articles in an effort to present a complete representation of the intricacies of "Original Medicare Parts A & B". Please see the hyperlinks below for media sources, author profiles and references.

(1) Medicare Trustees' Report ; Clarification on Medicare Parts B & C
https://en.wikipedia.org/wiki/Medicare_(United_States)
(See hyperlink for full text and references.)

(2) How Original Medicare (Parts A & B) Works
https://www.medicare.gov/what-medicare-covers/your-medicare-coverage-choices/how-original-medicare-works
(See hyperlink for full text and references.)

(3) Medicare Parts A & B = "Original Medicare"
https://www.medicare.gov/your-medicare-costs/part-a-costs
(See hyperlink for full text and references.)

(4) What is Medicare?
https://www.medicareresources.org/basic-medicare-information/what-is-medicare/
(See hyperlink for full text and references.)

(5) Original Medicare (Parts A & B)
https://www.bcbs.com/medicare/original-medicare?utm_medium=sem&utm_campaign=nmac_sem&utm_source=google_ad&gclid=EAIaIQobChMIubiJvbmD8AIVvOy1Ch3TFQ2MEAAYASAAEgK2pfD_BwE
(See hyperlink for full text and references.)

https://www.medicare.gov/what-medicare-covers/what-part-a-covers/how-hospice-works   (See hyperlink for full text and references.)

HOW HOSPICE WORKS

Medicare only covers your hospice care if the hospice provider is Medicare-approved. To find out if a hospice provider is Medicare-approved, ask one of these:

- Your doctor
- The hospice provider
- Your state hospice organization

- Your state health department

Your plan must help you locate a Medicare-approved hospice provider in your area. If you're in a Medicare Advantage Plan (like an HMO or PPO) and want to start hospice care, ask your plan to help find a Medicare-approved hospice provider.

If you qualify for hospice care, you and your family will work with your hospice team to set up a plan of care that meets your needs. You and your family members are the most important part of a team that may also include:

- Doctors
- Nurses or nurse practitioners
- Counselors
- Social workers
- Pharmacists
- Physical and occupational therapists
- Speech-language pathologists
- Hospice aides
- Homemakers
- Volunteers

A hospice doctor is part of your medical team. You can also choose to include your regular doctor or a nurse practitioner on your medical team as the attending medical professional who supervises your care.

In addition, a hospice nurse and doctor are on-call 24 hours a day, 7 days a week, to give you and your family support and care when you need it.

Your hospice benefit covers care for your terminal illness and related conditions. Once your hospice benefit starts, Original Medicare will cover everything you need related to your terminal illness. After your hospice benefit starts, you can still get covered services for conditions not related to your terminal illness.

Original Medicare will pay for covered services for any health problems that aren't part of your terminal illness and related conditions. However, you must pay the deductible and coinsurance amounts for all Medicare-covered services you get to treat health problems that aren't part of your terminal illness and related conditions.

Original Medicare will cover these services even if you choose to remain in a Medicare Advantage Plan or other Medicare health plan.

If you stay in your Medicare Advantage Plan, you can choose to get services not related to your terminal illness from either providers in your plan's network or other Medicare providers.

If you were in a Medicare Advantage Plan when you started hospice, you can stay in that plan by continuing to pay your plan's premiums. If you stop your hospice care, you're still a member of your plan and can get Medicare coverage from your plan after you stop hospice care. Check with your MA plan for their rules related to leaving hospice care - your Medicare Advantage Plan may not start again until the first of the following month.

If you weren't in a Medicare Advantage Plan when you started hospice care, and you decide to stop hospice care, you can continue in Original Medicare. If you're eligible, you can go back to hospice care at any time.

NOTE: If you start hospice care on or after October 1, 2020, you can ask your hospice provider for a list of items, services, and drugs that they've determined aren't related to your terminal illness and related conditions. This list must include why they made that determination. Your hospice provider is also required to give this list to your non-hospice providers or Medicare if requested.

The hospice benefit allows you and your family to stay together in the comfort of your home unless you need care in an inpatient facility. If your hospice team determines that you need inpatient care, they'll make the arrangements for your stay.

If your usual caregiver (like a family member) needs rest, you can get inpatient respite care in a Medicare-approved facility (like a hospice inpatient facility, hospital, or nursing home). Your hospice provider will arrange this for you. You can stay up to 5 days each time you get respite care. You can get respite care more than once, but only on an occasional basis (https://www.medicare.gov/Pubs/pdf/02154-medicare-hospice-benefits.pdf). Charges may apply depending on your plan.

If you need to get inpatient care at a hospital, your hospice provider must make the arrangements. The cost of your inpatient hospital care is covered by your hospice benefit, but paid to your hospice provider. They have a contract with the hospital and they work out the payment between them. However, if you go to the hospital and your hospice provider didn't make the arrangements, you might be responsible for the entire cost of your hospital care.

Hospice care is for people with a life expectancy of 6 months or less (if the illness runs its normal course). If you live longer than 6 months, you can still get hospice care, as long as the hospice medical director or other hospice doctor recertifies that you're terminally ill.

- You can get hospice care for two 90-day benefit periods, followed by an unlimited number of 60-day benefit periods.

- You have the right to change your hospice provider once during each benefit period.

- At the start of the first 90-day benefit period, your hospice doctor and your regular doctor (if you have one) must certify that you're terminally ill (with a life expectancy of 6 months or less). At the start of each benefit period after the first 90-day period, the hospice medical director or other hospice doctor must recertify that you're terminally ill, so you can continue to get hospice care.

NOTE: Only your hospice doctor and your regular doctor (if you have one) can certify that you're terminally ill and have 6 months or less to live. If your health improves or your illness goes into remission, you may no longer need hospice care.

You always have the right to stop hospice care at any time. If you choose to stop hospice care, you'll be asked to sign a form that includes the date your care will end.

You shouldn't be asked to sign any forms about stopping your hospice care at the time you start hospice. Stopping hospice care is a choice only you can make, and you shouldn't sign or date any forms until the actual date that you want your hospice care to stop.

Consider these questions when choosing your hospice care providers:

- Is the hospice provider certified and licensed by the state or federal government?

- Does the hospice provider train caregivers to care for you at home?

- How will your doctor work with the doctor from the hospice provider?

- How many other patients are assigned to each member of the hospice care staff?

- Will the hospice staff meet regularly with you and your family to discuss care?

- How does the hospice staff respond to after-hour emergencies?

- What measures are in place to ensure hospice care quality?

- What services do hospice volunteers offer? Are they trained?

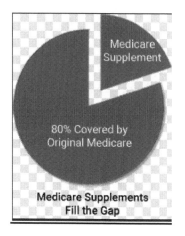

https://www.aarp.org/health/medicare-insurance/info-2017/choosing-right-medigap-plan   (See hyperlink for full text and references.)

Medigap Plans Help Bridge Gap
of Original Medicare Costs
Supplemental insurance will cover some deductibles and copays
by Dena Bunis, AARP, Updated 6 July 2020

If you decide to enroll in Original Medicare, one way you can help pay the extra costs the program doesn't cover is to buy a supplemental — or Medigap — insurance policy.

Medigap policies are sold by private insurers, but they are strictly regulated by states and the federal government. These plans are available for people enrolled in Medicare Parts A and B, not for those who elect a Medicare Advantage plan. Medigap plans pay for costs such as deductibles and copays and other charges that Medicare doesn't cover.

In 2010 the federal government standardized the types of Medigap plans, creating 10 options designated by A, B, C, D, F, G, K, L, M and N. Beginning in January, 2020 two of the more comprehensive and popular plans, C and F, stopped being available to people newly eligible for the program. That's because in 2015, Congress decided to prohibit Medigap from covering the annual deductible for Part B, which pays for doctor visits and other outpatient services.

Of the 10 Medigap plans, C and F currently pay that deductible, which is $198 for 2020. The difference between plans C and F is that C does not cover the 15 percent in excess charges that doctors who don't participate in Medicare are allowed to charge their patients; Plan F does.

Plan G is the closest in design to Plan F. It covers everything F does except the Part B deductible. And Plan D is the closest to Plan C. It covers everything C does except the Part B deductible and the excess charges that nonparticipating doctors are allowed to charge their Medicare patients.

It's been widely reported that Plan F is "going away," says Casey Schwarz, senior counsel for education and federal policy at the Medicare Rights Center. "That shorthand has caused a lot of panic," she says. "I think it's really important to highlight that for people who have been enrolled in Plan C and Plan F, there is absolutely nothing changing."

But if you turned 65 after Jan. 2020 or became disabled after the first of the year and want to buy a Medigap plan you will not be able to enroll in either C or F. Current Medicare enrollees and anyone who was eligible for Medicare before Jan. 1, 2020, still have those plans to choose from.

If you think a Medigap policy might be right for you, here is some basic information you'll need to know to make your decision.

The catch

And it's a big one. When you first enroll in Medicare (that is, during the seven-month initial enrollment period, or "IEP"), insurers offering Medigap policies cannot deny you coverage or charge you more for any preexisting condition. After that, anything goes. For example, if you don't buy a Medigap policy during your IEP but decide a year later that you want one, insurers may be able to turn you down based on your health status, or set prices higher due to a preexisting condition. How that works differs widely from state to state. "What's really important is that people find out what their rights are in their state," Schwarz emphasizes.

The message: To be guaranteed stable, ongoing Medigap coverage for years to come, the time to buy is when you first enroll in Medicare.

The choices

To compare your Medigap plan choices, go to **medicare.gov** and, under the Supplements & Other Insurance tab, click on How to Compare Medigap Policies. Details are there on a single chart.

Don't get confused by the way these policies are named. The letter designations of the Medigap policies have nothing to do with which Medicare program you chose.

Because the Medigap plans are standardized, an A or F plan sold by one insurer covers the same things as an A or F plan sold by another insurer. Medigap plans are consistent in all but three states — Massachusetts, Minnesota and Wisconsin have their own standard policies.

So how do the 10 policies differ? "Some are high deductible, some require higher cost-sharing, and some cover more costs," explains Mary Mealer, life and health manager at the Missouri Department of Insurance, Financial Institutions & Professional Registration. Consumers should "evaluate their individual situation as to what plan meets their needs and what they can afford," she advises.

What to focus on

The government's comparison chart shows 10 health care costs that could be covered by a Medigap policy. Some come into play more than others, so you should focus most on those big-ticket items. They include:

- Your 20 percent share of the cost of doctor visits
- Your 20 percent share of the cost of lab tests and other outpatient services
- The deductible for each time you are admitted to a hospital
- The coinsurance costs of hospital stays or stays in a skilled nursing facility after being in a hospital

There are other considerations, as well. For instance, while other plans cover 100 percent of Part B coinsurance, plans K and L have higher cost-sharing but also an out-of-pocket limit. Once you've paid that amount, they take care of 100 percent of covered services for the rest of the year. In 2020, the limit for the K plan is $5,880, and the limit for the L is $2,940. These limits increase each year, based on inflation.

Remember, Medigap does not cover prescription drugs or dental, vision or most other needs that Original Medicare doesn't cover.

What it will cost you

Nationwide, the average premium for the most popular Medigap F plan costs roughly $326 a month. There is also a high-deductible F plan ($2,340 for 2020), and that premium averages about $68 a month.

Premiums are based on three pricing systems and vary widely based on where you live.

- Community rated: The same monthly premium is charged to everyone who has this policy, regardless of age.
- Issue-age rated: This premium is based on your age when you first buy the policy. The younger you are, the lower the initial premium. Any premium increases in the future will not be based on your age.
- Attained-age rated: This premium is initially based on your current age but can rise as you get older.

Experts suggest that you ask a potential insurer which pricing system it uses before buying a Medigap policy. That way you'll know whether to expect increases as you age.

Additional considerations

Mealer suggests that consumers contact their state's insurance department before signing to make sure the agent and company selling the policy are licensed by the state and to find out that company's complaint record. Each state has a State Health Insurance Assistance Program that can help you find this information.

And remember, changing a Medigap policy can be hard. Give the policy one last read to see if it covers not just your current needs but potential future needs.

Editor's note: This story has been updated to reflect new 2020 rules.

Costs for Medigap

Costs for Medicare Supplement Insurance vary widely. The 2020 Medigap Price Index found that someone turning 65 could pay more than three times more for virtually identical coverage. Among the top ten metro areas, the lowest cost for a male age 65 was $109-per-month available in Dallas. The highest cost was $509-per-month in Philadelphia. (**https://en.wikipedia.org/wiki/Medigap**).

NOTE: Ah, yes! How do the 10 Medigap Supplemental policies differ? "Some are high deductible, some require higher cost-sharing, and some cover more costs". Consumers should "evaluate their individual situation as to what plan meets their needs and what they can afford." "And remember, changing a Medigap policy can be hard."

Every year the government publishes and mails to seniors a 125 page (8" x 11") "Medicare & You" handbook specific to each state. (Interpreters in several languages are available at 800-633-4227.) It addresses the rules, options and complexities of Medicare, Medigap, Medicare Advantage, etc. Tedious, overwhelming - - -

WITH "A CARD IN YOUR WALLET", one would never have to compare plans, decide what their needs are (as in, "do I think I'm going to get cancer like Mom or have a heart attack like Dad – or never need care because I take care of myself and may also be lucky"!) Or try to figure out "what I can afford". **Again we ask President Biden – why does it have to be so complicated?**

https://www.policygenius.com/medicare/medicare-part-c-plans/
(See hyperlink for full text and references.)

What is Medicare Part C?

By Derek Silva, Personal Finance Expert, December 3, 2021
1-855-869-0001 (50 W. 23ʳᵈ St, Flr 9, NY 10010)

Derek is a personal finance editor at Policygenius in New York City, and an expert in taxes. He has been writing about estate planning, investing, and other personal finance topics since 2017. He especially loves using data to tell a story. His work has been covered by Yahoo Finance, MSN, Business Insider, and CNBC.

Also called Medicare Advantage, Medicare Part C is private health insurance offered through Medicare.

Key Takeaways

- Medicare Part C plans are run by private insurance companies and work similarly to other private health insurance plans

- Plans often cover more benefits than traditional Medicare plans, including vision, dental, hearing, and prescription drug coverage

- Plans put an annual cap on out-of-pocket expenses, unlike standard Medicare

- Plans restrict you to a much smaller, local network of available doctors and health care providers

Medicare is a federal health insurance program that primarily serves Americans age 65 and older. It's also available to younger individuals with certain disabilities or health conditions. Medicare consists of multiple parts, which each cover different types of health services.

Medicare Part C, also called Medicare Advantage, is an alternative to traditional Medicare. It provides many of the same benefits but usually has additional coverage. Most Medicare Part C plans come with vision, dental, hearing, and prescription drug coverage, none of which are covered by Original Medicare (Part A and Part B).

People often choose to buy a Medicare Advantage plan because it covers more benefits than Original Medicare. However, that extra coverage comes at a price. For one, you cannot opt out of Original Medicare and so you need to continue paying its premiums on top of any Medicare Part C premiums.

Medicare Advantage is run by private insurance companies, and even though prices may be lower than traditional private health insurance, a lot of the complexities from private plans exist in Medicare Part C.

Medicare Advantage plans (sometimes called MA plans) also require you to use a local network of providers. You cannot sign up unless you live within a certain distance of a plan's network. With Original Medicare coverage, you can go to any health care provider in the country that accepts Medicare.

What is Medicare Part C?

Unlike traditional health insurance plans, Medicare is divided into four parts that each cover different services.

If you're already claiming Social Security benefits, then you will be automatically enrolled in Medicare Part A and Medicare Part B once you turn 65. These two parts are known as Original Medicare. (You can also sign up during several enrollment periods.) This is the traditional Medicare that people commonly talk about and it covers most of the care that people receive, such as hospital care, hospice care, routine doctor's visits, preventive care services, and lab work.

Medicare Part C, commonly called Medicare Advantage, is an alternative to Original Medicare. It provides nearly all the same benefits plus some extra coverage. Most Medicare Part C plans come with vision, dental, hearing and prescription drug coverage, none of which are covered by Original Medicare.

Medicare Part D offers prescription drug coverage that you can opt into if you only have parts A and B.

The Medicare program is run by the Centers for Medicare & Medicaid Services (CMS), a federal agency, but Medicare Advantage plans are run by private insurers. For that reason, Medicare Advantage plans often look similar to traditional health insurance plans. Prices are lower than regular private insurance, but the types of costs and the structure of plans are the same. So if you're interested in Medicare Advantage, it's useful to also brush up on the basics of how health insurance works.

Who is eligible for Medicare Part C?

You can purchase a Medicare Part C plan as long as you have enrolled in Original Medicare. You must also live in a particular Advantage plan's network to buy it.

What does Medicare Part C cover?

The law requires that Medicare Part C cover emergency care and other urgent care. Medicare Advantage plans also cover almost all of the services Original Medicare covers. That includes hospital care and other inpatient care that you can get through Medicare Part A. It also includes the outpatient care, like preventive care and lab services, that you receive from Medicare Part B.

Most Medicare Advantage plans also come with vision, dental, hearing, and prescription drug coverage. Medicare prescription drug plans that are part of Part C are known as Medicare Advantage Prescription Drug (MAPD) plans.

Some Medicare Advantage plans cover additional other services like transportation to doctor visits or adult day care services. Certain plans also tailor their benefits to chronically ill enrollees.

However, all of the benefits and services that go beyond what Original Medicare covers are optional. Insurers do not have to offer them and not all plans include them. Read the benefits information for a specific plan to see exactly what it covers.

No Medicare Advantage plan covers hospice care. However, Original Medicare (specifically Medicare Part A) still covers hospice care even if you primarily use Medicare Advantage.

How much does Medicare Part C cost?

Medicare Advantage prices vary greatly by plan, so how much you pay really depends on your individual plan. There are some particular costs you should pay attention to, though. In particular, let's cover the basics of your monthly premiums, copays, annual deductible, coinsurance, and maximum out-of-pocket limit.

Premiums

You have to enroll in Medicare Parts A and B to buy Medicare Part C, and you will always have to pay the Medicare Part B premium. The

Medicare Part B premium starts at $170.10 per month in 2022, but it may be higher if you earn a higher income.

Beyond that, prices can vary greatly by plan. Medicare Advantage premiums averaged $33 in 2020, according to data from the CMS compiled by Policygenius. At the same time, premiums can reach up to $481. Many Medicare Advantage plans have a $0 premium, but they still charge other costs, like copays.

Getting a plan with a larger network of doctors and hospitals will usually come with higher premiums than plans that offer a smaller, more local network.

Copays

A copay is a flat fee that you pay whenever you receive certain services. For example, a hospital stay for a surgery could come with a copay of $100 per day. If you stay three days, you will end up paying $300 in copays plus other costs the visit incurs.

Deductible

You will need to pay out of pocket for all your health care costs until you hit your deductible. Once you spend enough to hit the deductible, your insurance will begin to cover *some* of your costs.

Deductibles vary greatly by plan but your deductible may also vary within a plan, based on what services you receive. Note that copays typically don't count toward your deductible. Your deductible will also reset each year. So if you don't reach your deductible until December, you will need to start again from zero once January comes around.

Coinsurance

Insurance starts to pay some of your costs after you hit your deductible, but you will still need to pay for a portion of the costs. The percentage of the final bill that you have to pay is your coinsurance. Medicare Advantage coinsurance is typically 20%, but this varies by plan and some plans may not even have coinsurance.

Out-of-pocket limit

Once you spend a certain amount out of pocket each year, your insurance will step in to cover 100% of the remaining costs. The maximum you will ever have to spend out of pocket each year is your out-of-pocket limit or out-of-pocket maximum.

The Medicare program has maximum out-of-pocket limit that varies depending on what services you receive and whether you get them from an in-network or out-of-network health care provider. (We'll explain how your network works in the next section.)

If you have Medicare Part C, for services that Medicare Parts A and B cover, the maximum out-of pocket limit is $7,550 per year in 2021 if you go to in-network care providers. The limit is $11,300 per year for combined in-network and out-of-network costs.

Actual limits vary by plan because insurers can set their own limits, as long as they stay within these maximum legal limits. The average out-of-pocket limit for Medicare Advantage enrollees was $5,059 in 2019, according to the Kaiser Family Foundation.

How do Medicare Part C plans work?

Medicare Advantage plans all offer you care through a network of health care providers. Plans are divided into multiple types based on whether you can use providers outside of your network and how much you would have to pay for doing so. This is the same system that other (non-Medicare) private insurance plans use. Plans may not advertise very clearly what type they are, so make sure to check the plan details for more information.

The table below lays out the major features for each type of Medicare Advantage, and then we go into more detail on each one.

Primary care physician required?
HMO – Yes, in most cases
PPO – No
PFFS – No
SNP – Yes, in most cases
Out-of-network coverage?
HMO – Only in emergencies
PPO – Covered, but at a cost
PFFS – Usually covered, but at a cost
SNP – Sometimes
Referral necessary for specialist visit?
HMO – Yes
PPO – Yes, in most cases

PFFS – No

SNP – Only in emergencies or if you have ESRD (end-stage renal disease)

<u>Prescription Drug Coverage?</u>

HMO – Yes, in most cases

PPO – Yes, in most cases

PFFS – Sometimes

SNP – Yes

Health Maintenance Organization (HMO) Plans

Medicare Advantage HMOs are insurance plans that only cover services within your network of providers. If you go outside of that network, your insurance will not cover any medical expenses you incur. The only exception is for emergency services, which all plans must cover even if you go out of network.

The other major feature of a health maintenance organization is that you are required to select a primary care physician (PCP). Your PCP is the person who all your care goes through. For example, your insurance will not pay for you to see a specialist physician (like an ophthalmologist or surgeon) unless your primary care doctor refers you to that specialist.

One subset of HMO plans to note is an HMO point-of-service plans (HMOPOS). An HMOPOS allows you to get some services out-of-network for a higher copayment or coinsurance.

Preferred Provider Organization (PPO) Plans

A Medicare Advantage PPO offers more flexibility than an HMO because your insurance will usually cover out-of-network providers. It will cost you more than what you would pay if you went in-network, though. PPOs also don't require a primary care physician and they allow you to see a specialist without a referral.

Private Fee-For-Service (PFFS) Plans

A PFFS plan allows you to visit any Medicare-approved health care provider that agrees to treat you. Some PFFS plans have a network, but you can still go to out-of-network providers as long as they agree to treat you. It will cost you more to go out of network.

PFFS plans are appealing for some people because they give you more flexibility on where you receive care. However, providers can choose whether or not to accept your insurance each time you visit. So even if you've been to that provider before, they can opt not to treat you. This means you may actually have a harder time finding someone to treat you, depending on where you live. You should always ask ahead of time to see if a provider will take you as a patient.

In a PFFS plan, the insurer has more control over how much you pay for care. The other types of plans have to stick to prices set by Medicare. In general, PFFS plans have higher out-of-pocket costs than HMOs and PPOs.

Special Needs Plans (SNPs)

SNPs cover people who have specific conditions or characteristics. SNPs target specific types of consumers, and they tailor their plans — benefits, available providers, and list of prescription drugs — to better serve that target consumer. Conditions that SNPs may cover are diabetes, end-stage renal disease (ESRD), HIV/AIDS, chronic heart failure, and dementia.

All SNPs provide prescription drug coverage. Most require you to select a primary care physician, and most also require you to receive a referral if you want to visit a specialist (and have your insurance cover it). Some SNPs cover visits to out-of-network providers, but not all do. Check an individual plan's details.

Medical Savings Account (MSA) Plans

MSAs are a bit different from the types of plans above. An MSA works very similarly to a high-deductible health plan (HDHP) paired with a health savings account (HSA). With an MSA plan, Medicare will deposit money into an account that you can then use to pay for your health care services. Your insurance will not start to pay for your medical expenses until you spend enough to hit your deductible.

Deductibles vary by plan, but can be thousands of dollars. If you spend all of the money in your MSA before reaching your deductible, you will need to pay expenses out of pocket until you hit your deductible. (Though once you hit the deductible, insurance still won't cover 100% of your costs.) Make sure to take the high deductible into account before getting an MSA.

How to apply for Medicare Part C

First, enroll in Original Medicare (Medicare Part A and Medicare Part B). You cannot enroll in Medicare Part C until you do this. If you're on federal retirement benefits (meaning you have paid Medicare tax through your payroll taxes for at least 10 years) you're automatically enrolled in Medicare on the first day of the month you turn 65. You're also automatically enrolled once you've been receiving federal disability payments for 24 months regardless of your age.

If you're 65, but not receiving federal retirement benefits, you have to enroll for Medicare by visiting your local Social Security office, calling 1-800-772-1213, or filling out an online application through the Social Security Administration website at ssa.gov.

Once you're enrolled in Original Medicare, then you can shop for a Medicare Advantage plan. You can search for plans on the Medicare website and purchase the one you want directly from the insurer.

However, you can only enroll within a designated time period each year. New Medicare recipients have seven months to buy coverage, starting three months before the month you turn 65. This is your initial enrollment period. Outside of initial enrollment, these are the times you can purchase or make changes to a Medicare Advantage plan:

- Open Enrollment for Medicare Part C and Medicare Part D, which runs from Oct. 15 to Dec. 7 each year. This is also called the Annual Election Period (AEP).

- Special Enrollment, which follows an event such as moving or the loss of other health coverage. This is known as a Special Election Period (SEP).

- Medicare Advantage Disenrollment Period (MADP), a window from Jan. 1 to Feb. 14 each year where you can drop your Medicare Part C plan and revert back to Original Medicare.

Should I get a Medicare Part C plan?

Enrollment in Medicare Part C plans has been growing, largely because Advantage plans offer more benefits than standard Medicare plans. Medicare Advantage plans usually aren't the best option for low-income recipients because they can often qualify for other Medicare savings programs. Medicare Advantage also isn't generally necessary if you're still receiving employer-sponsored coverage.

Pros of Medicare Part C

- Provides coverage for services Original Medicare does not, like vision or dental

- Usually offers prescription drug coverage

- Caps out-of-pocket expenses, unlike traditional Medicare

Cons of Medicare Part C

- Likely have to pay two premiums, one for Medicare Part B and one for your Advantage Plan

- Many types of individual plans, each with their own rules on the coverage and costs for using out-of-network providers

- Your network of available health care providers is smaller than with Original Medicare plans

- Not all in-network providers are necessarily accepting new patients

- Can't be used in conjunction with employer-sponsored health care benefits that supplement Original Medicare

Policygenius (https://www.policygenius.com/about/): "Policygenius transforms the insurance journey for today's consumer, providing a one-stop platform where customers can compare options from top insurance carriers, get unbiased expert advice, buy policies, and manage their insurance portfolio in one seamless, integrated experience. Our proprietary technology platform integrates with the leading life, disability, and home and auto insurance carriers and delivers an exceptional digital experience for both consumers and insurance carriers. Since 2014, our content, digital tools, and experts have served as a resource for millions of people on their insurance journey, and we have sold more than $140 billion in coverage."

Tips to Find the Best Medicare Advantage Plan for Your Needs
By Rachael Zimlich, RN, BSN ; 7 June 2021

When you're choosing a Medicare Advantage plan, ask yourself:

• **How much did I spend on healthcare last year or the year before?** This may help determine your budget – how much you can afford to spend on premiums and out-of-pocket costs. Some plans do offer $0 premiums and deductibles, but others may charge a few hundred dollars.

• **What prescription drugs do I take or will I need?** If you take medication, you'll need to find an Advantage plan that includes prescription drug coverage or purchase a Part D plan. Be sure to search any plans drug lists (formulary) to confirm your medications are covered.

• **What types of coverage do I need?** Many Advantage plans include extra coverage such as dental, vision, and hearing. You can contact carriers to see what their plans have to offer.

• **What medical conditions do I have, and what are my long-term healthcare needs?** More than 40 percent of Americans have chronic health conditions. You'll also want to consider which plan will suit your long-term medical needs the best.

• **Does my healthcare provider accept Medicare or do they participate in an HMO network?** If keeping your current healthcare provider is important to you, you will need to know what Medicare plans they accept or participate in.

• **What is the CMS rating for the plans I'm considering?** The Centers for Medicare & Medicaid Services (CMS) uses a Five-Star Rating System to measure the quality of care provided by Medicare Advantage and Part D plans. The CMS star rating measures things like management of chronic conditions, availability of care, member experience and complaints, customer service, drug pricing, and more. CMS releases its star ratings every year.

https://eligibility.com/medicare/programs/dual-eligible-definition-qualifications   (See hyperlink for full text and references.)

What Is Medicare Dual Eligible and How Do I Qualify?

By Alex Enabnit, Licensed Insurance Agent and Medicare Expert Writer

Most Americans understand that when they turn 65, Medicare will become their main health insurance plan. However, many Americans are less familiar with another health care program, Medicaid, and what it means if they are eligible for both Medicare and Medicaid. If you are dual eligible, Medicaid may pay for your Medicare out-of-pocket costs and certain medical services that aren't covered by Medicare.

What is Medicaid?

Like Medicare, Medicaid is a health care coverage program funded by the federal government (aka taxpayers). It was established to help low-income individuals access health care coverage. Unlike Medicare, however, Medicaid is partially funded by state governments. This means that states have the flexibility to design their Medicaid programs to best meet the needs of their residents, as long as the program meets the minimum federal guidelines. As a result, Medicaid eligibility, services, and cost-sharing (the amount you pay alongside your insurance policies) will vary state-by-state, while the Medicare program is generally consistent across all states. (Cost sharing is the amount of your health care that you pay out of your own pocket. Typically, this includes deductibles, coinsurance, and copayments.)

Twelve million individuals are currently enrolled in both Medicaid and Medicare. These individuals are known as "dual eligible beneficiaries" because they qualify for both programs. As long as you meet the federal qualifications for Medicare eligibility and the state-specific qualifications for Medicaid eligibility, you will qualify as a dual eligible. To qualify for Medicare, individuals generally need to be 65 or older or have a qualifying disability.

Levels of Medicaid coverage

There are several levels of assistance an individual can receive as a dual eligible beneficiary. The term "full dual eligible" refers to individuals who are enrolled in Medicare and receive full Medicaid benefits. Individuals who receive assistance from Medicaid to pay for Medicare premiums or cost sharing are known as "partial dual eligible."

Full dual eligible coverage

Qualifications for Medicaid vary by state, but, generally, people who qualify for full dual eligible coverage are recipients of Supplemental Security Income (SSI). The SSI program provides cash assistance to people who are aged, blind, or disabled to help them meet basic food and housing needs. To qualify for SSI, you must be under a specified income limit. The maximum income provided by the federal government for SSI in 2020 is $783 per month for an individual and $1,175 per month for a couple. Additionally, your assets must be limited to $2,000 for an individual (or a child) and $3,000 for a couple. Qualifying assets typically include things like checking and savings accounts, stocks, real estate (other than your primary residence), and vehicles if you own more than one.

Partial dual eligible coverage

Individuals who are partial dual eligible typically fall into one of the following four Medicare Savings Program (MSP) categories.

1. **The Qualified Medicare Beneficiary (QMB) Program** helps pay for Medicare Part A and/or Part B monthly premiums, deductibles, coinsurance, and copayments. The monthly income limit is $1,084 for an individual or $1,457 for a couple. The resource limit is $7,860 for an individual or $11,800 for a couple.
2. **The Specified Low Income Medicare Beneficiary (SLMB) Program** helps pay for Medicare Part B premiums. The monthly income limit is $1,296 for an individual or $1,744 for a couple. The resource limit is $7,860 for an individual or $11,800 for a couple.
3. **The Qualifying Individual (QI) Program**, which may also be referred to as Qualified Individual, helps pay for Medicare Part B premiums. The monthly income limit is $1,456 for an individual or $1,960 for a couple. The resource limit is $7,860 for an individual or $11,800 for a couple.
4. **The Qualified Disabled Working Individual (QDWI) Program** pays the Part A premium for certain people who have disabilities and are working. The monthly income limit is $4,339 for an individual or

$5,833 for a couple. The resource limit is $4,000 for an individual or $6,000 for a couple.

Medicaid is known as the "payer of last resort." As a result, any health care services that a dual eligible beneficiary receives are paid first by Medicare, and then by Medicaid. For full dual eligible beneficiaries, Medicaid will cover the cost of care of services that Medicare does not cover or only partially covers (as long as the service is also covered by Medicaid). Such services may include but are not limited to:

- Nursing home care
- Care at an intermediate care facility
- Long-term institutional care
- Home health services
- Personal care services (available in some states)
- Other home and community-based services
- Transportation services
- Dental services (available in some states)
- Eye examinations for prescription glasses (available in some states)

The financial assistance provided to partial dual eligible beneficiaries is outlined in the table above.

People who qualify as dual eligible have several options for how their care is delivered, although the number of available options will vary at the state level.

Original Medicare: Some Medicare beneficiaries may choose to receive their services through the Original Medicare Program. In this case, they receive the Part A and Part B services directly through a plan administered by the federal government, which pays providers on a fee-for-service (FFS) basis. In this case, Medicaid would "wrap around" Medicare coverage by paying for services not covered by Medicare or by covering premium and cost-sharing payments, depending on whether the beneficiary is a full or partial dual eligible.

Medicare Advantage: Medicare Advantage plans are private insurance health plans that provide all Part A and Part B services. Many also offer prescription drug coverage and other supplemental benefits. Similar to how Medicaid works with Original Medicare, Medicaid wraps around the services provided by the Medicare Advantage plan and serves as a payer of last resort.

Medicaid Managed Care: Some states deliver care to the dual eligible population through Medicaid managed care programs. Others have established Medicaid managed care plans specific to the dual eligible population. Medicaid managed care is similar to Medicare Advantage, in that states contract with private insurance health plans to manage and deliver the care. In some states, the Medicaid managed care plan is responsible for coordinating the Medicare and Medicaid services and payments. In other states the payments related to Medicaid and Medicare are handled at the state/federal level, and the Medicaid managed care plan is only responsible for coordinating Medicaid services.

Dual Eligible Special Needs Plans (D-SNP): In some states, dual eligible beneficiaries may have the option of enrolling in a D-SNP, which is different from a traditional SNP or Special Needs Plan. These plans are specially designed to coordinate the care of dual eligible enrollees. Some plans may also be designed to focus on a specific chronic condition, such as chronic heart failure, diabetes, dementia, or End-Stage Renal Disease. These plans often include access to a network of providers who specialize in treating the specified condition. They may also include a prescription drug benefit that is tailored to the condition.

PACE (Programs of All-Inclusive Care for the Elderly): Similar to D-SNPs, PACE plans provide medical and social services to frail and elderly individuals (most of whom are dual eligible). PACE operates through a "health home"-type model, where an interdisciplinary team of health care physicians and other providers work together to provide coordinated care to the patient. PACE plans also focus on helping enrollees receive care in their homes or in the community, with the goal of avoiding placement in nursing homes or other long-term care institutions.

Programs and plans may be limited depending on your state and service area. Additional programs may also be available in some locations. To learn more about which type of plan is right for you, see your state's Medicaid website for contact information.

https://www.medicaidplanningassistance.org/dual-eligibility-medicare-medicaid/ (See hyperlink for full text and references.)

Dual Eligibility for Medicare and Medicaid: Requirements & Benefits for Long Term Care
Last updated: January 28, 2021

Differentiating Medicare and Medicaid

Persons who are eligible for both Medicare and Medicaid are called "dual eligibles", or sometimes, Medicare-Medicaid enrollees. While Medicare is a federal health insurance program for seniors and disabled persons, Medicaid is a state and federal medical assistance program for financially needy persons of all ages. Both programs offer a variety of benefits, including physician visits and hospitalization, but only Medicaid provides long-term nursing home care. Particularly relevant for the purposes of this article, Medicaid also pays for long-term care and supports in home and community based settings, which may include one's home, an adult foster care home, or an assisted living residence. That said, in 2019, Medicare Advantage plans (Medicare Part C) began offering some long-term home and community based benefits.

The Centers for Medicare and Medicaid Services, abbreviated as CMS, oversees both the Medicare and Medicaid programs. For the Medicaid program, CMS works with state agencies to administer the program in each state, and for the Medicare program, the Social Security Administration (SSA) is the agency through which persons apply.

Definition: Dual Eligible

To be considered dually eligible, persons must be enrolled in Medicare Part A, which is hospital insurance, and / or Medicare Part B, which is medical insurance. As an alternative to Original Medicare (Part A and Part B), persons may opt for Medicare Part C, which is also known as Medicare Advantage. (Original Medicare is managed by the federal government, while Medicare Advantage plans are managed by Medicare-approved private insurance companies). Via Medicare Advantage, program participants receive Medicare Part A, Part B, and often Part D, which is prescription drug coverage.

In addition, persons must be enrolled in either full coverage Medicaid or one of Medicaid's Medicare Savings Programs (MSPs): QMB, SLMB,

QI or QDWI.

Full coverage Medicaid covers physician visits, hospital services (in-patient and out-patient), laboratory services, and x-rays. Medicaid also pays for nursing home care, and often limited personal care assistance in one's home.

Benefits of Dual Eligibility

Persons who are enrolled in both Medicaid and Medicare may receive greater healthcare coverage and have lower out-of-pocket costs. Medicaid does cover some expenses that Medicare does not, such as personal care assistance in the home and community and long-term skilled nursing home care (Medicare limits nursing home care to 100 days). The one exception, as mentioned above, is that some Medicare Advantage plans cover the cost of some long term care services and supports. Medicaid, via Medicare Savings Programs, also helps to cover the costs of Medicare premiums, deductibles, and co-payments.

Long-Term Care Benefits

Medicaid provides a wide variety of long-term care benefits and supports to allow persons to age at home or in their community. Medicare does not provide these benefits, but some Medicare Advantage began offering various long term home and community based services in 2019. Benefits for long term care may include the following. This list is not exhaustive, and all benefits may not be available in all states.

- Adult Day Care / Adult Day Health
- Personal Care Assistance (at home, adult foster care homes, and assisted living facilities)
- Medical / Non-Medical Transportation
- Respite Care (to give the primary caregiver a break)
- Congregate Meals / Meal Delivery
- Home Health Aide / Skilled Nursing
- Home Modifications (widening of doorways, installation of ramps, addition of pedestal sinks to allow wheelchair access, etc.)
- Personal Emergency Response Systems
- Housekeeping / Chore Services
- Companion Services
- Transition Services (from nursing home back to home)
- Therapies (physical, occupational, and speech)
- Medication Administration

Both Medicaid and Medicare will provide Durable Medical Equipment, such as wheelchairs and walkers.

Eligibility Requirements for Medicare

Since Medicare is a federal program, eligibility is consistent across the states. Persons must be U.S. Citizens or legal residents residing in the U.S. for a minimum of 5 years immediately preceding application for Medicare. Applicants must also be at least 65 years old. For persons who are disabled or have been diagnosed with end-stage renal disease or Lou Gehrig's disease (amyotrophic lateral sclerosis), there is no age requirement. Eligibility for Medicare is not income based. Therefore, there are no income and asset limits.

Often, persons are not charged a monthly premium to receive Medicare Part A (hospitalization insurance). For premium free coverage, a person (or his or her spouse) must have worked a minimum of 10 years and paid into Medicare. If one has to pay the full monthly premium, it is $471. (This figure and the following Medicare figures are all current for 2021). Some persons who have worked, but have not met the full work requirements, are able to purchase Medicare Part A at a reduced rate of $259/month. The annual Part A in-patient hospitalization deductible is $1,484. After the deductible is met, one must pay a cost share (coinsurance) for services.

For Medicare Part B (medical insurance), enrollees pay a monthly premium of $148.50 in addition to an annual deductible of $203.

In order to enroll in a Medicare Advantage (MA aka "Medicare Part C") plan, one must be enrolled in Medicare Parts A and B. The monthly premium varies by plan, but is approximately $33/month. Not all MA plans charge a monthly premium, but for those that do, the premium is in addition to one's monthly Part A and Part B premiums, if applicable.

For Medicare Advantage plans that offer long-term home and community based services as a supplemental benefit, medical / functional requirements must be met to receive these benefits.

Becoming Medicaid Eligible

Please note that income and assets over the Medicaid limit(s) in one's state is not cause for automatic disqualification. This is because there are Medicaid-compliant planning strategies intended to lower one's countable income and / or assets in order to meet the limit(s). A word of caution: It is vital that assets not be given away a minimum of 5 years (2.5 years in California) prior to the date of one's Medicaid application. (New York is in the process of implementing a 2.5 year look back for long-term home and community based services). This is because Medicaid has a look-back period in which past transfers are reviewed to ensure an applicant (and / or an applicant's spouse) has not gifted assets or sold them under fair market value. If this rule has been violated, it is assumed the assets were transferred in order to meet Medicaid's asset limit and a penalty period of Medicaid disqualification will be calculated.

Note: Eldercare Resource Planning (415.854.8653) offers a comprehensive Medicaid planning package. Their service supports families in making informed choices about how and when they should help a loved one apply for Medicaid benefits.

https://en.wikipedia.org/wiki/Medicare_dual_eligible
(See hyperlink for full text and references.)

Medicare Dual Eligible
From Wikipedia, the free encyclopedia

Dual-eligible beneficiaries (**Medicare dual eligibles or "duals"**) refers to those qualifying for both Medicare and Medicaid benefits. Dual-eligibles make up 14% of Medicaid enrollment, yet they are responsible for approximately 36% of Medicaid expenditures. Similarly, duals total 20% of Medicare enrollment, and spend 31% of Medicare dollars. Dual-eligibles are often in poorer health and require more care compared with other Medicare and Medicaid beneficiaries.

Dual-eligibles may be categorized as full-benefit or partial-benefit. Those with full benefits may receive the entire range of Medicaid benefits; those with partial-benefits do not receive Medicaid-covered services, but Medicaid covers their Medicare premiums or cost-sharing, or both. Partial benefit dual-eligible beneficiaries have limited income and assets, but their income and assets are not low enough to qualify them for full Medicaid benefits in their state.

Dual-eligibles typically receive their Medicare and Medicaid benefits through each program separately. For Medicare benefits, beneficiaries may opt to enroll in Medicare's traditional fee-for-service (FFS) program or in a private Medicare Advantage (MA) plan (Medicare Part C), which is administered by a Managed Care Organization (MCO), under contract with the Centers for Medicare & Medicaid Services (CMS), the agency in the Department of Health and Human Services that administers the Medicare program and oversees state Medicaid programs. In addition, dual-eligibles may choose a type of MA plan called a dual-eligible special needs plan (D-SNP), which is designed to target the needs of this population.

Recently, Congress and CMS have placed greater emphasis on the coordination and integration of Medicare and Medicaid benefits for dual-eligible beneficiaries. Historically, one of the major challenges for the dually-eligible has been care coordination between Medicare and Medicaid. These two systems of care do not "talk to each other" systematically, so one physician that bills primarily through Medicare may not be familiar with benefits that are available through Medicaid. Additionally, since Medicaid benefits vary by state, it is difficult for care providers and consumers to understand the complexity that is inherent within the Medicaid system.

Because duals tend to be the most vulnerable, and often sickest, adults, their care has historically been expensive, totaling $319.5 billion in 2011. One proposed reason for this significant cost would be that many Medicaid programs, prior to the 2010 passage of the Affordable Care Act (ACA) used a fee-for-service model. Fee-for-service models are typically more costly because they allow providers to charge for the quantity of care they provide, rather than the quality.

In order to resolve these pain points, the ACA includes provisions that specifically address the coverage and care of duals. On a federal level, the Centers for Medicare and Medicaid Services (CMS) has established two new offices: The Federal Coordinated Health Care Office (FCHCO aka the "duals office") as well as the Center for Medicare and Medicaid Innovation (CMMI) in order to both strategize and monitor the type and quality of care afforded to duals. These offices focus on both monetary expenses as well as care innovation and quality for dual eligible beneficiaries.

MEDICARE SPECIAL NEEDS PLANS (SNPs)

SOURCES (See hyperlinks for full text and references.):

1. https://en.wikipedia.org/wiki/Special_needs_plan
2. https://www.cms.gov/Medicare/Health-Plans/SpecialNeedsPlans
3. https://www.medicare.gov/sign-up-change-plans/types-of-medicare-health-plans/special-needs-plans-snp
4. https://www.medicare.gov/sign-up-change-plans/types-of-medicare-health-plans/how-medicare-special-needs-plans-snps-work

A **Medicare Special Needs Plan** (or SNP, often pronounced "snip") is a Medicare Advantage (MA) Coordinated Care Plan (CCP) specifically designed to provide targeted care and limit enrollment to people with specific diseases or characteristics. Medicare SNPs tailor their benefits, provider choices, and drug formularies to best meet the specific needs of the groups they serve.

One type is the "exclusive SNP", which enrolls only those beneficiaries who fall into the special needs demographic. The other type is the "disproportionate share SNP", which enroll a greater percentage of the target special needs population as compared to a national percentage of the target population.

A special needs individual could be any one of the following:

1. An individual with a severe or disabling chronic condition, as specified by CMS,

2. People who live in certain institutions (like a nursing home) or who require nursing care at home, or

3. People who are eligible for both Medicare and Medicaid ("dual eligible").

A SNP may be any type of Medicare Advantage CCP, including either a local or a regional preferred provider organization (i.e., LPPO or RPPO) plan, a health maintenance organization (HMO) plan, or an HMO Point-of-Service (HMO-POS) plan.

SNPs are expected to follow existing MA program rules, including MA regulations at 42 CFR 422, as modified by guidance, with regard to Medicare-covered services and Prescription Drug Benefit program rules. All SNPs must provide Part D prescription drug coverage because special needs individuals must have access to prescription drugs to manage and control their special health care needs. SNPs should assume that, if no modification is contained in guidance, existing Part C and D rules apply.

The Medicare Modernization Act of 2003 (MMA) established an MA CCP specifically designed to provide targeted care to individuals with special needs. Congress identified "special needs individuals" as people in one of these groups, or a subset of one of these groups:

1. **Chronic Condition SNP (C-SNP):** Beneficiaries with chronic conditions, defined as individuals who have acquired one or more of 15 severe or disabling chronic conditions, including, but not limited to: cardiovascular disease, diabetes, congestive heart failure, osteoarthritis, mental disorders, ESRD, and HIV/AIDS.

2. **Institutional SNP (I-SNP):** Institutionalized beneficiaries, defined as those who reside or are expected to reside for 90 days or longer in a long term care facility (defined as either: skilled nursing facility (SNF)/NF, ICF or inpatient psychiatric facility), or those living in the community but requiring an equivalent level of care to those residing in a long term care facility.

3. **Dual Eligible SNP (D-SNP):** Dually eligible beneficiaries, defined as individuals who are entitled to Medicare Part A and/or Part B and are eligible for some form of Medicaid benefit.

CMS solicited public comments on chronic conditions meeting the clarified definition and convened the SNP Chronic Condition Panel in the fall of 2008. Panelists included six clinical experts on chronic condition management from three federal agencies — the Agency for Healthcare Research and Quality (AHRQ), the Centers for Disease Control and Prevention (CDC), and CMS.

After discussing public comments on a proposed list of SNP-specific chronic conditions, the panelists recommended, and CMS subsequently approved, the following 15 C-SNP-specific chronic conditions:

1. Chronic alcohol and other drug dependence
2. Autoimmune disorders limited to:
   - Polyarteritis nodosa
   - Polymyalgia rheumatic

- Polymyositis
- Rheumatoid arthritis
- Systemic lupus erythematosus
3. Cancer, excluding pre-cancer conditions or in-situ status
4. Cardiovascular disorders limited to:
   - Cardiac arrhythmias
   - Coronary artery disease
   - Peripheral vascular disease
   - Chronic Venous thromboemolic disorder
5. Chronic heart failure
6. Dementia
7. Diabetes mellitus
8. End-stage liver disease
9. End-stage renal disease (ESRD) requiring dialysis
10. Severe hematologic disorders limited to:
    - Apastic anemia
    - Hemophilia
    - Immune thrombocytopenic pupura
    - Myelodysplatic syndrome
    - Sickle-cell disease (excluding sickle-cell trait)
11. HIV/AIDS
12. Chronic lung disorders limited to:
    - Asthma
    - Chronic bronchitis
    - Emphysema
    - Pulmonary fibrosis
    - Pulmonary hypertension
13. Chronic and disabling mental health conditions limited to:
    - Bipolar disorders
    - Major depressive disorders
    - Paranoid disorder
    - Schizophrenia
    - Schizoaffective disorder
14. Neurological disorders limited to:
    - Amyotrophic lateral sclerosis (ALS)
    - Epilepsy
    - Extensive paralysis (i.e. hemiplegia, quadriplegia, paraplegia, monoplegia)
    - Huntingdon's disease
    - Multiple sclerosis

- Parkinson's disease
- Polyneuropathy
- Spinal stenosis
- Stroke-related neurologic deficit

15. Stroke

In most cases, SNPs may require you to have a primary care doctor. Or, the plan may require you to have a care coordinator to help with your health care. Generally, you must get your care and services from doctors or hospitals in the Medicare SNP network, except:

- Emergency or urgent care, like care you get for a sudden illness or injury that needs medical care right away

- If you have End-Stage Renal Disease (ESRD) and need out-of-area dialysis

Medicare SNPs typically have specialists in the diseases or conditions that affect their members. In most cases, you have to get a referral to see a specialist in SNPs. Certain services don't require a referral, like these:

- Yearly screening mammograms

- An in-network pap test and pelvic exam (covered at least every other year)

Plans should coordinate the services and providers you need to help you stay healthy and follow doctor's or other health care provider's orders.

If you have Medicare and Medicaid , your plan should make sure that all of the plan doctors or other health care providers you use accept Medicaid.

If you live in an institution, make sure that plan providers serve people where you live.

Where are Medicare SNPs offered?

Each year, different types of Medicare SNPs may be available in different parts of the country. Insurance companies decide where they'll do business, so Medicare SNPs may not be available in all parts of the country.

Insurance companies can decide that a plan will be available to everyone with Medicare in a state, or only in certain counties. Insurance companies may also offer more than one plan in an area, with different benefits and costs. Each year, insurance companies offering Medicare SNPs can decide to join or leave Medicare.

What do I pay in a Medicare SNP?

If you have Medicare and Medicaid, most of the costs of joining a Medicare SNP will be covered for you. Contact your Medicaid office for more information and to see if you qualify for Medicaid benefits. If you qualify, you can join a Medicare SNP at any time.

If you don't have both Medicare and Medicaid (or get other help from your state paying your Medicare premiums), your exact costs will vary depending on the plan you choose. In general, you'll pay the basic costs of having a Medicare Advantage plan.

What benefits and services are covered in Medicare SNPs?

Medicare SNPs cover the same Medicare services that all Medicare Advantage plans must cover. Medicare SNPs may also cover extra services tailored to the special groups they serve, like extra days in the hospital.

For example, a Medicare SNP may be designed to serve only people diagnosed with congestive heart failure. The plan might include access to a network of providers who specialize in treating congestive heart failure. It would also feature clinical case management programs designed to serve the special needs of people with this condition. The plan's drug formulary would be designed to cover the drugs usually used to treat congestive heart failure. People who join this plan would get benefits specially tailored to their condition, and have all their care coordinated through the Medicare SNP.

Contact your plan to learn exactly what benefits and services the plan covers.

What is a care coordinator in a Medicare SNP?

Some Medicare SNPs use a care coordinator to help you stay healthy and follow your doctor's orders. A care coordinator is someone who helps make sure people get the right care and information.

For example, a Medicare SNP for people with diabetes might use a care coordinator to help members do these things:

- Monitor their blood sugar
- Follow their diet
- Get proper exercise
- Schedule preventive services (like eye and foot exams)
- Get the right prescriptions to prevent complications

A Medicare SNP for people with both Medicare and Medicaid might use a care coordinator to help members access community resources and coordinate their different Medicare and Medicaid services.

When can/must I leave a Medicare SNP?

You can stay enrolled in a Medicare SNP only if you continue to meet the special conditions served by the plan.

Example: Mr. Johnson joined a Medicare SNP that only serves members with both Medicare and Medicaid. Mr. Johnson loses his Medicaid eligibility. Medicare requires Mr. Johnson's plan to disenroll him unless he becomes eligible for Medicaid again within the plan's grace period.

The grace period is at least one month long, but plans can choose to have a longer grace period. If you lose eligibility for the plan, you'll have a Special Enrollment Period to make another choice.

This Special Enrollment Period starts when your Medicare SNP notifies you that you're no longer eligible for the plan. It continues during the plan's grace period, and if you're disenrolled from the plan at the end of the grace period, it continues for 2 months after your coverage ends. It's very important to review your coverage options at this time to make sure you continue to have the Medicare health and prescription drug coverage you want.

https://www.cms.gov/Medicare/Health-Plans/SpecialNeedsPlans/I-SNPs

Institutional Special Needs Plans (I-SNPs)

Institutional Special Needs Plans (I-SNPs) are SNPs that restrict enrollment to MA eligible individuals who, for 90 days or longer, have had or are expected to need the level of services provided in a long-term care (LTC) skilled nursing facility (SNF), a LTC nursing facility (NF), a SNF/NF, an intermediate care facility for individuals with intellectual disabilities (ICF/IDD), or an inpatient psychiatric facility. A complete list of acceptable types of institutions can be found in the Medicare Advantage Enrollment and Disenrollment Guidance.

CMS may allow an I-SNP that operates either single or multiple facilities to establish a county-based service area as long as it has at least one long-term care facility that can accept enrollment and is accessible to the county residents. As with all MA plans, CMS will monitor the plan's marketing/enrollment practices and long-term care facility contracts to confirm that there is no discriminatory impact.

Institutional Equivalent SNPs

For an I-SNP to enroll MA eligible individuals living in the community, but requiring an institutional level of care (LOC), the following two conditions must be met:

1. A determination of institutional LOC that is based on the use of a state assessment tool. The assessment tool used for persons living in the community must be the same as that used for individuals residing in an institution. In states and territories without a specific tool, I-SNPs must use the same LOC determination methodology used in the respective state or territory in which the I-SNP is authorized to enroll eligible individuals.

2. The I-SNP must arrange to have the LOC assessment administered by an independent, impartial party (i.e., an entity other than the respective I-SNP) with the requisite professional knowledge to identify accurately the institutional LOC needs. Importantly, the I-SNP cannot own or control the entity.

Change of Residence Requirement for I-SNPs

If an I-SNP enrollee changes residence, the I-SNP must document that it is prepared to implement a CMS-approved MOC (Model of Care) at the enrollee's new residence, or in another I-SNP contracted LTC (long-term care) setting that provides an institutional level of care.

https://www.macpac.gov/subtopic/medicare-advantage-dual-eligible-special-needs-plans-aligned-with-medicaid-managed-long-term-services-and-supports/

Medicare Advantage Dual Eligible Special Needs Plans

MACPAC, 1800 M Street NW, Suite 650 South, Washington, DC 20036 (202.350.2000 ; https://www.macpac.gov/about-macpac/)

The Medicaid and CHIP Payment and Access Commission is a non-partisan legislative branch agency that provides policy and data analysis and makes recommendations to Congress, the Secretary of the U.S. Department of Health and Human Services, and the states on a wide array of issues affecting Medicaid and the State Children's Health Insurance Program (CHIP). The U.S. Comptroller General appoints MACPAC's 17 commissioners, who come from diverse regions across the United States and bring broad expertise and a wide range of perspectives in Medicaid and CHIP.

Dual eligible special needs plans (D-SNPs) are a type of Medicare Advantage plan designed to meet the specific needs of dually eligible beneficiaries. As of February 2021, D-SNPs were operating in 43 states and the District of Columbia with about 3 million dually eligible beneficiaries enrolled.

D-SNPs are required to contract with states but states are not required to contract with D-SNPs. The contracts must cover eight minimum MIPPA (Medicare Improvement for Patients and Providers Act) requirements, including:

- the Medicare Advantage organization's responsibilities — including financial obligations — to provide or arrange for Medicaid benefits;

- categories of eligibility for dually eligible beneficiaries to be enrolled under the D-SNP, including the targeting of specific subsets;

- Medicaid benefits covered under the D-SNP;

- cost-sharing protections covered under the D-SNP;

- information about Medicaid provider participation and how that information is to be shared;

- verification process of an enrollee's eligibility for both Medicare and Medicaid;

- service area covered under the SNP; and

- period of the contract.

States have authority under their MIPPA contract to add additional requirements for D-SNPs that further integrate care. Some states have maximized their MIPPA authority and are providing fully integrated care through D-SNPs.

FIDE SNP - Fully integrated dual eligible special needs plan. FIDE SNPs fully integrate care for dually eligible beneficiaries under a single managed care organization.

HIDE SNP - Highly integrated dual eligible special needs plan. HIDE SNPs have a higher level of integration than typical D-SNPs.

MLTSS - D-SNP affiliated with Managed Long-Term Services and Supports. States may integrate care for dually eligible beneficiaries enrolled in their MLTSS programs with D-SNPs.

https://www.state.nj.us/humanservices/dmahs/clients/d_snp.html

New Jersey Dual Eligible Special Needs Plan: Consumer and Provider Information
(Here is NJ's program as an example.)

New Jersey residents who have both Medicare and Medicaid, known as "Dual Eligibles," can enroll in a Dual Eligible Special Needs Plan (D-SNP, pronounced "dee-snip"). A D-SNP is a special kind of Medicare managed care plan that coordinates all covered Medicare and Medicaid managed care benefits in one health plan.

If you or a trusted family member or doctor heard about D-SNP health plans and would like to know more about them, please use this web page as a guide to get started. A free Guide about Special Needs Plans is available from Medicare, too.

Dual Special Needs Plan Features:
- A team of doctors, specialists, and care managers working together for you
- No co-payments, premiums or deductibles
- One health plan to coordinate all your Medicare and Medicaid managed care benefits

- All the same member rights available to Medicare and Medicaid recipients
- Extra Medicare benefits not available under other Medicare or Medicaid plans
- D-SNPs may require referrals before you make an appointment to see specialists

Coverage

Most D-SNP covered services are covered by Medicare, and a few are covered exclusively by Medicaid, including dental, vision, hearing aids and fittings, certain private duty nursing services, medical day care, personal care assistance, and long-term nursing facility stays.

Generally, when Medicaid covers health care services beyond the limits of Medicare, then Medicaid will pay for what Medicare does not.

https://bmchealthservres.biomedcentral.com/articles/10.1186/s12913-021-06228-3 (See hyperlink for full text and references.) Cite this article: https://bmchealthservres.biomedcentral.com/articles/10.1186/s12913-021-06228-3#citeas

The Impact of Dual Eligible Special Need Plan Regulations on Healthcare Utilization

BMC Health Services Research volume 21, Article number: 206 (2021)

Authors: Kimberly Danae Cauley-Narain, Jessica Harwood, Carol Mangione, O. Kenrik Duru & Susan Ettner

More than 3 million individuals referred to as dual-eligible beneficiaries receive both Medicare and Medicaid health insurance benefits as a consequence of low income and assets in conjunction with age ≥ 65 years or disability. Relative to Medicare-only beneficiaries, dual-eligible beneficiaries have a higher chronic disease burden, more functional impairments and more behavioral health conditions. Consequently, dual-eligible beneficiaries have higher levels of healthcare utilization than Medicare-only beneficiaries and account for a disproportionate share of both Medicare and Medicaid program spending. In 2013 dual-eligible beneficiaries were only 20% of the Medicare population but accounted for 34% of total program spending. Similarly, they made up 15% of Medicaid enrollment but generated 32% of total program costs.

While differences in need partially explain the higher health care utilization and costs among dual-eligible beneficiaries relative to Medicare-only beneficiaries, care fragmentation has also been shown to play a role. A high level of care fragmentation stems from receiving health care through both Medicare and Medicaid, separate programs with distinct funding streams, eligibility criteria, administrative processes, medical providers, covered services and accountability mechanisms.

Specifically, Medicare is a purely federal program which covers most acute care services such as inpatient and outpatient care, physician services, diagnostic and preventive care and since 2006, prescription medications. Medicaid, which covers Medicare premiums, patient cost-sharing requirements, and long-term services and supports such as home health and nursing home care, is operated by states with federal oversight and paid for with a mix of federal and state funding.

Medicaid and Medicare have traditionally had little incentive to coordinate care for dual-eligible beneficiaries. For example, Medicare has had little incentive to keep dual-eligible beneficiaries out of nursing homes since the costs would be borne primarily by states. Likewise, states have had little incentive to reduce hospitalizations among dual-eligible beneficiaries because hospitalization costs would be mainly absorbed by Medicare.

In 2003, the Medicare Modernization Act authorized Dual-Eligible Special Needs Plans (D-SNPs), managed care plans offered by private insurers and targeted specifically to dual-eligible beneficiaries, with the goal of aligning financial incentives across Medicare and Medicaid to promote care coordination and reduce costs. Insurers offering D-SNPs are paid a fixed monthly amount per person (capitated payment) by Medicare to provide the full range of Medicare services and coordinate Medicaid services among dual-eligible beneficiaries. D-SNPs are at financial risk for Medicare costs in excess of the capitated payment but they are permitted to retain a portion of the Medicare payment not spent on covered services for contractually mandated activities. When D-SNPs were initially authorized, there was no requirement to provide Medicaid benefits to beneficiaries and no specific Model of Care requirements (MOC). Consequently, the majority of D-SNPs did not have any formal relationship with state Medicaid agencies and did not provide a coordinated Medicare-Medicaid product.

In 2017, 2,060,218 dual-eligible beneficiaries were enrolled in D-SNPs.

Since the original authorization of D-SNPs, Congress has passed additional legislation with the aim of increasing quality of care, improving health outcomes and reducing healthcare costs among dual-eligible beneficiaries enrolled in D-SNPs. The Medicare Improvement Act for Patients and Providers (MIPPA) of 2008, as amended by the Patient Protection and Affordable Care Act (PP-ACA) of 2010, required all D-SNPs to have a contract with states in which they operated and specified minimum requirements for these contracts. The PP-ACA mandated that as of 2012, any new D-SNP would have to either provide Medicaid benefits in their capitated benefit package or arrange for Medicaid benefits to be provided through either a Medicaid Managed Care (MMC) plan or Medicaid FFS, depending on the requirements of the state.

Evidence has also shown that racial/ethnic minority beneficiaries, which constitute a disproportionate share of dual-eligible beneficiaries, are often enrolled in lower-performing managed care plans relative to non-minority beneficiaries. Consequently, augmented D-SNP care coordination and MOC requirements may have stronger beneficial effects on health outcomes among racial/ethnic minorities who experience significant health disparities.

Our finding of stronger D-SNP regulation effects on hospital utilization with increasing co-morbidity is particularly important because studies suggest that individuals with higher levels of co-morbidity are less likely to enroll in managed care plans and are more likely to leave these plans even in states with seamless conversion. Consequently, D-SNPs may be limited in the hospital utilization and healthcare costs reductions they can achieve. One study found that concerns about service restrictions and loss of access to trusted providers may be important drivers of enrollment decisions. Furthermore, implementing a pro-active strategy to retain this population once they have been enrolled will be important.

https://www.uhccommunityplan.com/dual-eligible/benefits/healthy-food-benefit   (See hyperlink for full text and references.)

A DUAL HEALTH PLAN COULD HELP YOU BUY HEALTHY FOOD AT NO COST
Last Updated Date: April 02, 2021

Good food is important for good health. But eating healthy can be hard on a limited budget. Knowing this, UnitedHealthcare created a new health benefit called "healthy food." Like the name says, the healthy food benefit helps people buy healthy food. It's included with most UnitedHealthcare Dual Health Plans for 2021.

Dual Health Plans are for people who qualify for both Medicaid and Medicare. Healthy food is one of many extra dual benefits you could get with a Dual Health Plan. See all the other benefits Dual Health Plans may offer.

The healthy food benefit is like having free food credit. It helps members make their food dollars go farther.

The healthy food benefit helps Dual Health Plan members stretch their monthly food budget. On the first day of every month, eligible members get a set amount of credits loaded onto a prepaid debit card. They shop for groceries, then use their debit card to pay. Any qualifying purchases are automatically taken off the total by using credits. There's no cost to members. So it really is like having free food credit.

Some Dual Health Plans give members as much as $60 monthly. Just think of it as being like free food credit. Then you can see how the healthy food benefit can help people with low income make their food dollars go farther.

https://populationhealth.humana.com/food-card-added-for-70000-members/   (See hyperlink for full text and references.)

Protected: Healthy Foods Access Made Easier with Food Benefit Card

Because food insecurity results in higher rates of chronic conditions, leading to increased medical costs and a reduced sense of overall well-being, Humana offered a Healthy Food Card Benefit with some 2020

Medicare Advantage plans in several states.

The benefit, for qualifying members with Dual-Eligible Special Needs Plans (DSNPs), can be used to purchase healthy groceries and comes in the form of a wallet card that is loaded with a cash benefit each month, either $25 or $50, depending on need and plan. The card can be used at various national retailers.

As the food card is a new benefit in 2020, we have many members just using it for the first time. Humana MarketPoint sales representative Lisa Ruskanen said one of her clients with the benefit is vision impaired and relies on public transportation or a caregiver to run errands.

"He's called me more than once this year saying that his caregiver tried to use the card but wasn't able to use it," she said. "He's always been very nice about it and explains he's not upset with me, but if this is a benefit in the plan and he's not able to use it, it's frustrating.

"I took advantage of the extra time we have during work at home/shelter in place and told him to make me a list and I would pick up the card and go shopping for him. I went to the store he normally goes to and purchased eggs, a gallon of milk, flour, butter, hot cereal, cheddar cheese, cranberry juice, and diet soda. The cashier ran the items through and then had me swipe the card. Everything worked exactly the way it was supposed to!"

Lisa said when she brought the items back to the member, he was happy to get those them and now has confidence to continue using it and to reach out to her if he encounters issues.

Humana understands the importance of healthy food to overall health. That's why we created the Healthy Foods Card to give members on eligible Dual-Eligible Special Needs Plans (DSNPs) a monthly $25 or $50 allowance to use towards groceries.

The Humana Healthy Foods Card helps members, who have this benefit as part of their Humana plan, to extend monthly food resources when financial barriers can otherwise limit access to an adequate food supply. The card will be offered with $25 or $50 allowance amounts per month.

NOTE: While more than 31 million people in the USA lacked health insurance in 2020, private health insurance companies were using some of their taxpayer revenues to provide monthly food allowances to certain "Medicare Advantage" beneficiaries. Why not "SNAP", that "helps low-income people buy nutritious food" (ssa.gov/pubs/EN-05-10101.pdf)?

An Overview of the Medicare Part D Prescription Drug Benefit
Published: Oct 14, 2020

Medicare Part D is a voluntary outpatient prescription drug benefit for people with Medicare, provided through private plans approved by the federal government. Beneficiaries can choose to enroll in either a stand-alone prescription drug plan (PDP) to supplement traditional Medicare A/B or a Medicare Advantage prescription drug plan (MA-PD), mainly HMOs and PPOs, that cover all Medicare benefits including drugs. In 2020, 46 million of the more than 60 million people covered by Medicare are enrolled in Part D plans. This fact sheet provides an overview of the Medicare Part D program, plan availability, enrollment, and spending and financing, based on data from the Centers for Medicare & Medicaid Services (CMS), the Congressional Budget Office (CBO), and other sources.

Beneficiaries with low incomes and modest assets are eligible for assistance with Part D plan premiums and cost sharing. Through the Part D Low-Income Subsidy (LIS) program, additional premium and cost-sharing assistance is available for Part D enrollees with low incomes (less than 150% of poverty, or $19,140 for individuals/$25,860 for married couples in 2020) and modest assets (less than $14,610 for individuals/$29,160 for couples in 2020). An estimated 13 million Part D enrollees received the Low-Income Subsidy in 2020.

The Part D defined standard benefit has several phases, including a deductible, an initial coverage phase, a coverage gap phase, and catastrophic coverage.

- The standard deductible is increasing from $435 in 2020 to $445 in 2021

- The initial coverage limit is increasing from $4,020 to $4,130, and

- The out-of-pocket spending threshold is increasing from \$6,350 to \$6,550 (equivalent to \$10,048 in total drug spending in 2021, up from \$9,719 in 2020).

For costs in the coverage gap phase, beneficiaries pay 25% for both brand-name and generic drugs, with manufacturers providing a 70% discount on brands and plans paying the remaining 5% of brand drug costs, and plans paying the remaining 75% of generic drug costs. For total drug costs above the catastrophic threshold, Medicare pays 80%, plans pay 15%, and enrollees pay either 5% of total drug costs or \$3.70/\$9.20 for each generic and brand-name drug, respectively.

Part D plans must offer either the defined standard benefit or an alternative equal in value ("actuarially equivalent") and can also provide enhanced benefits. Both basic and enhanced benefit plans vary in terms of their specific benefit design, coverage, and costs, including deductibles, cost-sharing amounts, utilization management tools (i.e., prior authorization, quantity limits, and step therapy), and formularies (i.e., covered drugs).

Plan formularies must include drug classes covering all disease states, and a minimum of two chemically distinct drugs in each class. Part D plans are required to cover all drugs in six so-called "protected" classes: immunosuppressants, antidepressants, antipsychotics, anticonvulsants, antiretrovirals, and antineoplastics.

In 2020, 46.5 million Medicare beneficiaries are enrolled in Medicare Part D plans, including employer-only group plans; of the total, just over half (53%) are enrolled in stand-alone PDPs and nearly half (47%) are enrolled in Medicare Advantage drug plans (Figure 4). Another 1.3 million beneficiaries are estimated to have drug coverage through employer-sponsored retiree plans where the employer receives a subsidy from the federal government equal to 28% of drug expenses between \$445 and \$9,200 per retiree (in 2021). Several million beneficiaries are estimated to have other sources of drug coverage, including employer plans for active workers, FEHBP, TRICARE, and Veterans Affairs (VA). Another 12% of people with Medicare are estimated to lack creditable drug coverage.

Financing for Part D comes from general revenues (71%), beneficiary premiums (16%), and state contributions (12%). The monthly premium paid by enrollees is set to cover 25.5% of the cost of standard drug coverage. Medicare subsidizes the remaining 74.5%, based on bids submitted by plans for their expected benefit payments. Higher-income Part D enrollees pay a larger share of standard Part D costs, ranging from 35% to 85%, depending on income.

In light of ongoing attention to prescription drug spending and rising drug costs, policymakers have issued several proposals to control drug spending by Medicare and beneficiaries.

Understanding how well Part D continues to meet the needs of people on Medicare will be informed by ongoing monitoring of the Part D plan marketplace, examining formulary coverage and costs for new and existing medications, assessing the impact of the new insulin model, and keeping tabs on Medicare beneficiaries' out-of-pocket drug spending.

https://en.wikipedia.org/wiki/Medicare_Part_D
(See hyperlink for full text and references.)

Medicare Part D
From Wikipedia, the free encyclopedia

Medicare Part D, also called the Medicare prescription drug benefit, is an optional U.S. federal-government program to help Medicare beneficiaries pay for self-administered prescription drugs through prescription drug insurance premiums (the cost of almost all professionally administered prescriptions is covered under optional Part B of United States Medicare).

Part D was originally proposed by President Bill Clinton in 1999, then by both political parties and Houses of Congress and President Bush during 2002 and 2003. The final bill was enacted as part of the Medicare Modernization Act of 2003 and went into effect on January 1, 2006.

The various proposals were substantially alike in that Part D was optional, it was separated from the other three Parts of Medicare in most proposals, and it used private pharmacy benefit managers on a regional basis to negotiate drug prices.

The differences included consistent benefits nationwide in the Clinton/Democratic proposals (as opposed to multiple options in the

Republican plans and the bill finally enacted) and a wide array of deductibles and co-pays (including the infamous "donut hole").

Eligibility and Enrollment

Individuals on Medicare are eligible for prescription drug coverage under a Part D plan if they are signed up for benefits under Medicare Part A and/or Part B.

Beneficiaries obtain the Part D drug benefit through two types of plans administered by private insurance companies or other types of sponsors:

- the beneficiaries can join a standalone Prescription Drug Plan (PDP) for drug coverage only

- or they can join a public Part C health plan that jointly covers all hospital and medical services covered by Medicare Part A and Part B at a minimum, and typically covers additional healthcare costs not covered by Medicare Parts A and B including prescription drugs (MA-PD). (NOTE: Medicare beneficiaries need to be signed up for both Parts A and B to select Part C whereas they need only A or B to select Part D.)

About two-thirds of all Medicare beneficiaries are enrolled directly in Part D or get Part-D-like benefits through a public Part C Medicare Advantage health plan. Another large group of Medicare beneficiaries get prescription drug coverage under plans offered by former employers or through the Veterans Administration. It is also possible that a former employer or union might sponsor a Part D plan for former employees/members (such plans are called Employer Group Waiver Plans).

Medicare beneficiaries can enroll directly through the plan's sponsor, or indirectly via an insurance broker or the exchange — called Medicare Plan Finder — run by the Centers for Medicare and Medicaid Services (CMS) for this purpose. The beneficiary's benefits and any additional assistance payments and rights are the same regardless of enrollment channel.

Beneficiaries already on a plan can choose a different plan or drop Part C/D during the annual enrollment period or during other times during the year under special circumstances. For some time, the annual enrollment period has lasted from October 15 to December 7 of each year but that is changing for Part C in 2019. In particular, low-income seniors on Social Security Extra Help/LIS and many middle-income seniors on state pharmaceutical assistance programs can choose a different plan or drop Part C/D more often than once a year.

Medicare beneficiaries who were eligible for but did not enroll in a Part D when they were first eligible and later want to enroll pay a late-enrollment penalty, basically a premium surtax, if they did not have acceptable coverage through another source such as an employer or the U.S. Veterans Administration. This penalty is equal to 1% of the national premium index times the number of full calendar months that they were eligible for but not enrolled in Part D and did not have creditable coverage through another source. The penalty raises the premium of Part D for beneficiaries, when and if they elect coverage.

In May 2018, enrollment exceeded 44 million, including both those on standalone Part D and those enrolled in a Part C plan that includes Part-D-like coverage. About 20% of those beneficiaries are on an EGWP drug plan where a former employer receives a Part D subsidy on his or her behalf. The latter two groups lack the same freedom of choice that the standalone Part D group has because they must use the Part D plan chosen by the Part C plan's sponsor or their former employer.

Plans Offered

All Medicare Part D plans are provided by private companies. As of May 2018, over 700 drug plan contracts had been signed between CMS and administrators, which in turn means multiple thousand plans because administrators can vary plans by county. Individual counties might have as few as three to as many 30 plans from which beneficiaries can choose. This allows participants to choose a plan that best meets their individual needs.

Plan administrators are required to offer a plan with at least the "standard" minimum benefit or one that is actuarially equivalent to the standard, and they may also offer plans with more generous benefits (e.g., no deductible during the initial spend phase). The terms "standard," "actuarially equivalent," and "more generous" relate to the plan's deductible/co-pay/formulary/"donut-hole"/pharmacy-preference aspects and has no direct relevance to the beneficiary other than increasing or decreasing personal choice. Each plan is approved by the CMS before being marketed.

(NOTE: It is often said the donut hole will be eliminated; that is not technically true. The "donut hole" is also called the gap phase of spending; at one time the co-pay in the gap was 100%. As of 2020, the "standard" co-pay in the gap became 25%, the same as in a "standard" initial spend phase policy. It is also important to note that relatively few people as a percent of the total number of people on Medicare are ever financially affected by either the donut hole or catastrophic phases of spending.)

Medicare offers an interactive online tool called the Medicare Plan Finder that allows for comparison of coverage and costs for all plans in a geographic area. The tool lets users enter a list of medications along with pharmacy preferences and Social-Security-Extra-Help/LIS and related status. The Finder can show the beneficiary's total annual costs for each plan along with a detailed breakdown of the plans' monthly premiums, deductibles and prices for each drug during each phase of spending (initial, gap, catastrophic). Plans are required to update this site with current prices and formulary information every other week throughout the year.

Costs to Beneficiaries

Beneficiary cost sharing (deductibles, coinsurance, etc.)

The Medicare Modernization Act (MMA) established a standard drug benefit that all Part D plans must offer. The standard benefit is defined in terms of the benefit structure and without mandating the drugs that must be covered. For example, in 2013, the standard benefit required payment by the beneficiary of a $325 deductible, then required 25% coinsurance payment by the beneficiary of drug costs up to an initial coverage limit of $2,970 (the full retail cost of prescriptions). Once this initial coverage limit is reached, the beneficiary has to pay the full cost of his/her prescription drugs up until the total out-of-pocket expenses reached $4,750 (excluding premiums and any expense paid by the insurance company) minus a 52.5% discount in this gap, referred to as the "Donut Hole". Once the beneficiary reaches the Out-of-Pocket Threshold, he/she becomes eligible for catastrophic coverage. During catastrophic coverage, he or she pays the greater of 5% coinsurance, or $2.65 for generic drugs and $6.60 for brand-name drugs. The catastrophic coverage amount is calculated on a yearly basis and a beneficiary who reaches catastrophic coverage by the end of the benefit year will start his or her deductible anew at the beginning of the next benefit year. Although uncommon, not all benefit years coincide with the calendar year. The donut-hole and catastrophic-coverage thresholds dropped slightly in 2014 and typically go up and down slightly between given years.

The standard benefit is not the most common benefit mix offered in Part D plans. Only 11% of plans in 2010 offered the defined standard benefit described above.

Plans vary widely in formularies and cost-sharing. Most eliminate the deductible and use tiered drug co-payments rather than coinsurance. The only out-of-pocket costs that count toward getting out of the coverage gap and into catastrophic coverage are True Out-Of-Pocket (TrOOP) expenditures. TrOOP expenditures accrue only when drugs on plan's formulary are purchased in accordance with the restrictions on those drugs. Monthly premium payments do not count towards TrOOP.

Under the Patient Protection and Affordable Care Act of 2010, the effect of the "Donut Hole" coverage gap was to be gradually reduced through a combination of measures including brand-name prescription drug discounts, generic drug discounts and a gradual increase in the percentage of out-of-pocket costs covered while in the donut hole. The "Donut Hole" will continue to exist after 2020 but its effect will be changed in some way yet to be determined, because plan administrators must treat out of pocket costs below the catastrophic level the same whether or not the insured is in the donut hole or not. That is, under the "standard benefit" design all prescriptions in all tiers could be subject to a 25% co-pay whereas as of 2014 many drugs in Tier 1 are available with no co-pay.

Most plans use specialty drug tiers, and some have a separate benefit tier for injectable drugs. Beneficiary cost sharing can be higher for drugs in these tiers.

Beneficiary Premiums

In 2014, the average (weighted) monthly premium paid by the beneficiary was around $30 a month. The average premium is a misleading statistic because it averages the premiums offered, not the premiums paid. Most insurers offer a very low-cost plan (e.g., $15 a month) that few choose. This lowers the average, but does not reflect what is happening in the market.

One option for those struggling with drug costs is the low-income subsidy (LIS). Beneficiaries with income below 150% of the poverty line are eligible for the low-income subsidy, which helps pay for all or part of the monthly premium, annual deductible and co-pays.

Excluded Drugs

While CMS does not have an established formulary, Part D drug coverage excludes drugs not approved by the Food and Drug Administration, those prescribed for off-label use, drugs not available by prescription for purchase in the United States, and drugs for which payments would be available under Part B.

Part D coverage excludes drugs or classes of drugs that may be excluded from Medicaid coverage. These may include:

- Drugs used for anorexia, weight loss, or weight gain

- Drugs used to promote fertility

- Drugs used for erectile dysfunction

- Drugs used for cosmetic purposes (hair growth, etc.)

- Drugs used for the symptomatic relief of cough and colds

- Prescription vitamin and mineral products, except prenatal vitamins and fluoride preparations

- Drugs where the manufacturer requires as a condition of sale any associated tests or monitoring services to be purchased exclusively from that manufacturer or its designee

While these drugs are excluded from basic Part D coverage, drug plans can include them as a supplemental benefit, provided they otherwise meet the definition of a Part D drug. However plans that cover excluded drugs are not allowed to pass those costs on to Medicare, and plans are required to repay CMS if they are found to have billed Medicare in these cases.

Part D plans may cover all benzodiazepines and those barbiturates used in the treatment of epilepsy, cancer or a chronic health disorder. These two drug classes were originally excluded, until their reassignment in 2008 by the Medicare Improvements for Patients and Providers Act.

Plan Formularies

Part D plans are not required to pay for all covered Part D drugs. They establish their own formularies, or list of covered drugs for which they will make payment, as long as the formulary and benefit structure are not found by CMS to discourage enrollment by certain Medicare beneficiaries. Part D plans that follow the formulary classes and categories established by the United States Pharmacopoeia will pass the first discrimination test. Plans can change the drugs on their formulary during the course of the year with 60 days' notice to affected parties.

The Plan's tiered co-pay amounts for each drug only generally apply during the initial period before the coverage gap.

The primary differences between the formularies of different Part D plans relate to the coverage of brand-name drugs.

Typically, each Plan's formulary is organized into tiers, and each tier is associated with a set co-pay amount. Most formularies have between 3 and 5 tiers. The lower the tier, the lower the co-pay. For example, Tier 1 might include all of the Plan's preferred generic drugs, and each drug within this tier might have a co-pay of $5 to $10 per prescription. Tier 2 might include the Plan's preferred brand drugs with a co-pay of $40 to $50, while Tier 3 may be reserved for non-preferred brand drugs which are covered by the plan at a higher co-pay, perhaps $70 to $100. Tiers 4 and higher typically contain specialty drugs, which have the highest co-pays because they are generally more expensive.

CMS funds a national program of counselors to assist all Medicare beneficiaries, including duals, with their plan choices. The program is called State Health Insurance Assistance Program (SHIP).

Background

It was clear that Canadian pharmacies were marketing prescription drugs to Americans at lower prices than U.S. based pharmacies. However, it became evident in April 2018 that the health risk of purchasing drugs from Canada could result in the sale of millions of counterfeit prescriptions being sold cross border.

As of January 30, 2007, nearly 24 million individuals were receiving prescription drug coverage through Medicare Part D (PDPs and MA-PDs combined), according to CMS. Medicare offers other methods of receiving drug coverage, including the Retiree Drug Subsidy. Federal retiree programs such as TRICARE and Federal Employees Health Benefits Program (FEHBP) or alternative sources, such as the Department of Veterans Affairs. Including people in these categories, more than 39 million Americans are covered for prescriptions by the federal government.

From a budget perspective, Part D is effectively three different programs:

- About 40% is spent for low-income Medicare beneficiaries (20% of those on Medicare overall) mentioned above and the drug costs of low income people on Part C. A very large percent of this first group is also on Medicaid.

- About 40% is premium support that allows middle-income Medicare beneficiaries and the rest of the people on Part C (about 40% of those on Medicare overall) get drug coverage.

- About 20% of the Part D budget covers re-insurance for catastrophic drug costs as described above. Part D pays 95% of costs over the True Out-Of-Pocket (TrOOP). This part of the budget helps about 1% of the people on Medicare who are very ill.

Cost Utilization

Medicare Part D Cost Utilization Measures refer to limitations placed on medications covered in a specific insurer's formulary for a plan. Cost utilization consists of techniques that attempt to reduce insurer costs. The three main cost utilization measures are quantity limits, prior authorization and step therapy. ("Step therapy" is a process in which a plan requires an individual to try, and prove ineffective, one or more specified lower-cost drugs before a higher-cost drug in the same therapeutic class is approved.)

Quantity limits refer to the maximum amount of a medication that may be dispensed during a given calendar period. For example, a plan may dictate that it will cover 90 pills of a given drug within a 30-day period.

A prior authorization requirement requires a health care worker to receive formal approval from a plan before it agrees to cover a specific prescription. It may be used by insurers for drugs that are often misused. Prior authorization helps ensure that patients receive correct medications.

Implementation Issues

- Plan and Health Care Provider goal alignment: PDP's and MA's are rewarded for focusing on low-cost drugs to all beneficiaries, while providers are rewarded for quality of care – sometimes involving expensive technologies.

- Conflicting goals: Plans are required to have a tiered exemptions process for beneficiaries to get a higher-tier drug at a lower cost, but plans must grant medically-necessary exceptions. However, the rule denies beneficiaries the right to request a tiering exception for certain high-cost drugs.

- Lack of standardization: Because each plan can design their formulary and tier levels, drugs appearing on Tier 2 in one plan may be on Tier 3 in another plan. Co-pays may vary across plans. Some plans have no deductibles and the coinsurance for the most expensive drugs varies widely. Some plans may insist on "step therapy", which means that the patient must use generics first before the company will pay for higher-priced drugs. Patients can appeal and insurers are required to respond within a short timeframe, so as to not further the burden on the patient.

- Standards for electronic prescribing for Medicare Part D conflict with regulations in many U.S. states.

Impact on Beneficiaries

A 2008 study found that the % of Medicare beneficiaries who reported forgoing medications due to cost dropped with Part D, from 15.2% in 2004 and 14.1% in 2005 to 11.5% in 2006. The percentage who reported skipping other basic necessities to pay for drugs also dropped, from 10.6% in 2004 and 11.1% in 2005 to 7.6% in 2006. The very sickest beneficiaries reported no reduction, but fewer reported forgoing other necessities to pay for medicine.

A parallel study found that Part D beneficiaries skip doses or switch to cheaper drugs and that many do not understand the program. Another study found that Part D resulted in modest increases in average drug utilization and decreases in average out-of-pocket expenditures. Further studies by the same group of researchers found that the net impact among beneficiaries was a decrease in the use of generic drugs.

A further study concludes that although a substantial reduction in out-of-pocket costs and a moderate increase in utilization among Medicare beneficiaries during the first year after Part D, there was no evidence of improvement in emergency department use, hospitalizations, or preference-based health utility for those eligible for Part D during its first year of implementation. It was also found that there were no significant changes in trends in the dual eligibles' out-of-pocket expenditures, total monthly expenditures, pill-days, or total number of prescriptions due to Part D.

A 2020 study found that Medicare Part D led to a sharp reduction in the number of people over the age of 65 who worked full-time. The authors say that this is evidence that before the change, people avoided retiring in order to maintain employer-based health insurance.

Criticisms

The federal government is not permitted to negotiate Part D drug prices with drug companies, as federal agencies do in other programs. The Department of Veterans Affairs, which is allowed to negotiate drug prices and establish a formulary, has been estimated to pay between 40% and 58% less for drugs, on average, than Part D. On the other hand, the VA only covers about half the brands that a typical Part D plan covers.

Part of the issue is that Medicare does not pay for Part D drugs, and so has no actual leverage. Part D drug providers are using the private insurer leverage, which is generally a larger block of consumers than the 40 million or so actually using Medicare parts A and B for medical care.

Although generic versions of [frequently prescribed to the elderly] drugs are now available, plans offered by three of the five [exemplar Medicare Part D] insurers currently exclude some or all of these drugs from their formularies. ... Further, prices for the generic versions are not substantially lower than their brand-name equivalents. The lowest price for simvastatin (generic Zocor) 20 mg is 706 percent more expensive than the VA price for brand-name Zocor. The lowest price for sertraline HCl (generic Zoloft) is 47 percent more expensive than the VA price for brand-name Zoloft."

— Families USA 2007 "No Bargain: Medicare Drug Plans Deliver High Prices"

Former Congressman Billy Tauzin, R–La., who steered the bill through the House, retired soon after and took a $2 million a year job as president of Pharmaceutical Research and Manufacturers of America (PhRMA), the main industry lobbying group. Medicare boss Thomas Scully, who threatened to fire Medicare Chief Actuary Richard Foster if he reported how much the bill would actually cost, was negotiating for a new job as a pharmaceutical lobbyist as the bill was working through Congress. 14 congressional aides quit their jobs to work for related lobbies immediately after the bill's passage.

In 2012, the plan required Medicare beneficiaries whose total drug costs reach $2,930 to pay 100% of prescription costs until $4,700 is spent out of pocket. (The actual threshold amounts change year-to-year and plan-by-plan, and many plans offered limited coverage during this phase.) While this coverage gap does not affect the majority of program participants, about 25% of beneficiaries enrolled in standard plans find themselves in this gap.

https://www.seniorliving.org/prescription-discount-cards/best/
(See hyperlink for full text and references.)

Best Prescription Discount Cards in 2021

The prevalence of discount prescription cards has caused quite a bit of competition between card offers and pharmacy prices, as more and more individuals are finding themselves uninsured or underinsured. Prescription drug cards are designed to help lower the cost of many of the most popularly prescribed medications. Savings will vary depending on the card and the pharmacy, but most users report savings ranging between 20 and 90 percent on prescriptions by simply utilizing the card.

We identified the top 10 prescription discount cards and narrowed it down to 6 of our favorites based on a number of criteria (GoodRX Gold, WellRx, America's Pharmacy, Choice Drug Card, SingleCare, ValpakRx, Optimum Perks and FamilyWize). We looked at affordability, service, ease of use, and other factors to rank the best prescription discount cards on the market.

GOODRX

GoodRx is an American healthcare company that operates a telemedicine platform and a free-to-use website and mobile app that track prescription drug prices in the United States and provide free drug coupons for discounts on medications. GoodRx checks more than 75,000 pharmacies in the United States. The website gets about fourteen million visitors a month. As of February 25, 2020, "millions of people" had downloaded the GoodRx app.

GoodRx was founded in Santa Monica, California in 2011. In 2017, GoodRx announced partnerships with major prescription drug companies in the country to negotiate lower prescription drug costs. In September 2019, GoodRx acquired the telemedicine company HeyDoctor and rebranded the telemedicine platform as GoodRx Care. The platform allows individuals to consult with a doctor online and obtain a prescription for certain types of medications at a cost of US$20 as of December 2019, regardless of insurance status. Medical testing services, which vary in price, are also offered through the platform.

The Santa Monica, California-based startup was founded in September 2011 by Trevor Bezdek and former Facebook executives Doug Hirsch and Scott Marlette. Marlette was one of the first 20 employees at Facebook and built Facebook's photo application. In 2005, Hirsch was the Vice President of Product at Facebook, working closely with Mark Zuckerberg. In 2017, Jordan Michaels joined as director of operations. In 2019, technology executive John Asalone joined as a General Manager to add Telehealth to GoodRx's comparison-shopping platform.

On February 25, 2020, Consumer Reports published an article stating that GoodRx shared user data – specifically, pseudonymized advertising ID numbers that companies use to track the behavior of web users across websites, the names of the drugs that users browsed, and the pharmacies where user sought to fill prescriptions – with Google, Facebook, and around 20 other internet-based companies. A few days after the Consumer Reports article was published, GoodRx published a statement saying it made changes to prevent user search data on medical conditions and pharmaceuticals from being shared with Facebook.

Related links:

How GoodRx Profits from Our Broken Pharmacy Pricing System
("In 2019, GoodRx collected an astounding $364 million in fees on $2.5 billion in consumer Rx spending.")

➢ https://www.drugchannels.net/2020/08/how-goodrx-profits-from-our-broken.html

SingleCare vs. GoodRx: Which Is Cheaper? ("Of course, you don't need to limit your comparison shopping to just these two services. You can also check out similar services RxSaver and Blink Health.")

➢ https://clark.com/health-health-care/singlecare-vs-goodrx-which-is-cheaper/

How is Medicare Paid For?

Medicare is a federally run health insurance program for the elderly, the disabled, and people with qualifying health conditions specified by Congress. The Centers for Medicare & Medicaid Services (CMS) is the federal agency that runs the Medicare program and handles its budget. (CMS is a branch of HHS: the Department of Health and Human Services.)

Medicare is funded by taxpayers via the Social Security Administration. The Medicare Trust Fund, comprising two separate funds held by the United States Department of the Treasury, supplies the money for Medicare payments. Money in the two trust funds comes from taxpayers as follows:

- The Hospital Insurance (HI) Trust Fund is financed mainly through the Medicare Tax (a payroll tax on earnings paid by employers and employees), the SE (self-employed) tax, income taxes on Social Security benefits, premiums from voluntary enrollees ineligible for free Medicare Part A coverage based on their earnings records, transfers from the general fund and the Railroad Retirement account, interest earned on trust fund investments and miscellaneous receipts. The HI trust fund had receipts of $306.6 billion and a balance of $200.4 billion at the end of 2018.

- The Supplemental Medical Insurance (SMI) Trust Fund is financed through general tax revenue authorized by Congress (such as individual income taxes, corporate taxes, and excise taxes), Part B and Part D premiums paid by Medicare enrollees, a small amount of interest on trust fund balances and miscellaneous receipts. The SMI trust fund received $449.1 billion in revenues and had $104.3 billion in assets at the end of 2018. Unlike the HI fund, no payroll taxes are dedicated to the SMI fund.

Money in the two Medicare Trust Funds can only go toward paying for Medicare. Those two separate funds each pay for different parts of the Medicare program.

- The **Hospital Insurance (HI) Trust Fund** pays for Medicare Part A benefits, which include inpatient hospital, nursing home, skilled nursing facility, hospice, and home health care. It also pays for

Medicare program administration such as costs for paying benefits, collecting Medicare taxes and fighting fraud and abuse.

- The **Supplementary Medical Insurance (SMI) Trust Fund** pays for Medicare Part B benefits (which include doctors' visits for outpatients, mental health, ambulances, and preventative care) and Medicare Part D prescription drug coverage. It also pays for Medicare program administration such as costs for paying benefits and fighting fraud and abuse.

FICA (Federal Insurance Contributions Act) Taxes

FICA (the Federal Insurance Contributions Act) requires all U.S. employers and employees to pay taxes on income to help fund the federal insurance programs of Social Security and Medicare. Your employer withholds a certain amount of every paycheck toward FICA taxes.

- The Old Age, Survivors and Disability Insurance (OASDI) is the official name for the Social Security program. The 12.4% FICA tax is commonly referred to as the Social Security tax. FICA taxes into the Social Security system are 6.2% of an employee's wages and levied only on the first $147,000 in earnings (2022). Employers match the 6.2% payment. These funds do not pay for Medicare.

- The FICA Medicare Tax (also known as the Hospital Insurance or HI tax) funds Medicare Part A, and is levied on every penny you earn. All employees must pay at least 1.45% of their wages in Medicare taxes. Additionally, employers pay 1.45%, bringing the total to 2.9% of your income. If you're self-employed, you pay the entire 2.9%.

The Additional Medicare Tax

If you have a high income, you may have to pay an extra tax called the Additional Medicare Tax. This surtax is 0.9% of your income, paid on IRS Form 8959 (1.45% + 0.9% = 2.35% but no employer match on the 0.9%).

If you're self-employed

Employers are required to withhold FICA taxes from employee paychecks. Self-employed individuals pay the Self-employment (SE) Tax instead of FICA taxes. The SE Tax is the same as the combined employee/employer FICA taxes: 12.4% for Social Security tax and 2.9%

for Medicare tax.

Self-employed individuals must pay the entire 2.9% tax on self-employed net earnings because they are both employer and employee – they don't have an employer to pay half. But they can deduct the "employer" half of the taxes on their tax returns. If you're self-employed, you'll need to pay estimated taxes to cover the self-employment tax.

Revisions resulting from the 2010 Patient Protection and Affordable Care Act (PPACA) legislation

In the Affordable Care Act legislation of 2010 (PPACA), another surtax was then added to Part D premium for higher-income seniors to partially fund the Affordable Care Act, and the number of Part B beneficiaries subject to the 2006 surtax was doubled, also partially to fund PPACA.

Medicare Costs You Pay Once You Start Using Medicare

- Medicare Part A (hospital insurance) is paid through the HI Trust Fund. It provides coverage if you're hospitalized. You pay no premiums for this coverage if you paid into Social Security for at least 10 years. Most people qualify for premium-free Part A, but those who don't will have premiums of up to $471. Recipients will still have out-of-pocket costs even if they are eligible for free Medicare Part A, including a $1,556 deductible (in 2022) for each "benefit period". A "benefit period" begins upon admission to a hospital or skilled nursing facility and ends 60 days after a person stops receiving care related to the stay.

- Medicare Part B (outpatient insurance) is paid through the SMI Trust Fund. It provides coverage for doctor visits and other outpatient costs such as medical equipment and physical therapy. It also covers some preventive costs such as glaucoma screening, diabetes testing, and colon and prostate cancer screening. You must pay a monthly premium for Part B. In 2022, Medicare Part B recipients paid monthly premiums of $170.10 to $578.30.

- The Medicare Part C ("Medicare Advantage") program uses the same two trust funds (HI and SMI) as well as a proportion determined by the CMS reflecting that Part C beneficiaries are fully on Parts A and B of Medicare just as all other beneficiaries. Payments to private insurers that manage Part C Medicare

Advantage plans are calculated and paid by CMS based upon an annual bidding process.

- Medicare Part D prescription drug coverage is funded through the SMI Trust Fund and the premiums that Part D beneficiaries pay. It is a separate policy you buy from a private insurer if you want it. Each private insurer has its own plan. You pay a monthly premium for Part D coverage and you may also have an annual deductible of no more than $480 (for 2022), if there is any deductible at all. Once you cover the deductible, your plan will then pay some or all of your drug costs, but only for the first $4,430 in total drug costs per year. Once you reach $4,430 you are in the "donut-hole", where you will pay 25% of costs that fall within $4,430 and $7,050 and receive a 75% discount on both brand-name and generic drugs (70% from prescription drug manufacturers, 5% from your insurer). Once your annual costs are above $7,050, you move into the Catastrophic Benefit Period, with Medicare paying most costs. If your income (2022) is above $91,000 if you file individually or $182,000 if you're married and file jointly, you'll pay an extra amount in addition to your plan premium (a recent ACA surcharge sometimes called "Part D-IRMAA"). You'll also have to pay this extra amount if you're in a Medicare Advantage Plan that includes drug coverage. Social Security will contact you if you have to pay Part D IRMAA, based on your income. The extra amount you have to pay ($12.40 - $77.90 per month) isn't part of your plan premium. You don't pay the extra amount to your plan. Most people have the extra amount taken from their Social Security check. If the amount isn't taken from your check, you'll get a bill from Medicare or the Railroad Retirement Board. You must pay this amount to keep your Part D coverage. You'll also have to pay this extra amount if you're in a Medicare Advantage Plan that includes drug coverage. You're required to pay the Part D IRMAA, even if your employer or a third party (like a teacher's union or a retirement system) pays for your Part D plan premiums. If you don't pay the Part D IRMAA and get disenrolled, you may also lose your retirement coverage and you may not be able to get it back.

An Overview of How Medicare Part C (Medicare Advantage) is Funded

Medicare Advantage (Medicare Part C) is a private health insurance program that is funded separately from traditional Medicare Parts A, B and D, and funded from two different sources.

- The main source is the federal agency CMS (Centers for Medicare & Medicaid Services) that runs the Medicare program.

- Monthly premiums from beneficiaries provide additional funding.

Medicare pays private insurance companies a fixed monthly amount to manage each beneficiary's expected healthcare costs.

The Medicare Part C ("Medicare Advantage") program uses the same two trust funds (HI and SMI) as well as a proportion determined by the CMS reflecting that Part C beneficiaries are fully on Parts A and B of Medicare just as all other beneficiaries, but that their medical needs are paid for through a sponsor (most often an integrated health delivery system or spin out) to providers rather than "fee for service" (FFS) through an insurance company called a Medicare Administrative Contractor to providers.

Advantage plans pay for the services otherwise covered by Medicare parts A and B. Depending on the specific Advantage plan, they may also pay for some additional services.

Medicare pays into Advantage plans monthly an amount that covers the Part A and Part B costs of beneficiaries. If a plan also offers prescription drug coverage, Medicare provides a separate payment.

The amount of the monthly payments depends on two main factors:

- the anticipated costs of healthcare in the county where each beneficiary lives, which influences the CMS procedure called the bidding process

- the expected healthcare costs of the beneficiaries, which governs how Medicare raises or lowers the rates, in the CMS system known as risk adjustment

Medicare Advantage Bidding Process

The Advantage plan bidding process involves two steps:

- First, each private insurer plan submits a bid to Medicare, based on the estimated cost of Part A and Part B benefits per person.

- Next, Medicare compares the amount of the bid against the benchmark. The benchmark is a percentage of costs of average Medicare spending per individual.

Each county in the United States has its own benchmark. It reflects the practice patterns of resident healthcare providers that bill Medicare. Practice patterns differ among counties, so their benchmarks also differ.

- When the plan's bid is greater than the benchmark, the person enrolled in the Advantage plan pays the difference between the two amounts. This payment is a monthly premium. A person pays this in addition to the Medicare Part B premium.

- If the bid is lower than the benchmark, the plan gets a rebate from Medicare that is a percentage of the difference between the bid and the benchmark. Plans that receive rebates are expected to use a portion of the rebates to fund supplemental benefits or to reduce premiums.

Medicare Advantage Base Rate and Risk Adjustment Rate

Medicare uses the bid and the benchmark to determine the base rate.

- When the bid is lower than the benchmark, the bid becomes the base rate.

- In contrast, when the bid is higher than or equal to the benchmark, the benchmark becomes the base rate.

After the establishment of the base rate, Medicare uses risk adjustment to change the rate to reflect the anticipated healthcare costs of a person enrolled in a plan.

- For example, if someone has a risk score of 1.0, it means that their expected costs are equal to those of an individual with average health.

- A risk score of 0.5 indicates that the expected costs are half of those of the average person, while a risk score of 2.0 indicates the expected costs are double those of the average person.

Percentage of Medicare spending on Advantage plans

In 2019, Medicare payments to Medicare Advantage plans to fund Part A and Part B benefits were $250 billion, according to the Kaiser Family Foundation. This represents 33% of Medicare's total spending.

On average, across the country, 34% of people with Medicare chose to enroll in Advantage plans during 2019. The percentage of residents who have these plans varies widely by state, from 1% in Alaska to 43% in Minnesota and Florida.

If there is a nationwide rise in people choosing Medicare Advantage over original Medicare parts A and B, the percentage of total Medicare spending on the plans may also rise.

Solvency and Budget Pressures

As of July 2020, Medicare covered approximately 62.4 million people, but the number of beneficiaries is outpacing the number of people who pay into the program. This has created a funding gap. Stagnant wages in recent years have exacerbated the problem because the revenue from payroll taxes isn't enough keep up with the cost of running Medicare.

Retirement of the Baby Boom generation is projected to increase enrollment to more than 80 million by 2030. Baby-boomers are projected to have longer life spans, which will add to the future Medicare spending. In addition, the number of workers per enrollee will decline from 3.7 to 2.4 and overall health care costs in the nation will rise, posing substantial financial challenges to the program.

Because of the two Trust funds and their differing revenue sources (one dedicated and one not), the Trustees analyze Medicare spending as a percent of GDP rather than versus the Federal budget. In 2018, Medicare spending was just over $740 billion, about 3.7% of U.S. gross domestic product and over 15% of total US federal spending. Medicare spending is projected to increase to just over $1.2 trillion by 2026, to 4.7% of GDP.

Total Medicare income is estimated to be $793.5 billion in 2019, while total Medicare spending is estimated to reach $796.6 billion.

The 2019 Medicare Trustees Report estimates that spending as a percent of GDP will grow to 6% by 2043 (when the last of the baby boomers turns 80) and then flatten out to 6.5% of GDP by 2093. In response to these financial challenges, Congress made substantial cuts to future payouts to providers (primarily acute care hospitals and skilled nursing facilities) as part of PPACA in 2010 and the Medicare Access and CHIP Reauthorization Act of 2015 (MACRA) and policymakers have offered many additional competing proposals to reduce Medicare costs further.

The Hospital Insurance (HI) Trust Fund faces long-term deficits. According to the intermediate assumptions of the 2019 Trustees Report, the HI Trust Fund (that funds Medicare Part A, which is premium-free to most enrollees) is projected to be exhausted by 2026. These pressures, now and in the future, will force lawmakers to find ways to finance promised benefits or cut services or provider payment rates.

The Supplemental Medical Insurance (SMI) Trust Fund, which funds Medicare Part B and Part D, remains solvent, since the majority of beneficiaries pay premiums to participate.

Cost reduction is influenced by factors including reduction in inappropriate and unnecessary care by evaluating evidence-based practices as well as reducing the amount of unnecessary, duplicative, and inappropriate care. Cost reduction may also be effected by reducing medical errors, investment in healthcare information technology, improving transparency of cost and quality data, increasing administrative efficiency, and by developing both clinical/non-clinical guidelines and quality standards.

For now, it's unclear what will happen with Medicare Part A funding. Congress may act in the future to address the funding shortfall. For instance, they could raise the Medicare tax or the age when Americans are eligible for benefits.

Information in this chapter is extracted from the following articles in an effort to present a complete representation of the intricacies of "How Medicare Is Paid For". Please see the hyperlinks below for full text, media sources, author profiles and references.

(1) Medicare A, B, C & D Funding
- **https://en.wikipedia.org/wiki/Medicare_(United_States)**
  (See hyperlink for full text and references.)

(2) How is Medicare Funded?
- https://www.medicare.gov/about-us/how-is-medicare-funded
  (See hyperlink for full text and references.)

(3) Part D IRMAA
- https://www.medicare.gov/drug-coverage-part-d/costs-for-medicare-drug-coverage/monthly-premium-for-drug-plans
  (See hyperlink for full text and references.)

(4) What is the Medicare Trust Fund and How is it Financed?
- https://www.taxpolicycenter.org/briefing-book/what-medicare-trust-fund-and-how-it-financed
  (See hyperlinks for full text and references.)

(5) How is Medicare Funded?
By Derek Silva, November 11, 2020 (Derek is a personal finance editor at Policygenius in New York City, and an expert in taxes. He has been writing about estate planning, investing, and other personal finance topics since 2017. His work has been covered by Yahoo Finance, MSN, Business Insider, and CNBC.)
- https://www.policygenius.com/medicare/how-is-medicare-funded/
  (See hyperlink for full text and references.)

(6) How is Medicare Advantage Funded?
Medically reviewed by Ayonna Tolbert, PharmD
Written by Mary West on May 21, 2020
- https://www.medicalnewstoday.com/articles/how-is-medicare-advantage-funded   (See hyperlink for full text and references.)

HEALTH SAVINGS ACCOUNT
From Wikipedia, the free encyclopedia

A Health Savings Account (HSA) is a tax-advantaged medical savings account available to taxpayers in the United States who are enrolled in a high-deductible health plan (HDHP). The funds contributed to an account are not subject to federal income tax at the time of deposit. Unlike a Flexible Spending Account (FSA), HSA funds roll over and accumulate year to year if they are not spent. HSAs are owned by the individual, which differentiates them from company-owned Health Reimbursement Arrangements (HRA) that are an alternate tax-deductible source of funds paired with either high-deductible health plans or standard health plans. HSA funds may be used to pay for qualified medical expenses at any time without federal tax liability or penalty.

Proponents of HSAs believe that they are an important reform that will help reduce the growth of health care costs and increase the efficiency of the health care system. According to proponents, HSAs encourage saving for future health care expenses, allow the patient to receive needed care without a gatekeeper to determine what benefits are allowed, and make consumers more responsible for their own health care choices through the required high-deductible health plan. Opponents observe that the structure of HSAs complicates the decision of whether to obtain medical treatment, by setting it against tax liability and retirement-saving goals. There is also debate about consumer satisfaction with these plans.

COMPARED TO MEDICAL SAVINGS ACCOUNTS

Health Savings Accounts are similar to Medical Savings Account (MSA) plans that were authorized by the federal government before health savings account plans. Health savings accounts can be used with some high-deductible health plans. Health savings accounts came into being after legislation was signed by President George W. Bush on December 8, 2003. The law went into effect on January 1, 2004.

Health Savings Accounts differ in several ways from Medical Savings Accounts. Perhaps the most significant difference is that employers of all sizes can offer a Health Savings Account and insurance plan to employees. Medical Savings Accounts are limited to the self-employed and employers with 50 or fewer employees.

CRITICISM

Some consumer organizations, such as Consumers Union, and many medical organizations, such as the American Public Health Association, oppose Health Savings Accounts because, in their opinion, they benefit only healthy, younger people, and make the health care system more expensive for everyone else.

Critics contend that low-income people, who are more likely to be uninsured, do not earn enough to benefit from the tax breaks offered by Health Savings Accounts. These tax breaks are too modest, when compared to the actual cost of insurance, to persuade significant numbers to buy this coverage.

https://en.wikipedia.org/wiki/Flexible_spending_account
(See hyperlink for full text and references.)

FLEXIBLE SPENDING ACCOUNT
From Wikipedia, the free encyclopedia

In the United States, a Flexible Spending Account (FSA), also known as a Flexible Spending Arrangement, is one of a number of tax-advantaged financial accounts, resulting in payroll tax savings. One significant disadvantage to using an FSA is that funds not used by the end of the plan year are forfeited to the employer, known as the "use it or lose it" rule. Under the terms of the Affordable Care Act, however, a plan may permit an employee to carry over up to $550 into the following year without losing the funds but this does not apply to all plans and some plans may have lower limits.

The most common type of flexible spending account, the Medical Expense FSA (also Medical FSA or Health FSA), is similar to a Health Savings Account (HSA) or a Health Reimbursement Account (HRA). However, while HSAs and HRAs are almost exclusively used as components of a consumer-driven health care plan, medical FSAs are commonly offered with more traditional health plans as well. In addition, funds in an HSA are not lost when the plan year is over, unlike funds in an FSA. Paper forms or an FSA debit card may be used to access the account funds.

HEALTH FSA

The most common type of FSA is used to pay for medical and dental expenses not paid for by insurance, usually deductibles, copayments, and coinsurance for the employee's health plan. As of January 1, 2011, over-the-counter medications are allowed only when purchased with a doctor's prescription, except for insulin. Over-the-counter medical devices, such as bandages, crutches, and eyeglass repair kits, are allowable. Generally, allowable items are the same as those allowable for the medical tax deduction, as outlined in IRS publication 502.

Prior to the enactment of the Patient Protection and Affordable Care Act, the Internal Revenue Service permitted employers to enact any maximum annual election for their employees. The Patient Protection and Affordable Care Act amended Section 125 such that FSAs may not allow employees to choose an annual election in excess of a limit determined by the Internal Revenue Service. The annual contribution limit for 2018 was $2,650. Employers have the option to limit their employees' annual elections further. The limit is applied to each employee, without regard to whether the employee has a spouse or children. Non-elective contributions made by the employer that are not deducted from the employee's wages are not counted against the limit. An employee employed by multiple unrelated employers may elect an amount up to the limit under each employer's plan. The limit does not apply to Health Savings Accounts, Health Reimbursement Arrangements, or the employee's share of the cost of employer-sponsored health insurance coverage.

Also, one cannot have a Healthcare FSA if he or she has a High Deductible Health Plan (HDHP) with a Health Savings Account (HSA). In cases where an employee has a HDHP with a HSA, they are eligible for a Limited Expense FSA (LEX) (also called Limited Purpose FSA). These FSAs may be used to reimburse dental and vision expenses, regardless of any plan deductible; at the employer's discretion, eligible medical expenses incurred after the deductible is met may also be reimbursable.

In 2020, the Consolidated Appropriations Act of 2021 contained provisions to allow employees to roll over the remainder of their accounts from 2020 into 2021 and from 2021 into 2022.

The FSA debit card was developed to eliminate "double-dipping", by allowing employees to access the FSA directly. However, the substantiation requirement itself did not go away, and has even been expanded on by the IRS for the debit-card environment; therefore, withdrawal issues still remain for FSAs. These withdrawal issues have led to creative solutions by e-commerce companies who created an entire website dedicated to FSA-eligible items and accepting all FSA debit cards, and other websites which created a small portion of their website dedicated to FSAs.

According to Celent, as of May 2006, there were approximately 6 million debit cards in the market tied to FSA accounts, representing 25% of the FSA participating community.

ADVANTAGES AND DISADVANTAGES

Pre-funding and risks incurred by the employee and employer

One consideration regarding medical FSAs is that the participating employee's entire annual contribution is available at the start of the plan year, commonly January 1, or after the first contribution to the FSA is received by the FSA vendor, depending on the plan. Therefore, if the employee experiences a qualifying event during the first period, the entire amount of the annual contribution can be claimed against the FSA benefits. If the employee is terminated, quits, or is unable to return to work, he or she does not have to repay the money to the employer.

The employee contributes to the FSA in small increments throughout the year (for example, 1/26 of the annual amount if one is paid every two weeks), but taken together, all employees of a company contribute the full average amount during any given period, and no real risk is incurred by the employer. In addition, instead of paying payroll taxes to the government, the employer typically pays only a small administrative fee to the plan of $4-$10 per month per participating employee. This is much less than the employer would have paid for its share of payroll taxes. In addition, any money that is not used by the end of the plan year (or grace period) is returned to the employer. This is estimated to be up to 14% of the total employee contributions, which can be a substantial boon to the employer's bottom line.

If a company plans to lay off some employees, and announces such plans, then if multiple employees use their entire flexible benefit before they are terminated, that may cause the company to have to reimburse the plan. Typically, however, employers do not announce layoffs for specific employees with enough notice for employees to use the available benefits, and employees may actually lose their contributions in addition to being laid off.

An employee does not continue to contribute to the plan upon termination of employment. Thus, one could use the entire amount on day one of the plan year, terminate employment on day two of the plan year, and contributions would have been none or negligible (e.g., perhaps 1/26 in the case of biweekly contributions). The "free" money is not taxable because the IRS views these plans as health insurance plans for tax purposes. According to IRS section 125, benefits received from a health insurance plan are not considered taxable income.

The same reasons that make pre-funding a possible benefit to an employee participating in a plan make them a potential risk to employers setting up a plan. The employer has to make up the difference that the employee has spent from the flexible spending account but not yet contributed if other employees' contributions do not account for the money spent.

Over-the-counter drugs and medical items

Another FSA feature introduced in 2003 is the ability to pay for over-the-counter (OTC) drugs and medical items. In addition to substantially expanding the range of "FSA-eligible" purchases, adding OTC items made it easier to "spend down" medical FSAs at year-end to avoid the "use it or lose it" rule.

However, substantiation has again become an issue; generally, OTC purchases require either manual claims or, for FSA debit cards, submission of receipts after the fact. Most FSA providers require that receipts show the complete name of the item; the abbreviations on many store receipts are incomprehensible to many claims offices. Also, some of the IRS rules on what is and isn't eligible have proven rather arcane in practice. The recently developed Inventory Information Approval System (IIAS) separates eligible and ineligible items at the point-of-sale and provides for automatic debit-card substantiation.

Effective January 1, 2020, over-the-counter medicines are allowable without a prescription or a note from a physician. In addition, menstrual care products are also allowable. The change was made as part of the Coronavirus Aid, Relief, and Economic Security Act (CARES Act).

Eligible Medical Item List

The IIAS system references a master eligibility list of FSA eligible products at the point of sale. The Special Interest Group for IIAS Standards (SIG-IS) maintains this eligibility list and updates it on a monthly basis.

The FSA Eligibility List includes items within eligible healthcare product categories determined by the IRS. Health Savings Accounts share the same medical item eligibility list as FSAs.

Any money left unspent at the end of the coverage period is forfeited and can be applied to future plan administrative costs or can be equally allocated as taxable income among all plan participants; this is commonly known as the "use it or lose it" rule. Under most plans, the "coverage period" generally ceases upon termination of employment whether initiated by the employee or the employer, unless the employee continues coverage with the company under COBRA or other arrangement. A possibility, especially in the case of unexpected, immediate layoff, is that should an employee have unused contributions in an FSA and no additional qualifying claims during the coverage period the employee will have the added insult of "losing" these funds. On the other hand, if the payroll taxes saved on the employee's contributions exceeds the amount the employee forfeited, then the employee has still saved money overall.

A second requirement is that all applications for refunds must be made by a date defined by the plan. If funds are forfeited, this does not eliminate the requirement to pay taxes on these funds if such taxes are required. For example, if a single person elects to withhold $5,000 for child care expenses and marries a non-working spouse, the $5,000 would become taxable. If this person did not submit claims by the required date, the $5,000 would be forfeited but taxes would still be owed on the amount.

Also, the annual contribution amount must remain the same throughout the year unless certain qualifying events occur, such as the birth of a child or death of a spouse.

Effective 2013 plan years, employers may amend their plan documents to allow participants to carry over up to $500 of unused amounts to the following plan year. (The limit was increased to $550 as of January 1, 2020.) Doing so allows participants to spend the carryover amounts on qualifying medical expenses incurred during the following plan year. A carryover of unused amounts does not affect the indexed $2,500 annual limit. A plan year may allow either a rollover or a grace period for unused amounts for the same plan year but not both. Carryovers only apply for qualifying medical expenses; plans may not allow participants to carry over unused amounts for dependent care or other expenses. The carryover amount does not reduce the participant's maximum FSA contribution for the next plan year. Accordingly, a person who carries over $550 to the next plan year and who also contributes $2,500 to their FSA for that plan year may be able to receive reimbursements from his or her FSA for up to $3,050 of eligible medical expense during that plan year. In order for an individual to be able to carry over unused amounts, the plan must be amended to permit this type of a carryover.

Employers in California that sponsor flexible spending accounts must notify participants of any "deadline to withdraw funds" before the end of the plan year. The law is effective for plan years beginning on or after January 1, 2020.

Effective January 1, 2013, the Patient Protection and Affordable Care Act (PPACA) essentially required flexible spending accounts to limit employees' annual elections to no more than $2,500, with small increases each year based on inflation. Over-the-counter medications became ineligible expenses as well.

What Is Medical Payments Coverage?

Published November 2017   (Have questions about medical payments coverage? Talk to a local Allstate agent, who can help you with your state's requirements and coverage limits.)

Medical Payments Coverage is part of an auto insurance policy. It may help pay your or your passengers' medical expenses if you're injured in a car accident, regardless of who caused the accident. This coverage is optional and not available in all states. Medical Payments Coverage is sometimes called Medical Expense Coverage, or just "Med Pay."

What does Medical Payments cover?

If you're injured in a car accident, medical payments coverage may help pay the following expenses for you or your passengers:

- Health insurance deductibles and co-pays
- Doctor or hospital visits
- Surgery, X-rays or prostheses
- Ambulance and emergency medical technician fees
- Professional nursing services

What's the difference between Liability Coverage and Medical Payments Coverage?

Medical payments coverage is optional. So, if you cause a car accident and don't have medical payments coverage, you would have to pay out of your own pocket for your medical bills.

On the other hand, auto liability coverage is required by law in most states. Your auto liability coverage will not pay for your or your passengers' medical bills after a car accident.

If you cause a car accident, the bodily injury liability portion of your car insurance coverage helps pay for the other party's medical expenses. Likewise, if another driver is at fault for an accident that injures you, their auto liability coverage may help pay for your medical bills.

What's the difference between Personal Injury Protection (PIP) and Medical Payments Coverage?

Like Medical Payments Coverage, Personal Injury Protection (PIP) helps pay for your or your passengers' medical expenses after a car accident, regardless of who caused the accident.

But, there are three main differences between PIP and Medical Payments Coverage:

- PIP is available in "no-fault" states. Medical Payments Coverage is offered in states that aren't "no-fault." (Medical Payments Coverage is only available in states that do not have PIP.)

- PIP is sometimes required, and sometimes optional, depending on state law. Medical Payments Insurance is always an optional coverage.

- PIP helps cover expenses such as lost wages or child care if you're unable to perform essential services due to injuries after a car accident. Medical Payments Insurance does not cover essential services.

Medical Payments Coverage Limits

Medical Payments Insurance has a coverage limit, which is the maximum amount your insurer will pay for a covered loss. You can choose your limit when you buy coverage. Remember, any medical expenses that exceed your coverage limit are your responsibility.

If you need help choosing a coverage limit that fits your needs, you may want to think about the cost of short-term emergency medical expenses after a car accident. For example, say you had to go to the emergency room with injuries after an accident. Your health insurance might pay for some of the ER visit, but your health coverage may require you to pay a $2,000 deductible and a co-insurance payment for the emergency medical services.

That's where medical payments coverage on your car insurance policy may help. In the above scenario, if you had selected a coverage limit of $3,000, your medical payments insurance could help pay your health insurance deductible and some of your co-pay for your ER visit.

https://www.dol.gov/general/topic/health-plans/cobra
(See hyperlink for full text and references.)

COBRA:
CONTINUATION of
HEALTH COVERAGE

The Consolidated Omnibus Budget Reconciliation Act (COBRA) gives employees and their families who lose their health benefits the right to choose to continue group health benefits provided by their employer's group health plan for limited periods of time under certain circumstances such as voluntary or involuntary job loss, reduction in the hours worked, transition between jobs, death, divorce, and other life events. Qualified individuals may be required to pay the entire premium for coverage up to 102% of the cost to the plan.

COBRA continuation coverage laws are administered by several agencies:

- The Departments of Labor and Treasury have jurisdiction over private-sector group health plans.

- The Department of Health and Human Services administers the continuation coverage law as it applies to state and local governmental health plans.

- The Labor Department's interpretive responsibility for COBRA is limited to the disclosure and notification requirements of COBRA.

- If you need further information on your rights under a private sector plan, or about ERISA generally, contact the U.S. Department of Labor Employee Benefits Security Administration (EBSA) electronically at askebsa.dol.gov or call toll free 1-866-444-3272.

- The Internal Revenue Service, Department of the Treasury, has issued regulations on COBRA provisions relating to eligibility, coverage and payment. Both the Departments of Labor and Treasury share jurisdiction for enforcement of these provisions.

- The Centers for Medicare and Medicaid Services offer information about COBRA provisions for public sector employees. You can write them at this address: Centers for Medicare and Medicaid

Services 7500 Security Boulevard Mail Stop C1-22-06 Baltimore, MD 21244-1850.

FAQs - Frequently Asked Questions about COBRA

https://www.dol.gov/sites/dolgov/files/EBSA/about-ebsa/our-activities/resource-center/faqs/cobra-continuation-health-coverage-consumer.pdf (See hyperlink for answers.)

Q1: What is COBRA continuation health coverage?

Q2: What does COBRA do?

Q3: What group health plans are subject to COBRA?

Q4: Are there alternatives for health coverage other than COBRA?

Q5: Who is entitled to continuation coverage under COBRA?

Q6: How do I become eligible for COBRA continuation coverage?

Q7: How do I find out about COBRA coverage?

Q8: How long do I have to elect COBRA coverage?

Q9: If I waive COBRA coverage during the election period, can I still get coverage at a later date?

Q10: Under COBRA, what benefits must be covered?

Q11: How long does COBRA coverage last?

Q12: Can continuation coverage be terminated early for any reason?

Q13: Can I extend my COBRA continuation coverage?

Q14: Is a divorced spouse entitled to COBRA coverage from their former spouses' group health plan?

Q15: Who pays for COBRA coverage?

Q16: What is the Health Coverage Tax Credit and can it help me pay for COBRA?

Q17: If I did not make the premium payment on time and my coverage was canceled what can I do?

Q18: How do I file a COBRA claim for benefits?

Q19: Can I receive COBRA benefits while on FMLA leave?

Q20: I have both Medicare and COBRA coverage, how do I know which will pay my benefits?

Q21: Am I eligible for COBRA if my company closed or went bankrupt and there is no health plan?   (Short Answer: No)

Q22: I am a federal employee. Can I receive benefits under COBRA?

Q23: Where can I go if I have questions or want more information on COBRA?

<u>And OUR Question, Congress</u>:

Why do we have to have so many questions just to have predictable, cost-effective health coverage if we lose our job?

If we each had "a card in our wallet" from birth, all of this would go away!

Health coverage should not be tied to our place of employment!

https://www.singlepayeraction.org/2021/03/09/kay-tillow-on-the-downside-of-medicare-advantage-and-the-upside-of-single-payer/
(See hyperlink for full text and references.)

The Downside of Medicare Advantage and the Upside of Single Payer

By Kay Tillow for SinglePayerAction.org ; 9 March 2021
Tillow is a labor and single payer organizer
based in Louisville, Kentucky.

Almost 40 percent of all Medicare beneficiaries are now on private Medicare Advantage plans.

"It is true that a person may be able to lower monthly costs by enrolling in one of these plans," Kay Tillow wrote last year in an article titled "Beyond the Medicare Advantage Scam".

"That's a powerful incentive in a time when the majority of seniors live on tight budgets, many just an inch from disaster."

"The laws and regulations allow these insurance companies to lure seniors away from traditional Medicare, and members of Congress of both parties should be held responsible."

"You may be okay for a time and save money monthly – as long as you don't get sick. Once you need to use the plan, you will discover the problems that come from being in a for-profit plan that makes more when it denies you care. Your choice of physicians will be restricted to a list. The specialist you need may not be anywhere near where you live. The hospitals and rehabs centers will be limited. The post-hospitalization facility available to you is likely to be the one with the worst reputation. The drugs you need may now cost a fortune."

Tillow points out that if the patient tries to escape these exorbitant costs by returning to traditional Medicare and a prescription plan, the patient will need a supplemental Medigap plan to handle the twenty percent in copays and deductibles.

But the patient now has a pre-existing condition. When seniors first sign up for a Medicare plan, they are protected by law against discrimination for pre-existing conditions in the purchase of a Medigap plan. But when a person tries to change back to traditional Medicare later, that protection is gone. Only four states have regulations to prohibit such practices.

"Medicare Advantage plans are run by private for-profit insurers," Tillow told *Corporate Crime Reporter* in an interview last week. "And profits within the health care system work against patients. When you deny care, profits go up. We have the fox in the hen house. Those who are against the patients control how the patients are treated. They are very sharp at setting up systems. There are people who have lower monthly premiums because they are in Medicare Advantage. But what they will find is once they get sick that advantage goes away because the barriers go up to the care they need. They can't see the doctor they need or get to the hospital that they need. Those things work against the patient's care."

"Patients then find themselves in a plan that doesn't work for them and they go back to traditional Medicare. That's how the private insurers want it. When you are in good health and we can just profit from you and don't have to pay out for your care, we want you. But we want you to have incentives to leave once you get sick. That's the way it works. We the public pay about $1,000 annually per person more for everybody in Medicare Advantage. And yet the patients in Medicare Advantage are the healthiest patients. We should be paying less for them."

"You can't regulate enough around these foxes. We just have to get them out of the house because they are going to eat the chickens as long as they are in there."

We now have a lot of people who say they are for Medicare for All. And if you dig underneath, you find they are for lots of other steps between now and then. We have to change that idea that this is not urgent, that somehow we can do other things."

"Many people say – I'm for Medicare for All, but that may be years down the road – so in the meantime let's do the public option. The public option won't help because it maintains the private insurance industry within the system. It doesn't make it better and it deflects the pressure of the movement to get change".

"What we saw was the Democrats lost their majority and the ACA did not gain in popularity. For a long time, it was under fifty percent. And it is probably just barely above that now. It doesn't fix the problem. It doesn't cover everybody. It is unjust and unfair. Some people get subsidies, some people don't. Some people get Medicaid, some people don't. You get on Medicaid then you get a job and you lose your Medicaid. You get an employer based plan, the employer changes your plan and your deductible is $3,000. There is nothing that is stable about it."

"We have to push for the plan that will solve the problem. This is nonsense to go to the public option or in an emergency cover all the bills. You leave the insurance industry in there and we will still have all of the problems. Inherent in profit is the discrimination we suffer.

We have to get the profit out of the health care system. No one should make a business out of killing people. No one should make a business out of increasing the suffering. And that is precisely what they do.

We have all of these mechanisms in our health care system for keeping people from getting care. They claim it will keep the costs down. You have a deductible that is high. It means you can't afford it when your child needs emergency care and you don't go to the emergency room because there is a thousand dollar deductible. And you think – maybe the kid can live without it because the family's budget will be wrecked by it."

"Even people on Medicare go into bankruptcy. We are the only country in the industrialized world where you go bankrupt over your medical bills. It's a crime. It's an abomination. People in the Congress can't just say – oh well, the time isn't right. We don't yet have majority support. Well, work to get majority support. We need this."

We have the people with us. If we have any democracy left, we ought to be able to have the democratic will to push the people's Congress to do what it rightly ought to do for the welfare of the people.

See also https://www.singlepayeraction.org/: Liz Fowler Defending Trump Program to Privatize Medicare (16 January 2022)

https://publicintegrity.org/health/why-medicare-advantage-costs-taxpayers-billions-more-than-it-should/ -
This article was originally published by the Center for Public Integrity (https://publicintegrity.org/), a nonprofit investigative news organization based in Washington, D.C.

WHY MEDICARE ADVANTAGE COSTS TAXPAYERS BILLIONS MORE THAN IT SHOULD

By Fred Schulte, Erin Duncan and David Donald
for The Center for Public Integrity
Medicare Advantage Money Grab, Part 1 of 3
4 June 2014, Updated 14 January 2015

In South Florida, one of the nation's top privately-run Medicare insurance plans faces a federal investigation into allegations that it overbilled the government by exaggerating how sick some of its patients were.

In the Las Vegas area, private health care plans for seniors ran up more than $100 million in added Medicare charges after asserting patients they signed up also were much sicker than normal — a claim many experts have challenged.

In Rochester, New York, a Medicare plan was paid $41 million to treat people with serious diseases — even though the plan couldn't prove the patients in fact had those diseases.

These health plans and hundreds of others are part of Medicare Advantage, a program created by Congress in 2003 to help stabilize health care spending on the elderly. But the plans have sharply driven up costs in many parts of the United States — larding on tens of billions of dollars in overcharges and other suspect billings based in part on inflated assessments of how sick patients are, an investigation by the Center for Public Integrity has found.

Dominated by private insurers, Medicare Advantage now covers nearly 16 million Americans at a cost expected to top $150 billion this year. Many seniors choose the managed-care Medicare Advantage option instead of the traditional government-run Medicare program because it fills gaps in coverage, can cost less in out-of-pocket expenses and offers extra benefits, such as dental and eye care.

But billions of tax dollars are misspent every year through billing errors linked to a payment tool called a "risk score," which is supposed to pay Medicare Advantage plans higher rates for sicker patients and less for those in good health.

Government officials have struggled for years to halt health plans from running up patient risk scores and, in many cases, wresting higher Medicare payments than they deserve, records show.

The Center's findings are based on an analysis of Medicare Advantage enrollment data from 2007 through 2011, as well as thousands of pages of government audits, research papers and other documents.

Federal officials who run the Medicare program repeatedly refused to be interviewed or answer written questions.

Among the findings:

Risk score errors triggered nearly $70 billion in "improper" payments to Medicare Advantage plans from 2008 through 2013 — mostly overbillings, according to government estimates. Federal officials refused to identify health plans suspected of overcharging Medicare, citing agency policy that keeps many business records confidential. The Center is suing to make these records public.

Risk scores of Medicare Advantage patients rose sharply in plans in at least 1,000 counties nationwide between 2007 and 2011, boosting taxpayer costs by more than $36 billion over estimated costs for caring for patients in standard Medicare.

In more than 200 of these counties, the cost of some Medicare Advantage plans was at least 25 percent higher than the cost of providing standard Medicare coverage. The wide swing in costs was most evident in five states: South Dakota, New Mexico, Colorado, Texas and Arkansas.

Some academic experts and researchers believe the increase in risk scores is more likely to reflect aggressive billing than a rapid deterioration in patients' health.

Industry executives don't dispute that billing errors occur. But they deny that they charge too much, arguing they only want to be paid fairly for their services.

Clare Krusing, director of communications for America's Health Insurance Plans (AHIP), said that the industry trade group is "working together" with federal health officials to improve reporting of risk score data.

In the South Florida case, <u>government lawyers have been investigating Humana</u>, Inc. for several years <u>as they try to determine if the company and some of its medical clinics manipulated the complex Medicare Advantage billing system</u>. Humana says it is cooperating with the investigation.

In a separate civil case, a former Bush administration health official alleges in a whistleblower lawsuit unsealed earlier this year that two Puerto Rico health plans cheated Medicare out of as much as $1 billion by inflating patient risk scores. The plans, which at the time were owned by a subsidiary of New-Jersey based Aveta, Inc., denied the allegations.

Government audits and research reports have warned for years that <u>Medicare's risk scoring formula breeds overbilling, but efforts to hold the industry accountable have met with little success</u>. Federal officials have yet to recoup hundreds of millions of dollars in suspected overpayments to health plans that date back as far as 2007.

Excellus Health Plan, the Rochester, New York, health plan that federal auditors said may have overbilled by as much as $41 million in 2007 for treating patients with serious diseases, paid but a fraction of that amount back years later. A company spokesman said the plan settled the matter by paying the government $157,777 in December 2013.

<u>Some critics expect little to change unless federal officials disclose Medicare Advantage plans' full service and billing histories — as they have recently done with Medicare fees paid to more than 880,000 individual doctors and others.</u>

"The [Medicare Advantage] plans don't want the data out," said Dr. Brian Biles, a professor in the Department of Health Policy at George Washington University, whose Freedom of Information Act lawsuits shook loose limited enrollment records used in this project. (Biles assisted Center for Public Integrity reporters with the analysis.)

Dr. David Wennberg, a Dartmouth Institute researcher who has studied the payment issue, said that with billions of tax dollars at stake federal officials need to hit the "reset button" on risk scoring.

Wennberg said Medicare Advantage "is a very large program with lots of money flowing through it. There are always vested interests in protecting the status quo."

Health care politics

The Affordable Care Act, or Obamacare, orders deep rate cuts in Medicare Advantage, partly to cover millions of uninsured people. That's consistent with an early Obama administration promise to reduce payments to the health insurers.

But support for Medicare Advantage in Congress has snowballed as it has attracted more and more seniors who are happy with their care and the price they pay for it. Earlier this year, the insurance industry mounted a fierce media campaign to block the rate cuts, enlisting support from more than 200 members of Congress and forcing the administration to partially back off.

The debate over how best to pay Medicare Advantage health plans — and how to curb overcharging — has been contentious for years.

As far back as the 1980s, Congress hoped that carving a bigger role for managed care plans like Medicare Advantage would help curtail overall Medicare spending and ward off waste and fraud that can pop up when doctors and hospitals are paid for each and every service they perform.

To that end, Medicare decided to pay health plans a set monthly rate for patients regardless of how much care they needed. But some health plans stacked the deck by signing up people who were healthier than average, a marketing ploy known in insurance circles as "cherry picking."

That led to a "lot of game playing" and "dumping patients who were ill," said Laurence Bishoff, a Boston health care consultant.

Congress thought it saw a remedy in the Medicare Modernization Act of 2003. The law created Medicare Advantage and phased in "risk adjusted" payments starting a year later.

Thomas Scully, who helped get the program running under President George W. Bush, said rates were generous in hopes of enticing insurers to expand their Medicare business and not shy away from people in poor health. "We very intentionally tried to overpay them a little bit," said Scully, now a Washington lobbyist with numerous health care industry clients.

Health status was added to other factors such as sex, race and age in setting rates. Plans that took on the greatest risk by accepting the sickest patients were paid the most.

But turning to risk scores as the way to adjust payments ushered in a new form of Medicare billing abuse: Some health plans misstated how sick their patients were or failed to document they had treated illnesses Medicare paid them to treat, the Center's investigation found.

By 2009, government officials were estimating that just over 15 percent of total Medicare Advantage payments were inaccurate, about $12 billion that year.

By the end of 2013, officials reported the error rate had dropped to nine percent, which still added up to $11.8 billion for the year. Nearly 80 percent of that — $9.3 billion — was overcharges, records show.

The Medicare Advantage billing error rate has averaged 12 percent over the past six years, at times outpacing that of standard government-run Medicare, which federal officials assert is highly vulnerable to billing fraud and abuse.

Medicare Advantage has faced much less scrutiny. The federal Centers for Medicare and Medicaid Services didn't try to recoup overpayments until 2012, eight years after phasing in risk scoring. And when it did, it won back only $3.4 million — a tiny fraction of the estimated losses, according to government records. Though the agency is beefing up collection efforts starting this year, most health plans won't see federal auditors for years.

Malcolm Sparrow, a professor at Harvard University's John F.

Kennedy School of Government and health fraud expert, said officials are "asking for trouble" by allowing health plans to generate the data on which risk scores and their revenues are based. "You want to make sure this is audited rigorously," Sparrow said. "It's much more expensive [to taxpayers] not to."

Federal probe

Four of the ten major Medicare Advantage plans with the highest average risk scores nationally are in Puerto Rico.

Medicare Advantage plans, which control 70 percent of the island market, argue their patients are poorer and sicker than average. They also say that cuts required under the Affordable Care Act have hit them hard, prompting cuts in benefits and higher premiums for patients who can ill afford to pay more.

Risk scores at the two Aveta-related health plans, MMM Healthcare and Preferred Medical Choice, shot up by an average of 11 percent from 2007 through 2011. Nationwide, the growth rate averaged three percent over the same period. The company had no comment.

San Juan-based Medical Card System, known by the initials MCS, reported a 5 percent rise in the scores over the same time — nearly twice the national average.

The billing practices also have attracted legal scrutiny. The whistleblower lawsuit filed against Aveta by former executive Jose R. "Josh" Valdez alleges that the company overbilled Medicare by as much as $1 billion by inflating risk scores.

Valdez alleges that Aveta paid its stockholders a $100 million dividend during the time that it was overcharging Medicare.

MCS has faced its troubles over risk scores, too.

Federal agents searched the MCS tower headquarters on Oct. 13, 2011. MCS said in a 2012 financial statement that it had received four grand jury subpoenas as part of a U.S. Attorney's Office investigation of its "risk adjustment data reporting."

MCS said the company conducted an "internal review" that found no wrongdoing, but prompted it to return an "immaterial" amount of money to Medicare.

In an April interview inside the MCS tower in San Juan's Hato Rey financial district, Chief Executive Officer Jim O'Drobinak said the federal probe has ended and MCS has been cleared.

"Nothing came of it," he said, blaming the investigation on a "disgruntled former employee." Law enforcement sources confirmed that the investigation has been closed.

Dr. Inés Hernández, MCS chief medical officer, said that the health plan has moved aggressively to treat patients in their homes and identify diseases so they can be treated in the early stages.

"We're not just getting information for risk scores," she said.

But CMS officials have been concerned that home visits and other health assessments by health plans can contribute to higher risk scores — and drive up costs without benefiting patients by providing them with more care.

Over/under

Congressional auditors and some lawmakers have asserted for years that overpayments to Medicare Advantage plans may be much higher than federal officials have acknowledged.

Among the most steadfast critics is <u>Rep. Henry Waxman, D-Calif</u>. In a March 6, 2009, letter to an agency official, he <u>argued that Medicare Advantage plans were a bad deal for taxpayers because each illness they discover, "whether it is treated or not can increase the payment the plan receives from CMS."</u>

Waxman, who then chaired the House Energy and Commerce Committee, criticized health plans for figuring out how to "manipulate" risk scores to wrest money they didn't deserve from Medicare.

CMS officials have conceded that risk scores rose much faster for Medicare Advantage patients than for those in standard Medicare and that the rise couldn't be explained away by saying that the health plan members were sicker.

Starting in 2010, they stepped in and cut payments to Medicare Advantage plans to offset rising risk scores.

Yet in January 2012 the Government Accountability Office, the watchdog arm of Congress, said that the cuts weren't deep enough and opined that Medicare could have saved as much as $3 billion a year by reducing risk scores further.

A year later, the GAO went a step further. A January 2013 report said CMS made "excess payments" to Medicare Advantage plans of between $3.2 billion and $5.1 billion between 2010 and the end of 2012 because risk scores were higher than justified.

The Center for Public Integrity data analysis found that Medicare Advantage can cost the government as much as 25 percent more than standard Medicare in some areas.

The data analysis also found that seemingly tiny variations in risk scores can boost taxpayer costs enormously — especially in health plans that are growing fast.

Industry officials have a different take.

They argue that their members tend to have lower incomes than the elderly population as a whole and have a higher risk of needing expensive medical care.

"They have looked healthier because of incompleteness of this data," said John Gorman, a former federal health official who is now a prominent Medicare Advantage consultant.

Others blame the sheer complexity of risk-scoring for causing confusion about billing.

Jim Redmond, a vice president at Excellus Health Plan, which federal auditors in 2012 said couldn't always document illnesses it was paid to treat, denied any impropriety. He said the billing system was "established with good intentions" but "didn't fully recognize" how difficult it would be for health plans to oversee.

"We have more than 18,000 physicians submitting claims to us every day. We audit a portion of the claims and medical records for accuracy, completeness and consistency," Redmond wrote in an email.

"However, the medical delivery system would grind to a halt if we made every provider submit all of the documentation for each and every claim they file on behalf of members."

Court records show that the billing system's complexity has stymied government investigators reviewing a whistleblower lawsuit filed in 2010 by physician Olivia Graves against Humana.

Graves, who has practiced in South Florida for more than three decades, alleges that a Humana-owned clinic diagnosed patients with conditions such as diabetes with complications, which boosted Medicare payments. She alleged that those diagnoses were "not supported by the medical records." Her suit alleges that Humana knew about the alleged overcharging and did nothing to stop it.

The U.S. Attorney's Office declined to join the South Florida case even though a federal judge granted it 11 requests for more time to investigate. They argued lawyers and other government personnel "had little or no experience in the applicable regulations and operations of the [Medicare Advantage] program" However, government lawyers said their investigation is continuing.

The case was unsealed in May and is pending.

Humana also faces other investigations into allegations that it overbilled the government, including a criminal investigation by the Department of Justice in Washington and a criminal case involving the U.S. Attorney's branch office in West Palm Beach, Florida, according to court records. Humana spokesman Tom Noland said "Humana to our knowledge is not the subject of a criminal investigation."

'Black box'

Many researchers are hoping that CMS will make public detailed Medicare Advantage billing and service data that might allow them to assess how well risk scoring is doing in predicting costs. They also want to study industry claims that they are treating lower income and sicker patients. But that's not yet possible because CMS has shown little interest in making Medicare Advantage data public.

That's quite a different stance than the agency took in April, when it released detailed information about how much individual doctors were paid by Medicare. The decision drew criticism from the American Medical Association, which has argued that it violated the privacy of doctors. CMS principal deputy administrator Jonathan Blum, who left the agency in May, previously announced on his blog that data "can shine a light on how care is delivered in the Medicare program."

Sparrow, the fraud expert from Harvard, said that it should be easier for the government to cough up information about huge health care corporations than about individual physicians. The doctor billing data covers about $77 billion in taxpayer spending for 2012, about half the Medicare Advantage price tag.

"Anything that starts with a 'b' seems like a lot of money to me." Sparrow said, adding that Medicare Advantage financial data and other records "ought to be a matter of ordinary public record."

Medicare Advantage is a "black box," added James Cosgrove, who heads health investigations for the GAO, the audit arm of Congress.

"We know what services they say they will provide ... but we never know exactly what services are being provided," Cosgrove said.

https://www.fiercehealthcare.com/payer/big-name-payers-earned-35-7-billion-2019-here-s-one-common-thread-their-reports
(See hyperlink for full text and references.)

Health Insurers' Profits Topped $35B Last Year: Medicare Advantage is the Common Thread
By Paige Minemyer ; 24 February 2020

Big-name health insurers raked in $35.7 billion in profit in 2019.

The common theme in their financial success? Growth in Medicare Advantage (MA).

Of the seven biggest national insurers, all but one saw notable growth in their MA enrollment by the end of 2019. Many were projecting even bigger expansion to come in 2020.

UnitedHealth Group was once again the most profitable company on the list, netting $13.8 billion in profit across 2019. By comparison, the second-place finisher, CVS, earned $6.6 billion in profit for the year.

CVS edged out UnitedHealth in revenue, however, posting $256.8 billion in annual revenue. UnitedHealth earned $242.2 billion in revenue for the year.

While those two companies led the way by a substantial margin for the industry, Cigna's growth was the most explosive thanks in large part to its ongoing integration with Express Scripts. The insurer's profits nearly doubled within a year, from $2.6 billion in 2018 to $5.1 billion in 2019. Its revenues also skyrocketed, jumping from $48.1 billion in 2018 to $140.2 billion in 2019.

Other plans generally held steady, posting less flashy gains in their year-end reports. All saw an increase in their annual profits. Anthem, for example, saw its revenue grow from $92.1 billion in 2018 to $104.2 billion and profits increase from $3.8 billion in 2018 to $4.8 billion last year.

Humana reported $64.9 billion in revenue for 2019, an increase from $56.9 billion the year before, and earned $2.7 billion in profit for the year, up from $1.7 billion the year prior.

Centene Corporation posted similar gains, with profits increasing from $1.4 billion in 2018 to $1.9 billion and revenues growing from $60.1 billion to $74.6 billion.

Molina, which has continued to emerge from a financial quagmire, reported $737 million in profit for 2019 on $16.2 billion in revenue, up from profits of $707 million on revenue of $17.6 billion in 2018.

While a number of health plans saw their Medicare Advantage enrollment increase in 2019, they're truly eyeing 2020 as a big year for expansion.

UnitedHealthcare saw a Medicare Advantage membership boost from 1.9 million to 2.1 million in 2019. However, the insurer is planning for much bigger things in 2020 - in its guidance, it estimates adding 700,000 new members in Medicare.

Humana estimates 9.2% growth in its Medicare Advantage membership for 2020, adding between 270,000 and 330,000 people to its plans. It reported nearly 5.3 million Medicare Advantage members at the end of 2019.

Cigna views the market as a critical opportunity for expansion, and although its membership in Medicare trails UnitedHealthcare, Humana, Aetna and Anthem by a wide margin, the insurer grew its footprint significantly for the 2020 plan year. That growth is set to continue.

Reader: Have you noticed all the unsolicited phone calls and all the ads on TV about "Medicare Advantage"? **"Medicare for All" would stop all that!!!**

https://www.thenation.com/article/archive/insurance-health-care-medicare/
(See hyperlink for full text and references.) Used with permission.

The 'Public Option' on Health Care
Is a Poison Pill
(Part 1 of 2: The Public Option)
By David U. Himmelstein and Steffie Woolhandler
Co-Founders, PNHP ; 7 October 2019
Some Democratic candidates are pushing it as a free-choice version of Medicare for All. That's good rhetoric but bad policy.

Health care reform has been the most hotly contested issue in the Democratic presidential debates.

Bernie Sanders and Elizabeth Warren have been pushing a single-payer Medicare for All plan, under which a public insurer would cover everyone. They would ban private insurance, except for items not covered by the public plan, such as cosmetic surgery or private rooms in hospitals.

The other Democratic contenders favor a "public option" reform that would introduce a Medicare-like public insurer but would allow private insurers to operate as well. They tout this approach as a less traumatic route to universal coverage that would preserve a free choice of insurers for people happy with their plans.

And some public option backers go further, claiming that the system would painlessly transition to single payer as the public plan outperforms the private insurers.

That's comforting rhetoric. But the case for a public option rests on faulty economic logic and naive assumptions about how private insurance actually works.

Private insurers have proved endlessly creative at gaming the system to avoid fair competition, and they have used their immense lobbying clout to undermine regulators' efforts to rein in their abuses. That has enabled them to siphon hundreds of billions of dollars out of the health care system each year for their own profits and overhead costs while forcing doctors and hospitals to waste billions more on billing-related paperwork. Those dollars have to come from somewhere.

If private insurers required their customers to pay the full costs of private plans, they wouldn't be able to compete with a public plan like the traditional Medicare program, whose overhead costs are far lower.

But this is not the case: In fact, taxpayers – including those *not* enrolled in a private plan – pick up the tab for much of private insurers' profligacy. And the high cost of keeping private insurance alive would make it prohibitively expensive to cover the 30 million uninsured in the United States and to upgrade coverage for the tens of millions with inadequate plans.

Public Option Proposals Come in Three Main Varieties:

§ A Simple Buy-in. Some proposals, including those by Joe Biden and Pete Buttigieg, would offer a Medicare-like public plan for sale alongside private plans on the insurance exchanges now available under the Affordable Care Act. These buy-in reforms would minimize the need for new taxes, since most enrollees would be charged premiums. But tens of millions would remain uninsured or with coverage so skimpy, they still couldn't afford care.

§ Pay or play. This variant (similar to the plan advanced by the Center for American Progress and endorsed by Beto O'Rourke) would offer employers a choice between purchasing private insurance or paying a steep payroll tax (about 8 percent). Anyone lacking employer-paid private coverage would be automatically enrolled in the public plan. The public option would be a good deal for employers who would otherwise have to pay more than 8 percent of their payroll for private coverage — for example, employers with older or mostly female workers (who tend to use more care and incur high premiums) or with lots of low-wage workers (for whom 8 percent of payroll is a relatively small sum). But many firms employing mostly young, male, or highly paid workers (e.g., finance and tech) would likely stay with a private insurer.

§ Medicare Advantage for All. The public option approach favored by Kamala Harris would mimic the current Medicare Advantage program. Medicare Advantage plans are commercial managed care products currently offered by private insurers to seniors. The Centers for Medicare and Medicaid Services (CMS), the federal agency that administers Medicare, collects the taxes that pay for the program and passes the funds ($233 billion in 2018) along to the insurance companies. Under this approach, the public option would operate alongside the private Medicare Advantage plans and compete with them, as the traditional fully public Medicare program currently does.

Because a public option would leave the current dysfunctional payment approach in place, it would sacrifice most of the savings available via single-payer reform. The bottom line is that a public option would either cost much more or deliver much less than single payer.

A final point: While allowing private insurers to compete with a public plan amounts to a poison pill, the same isn't true for supplemental private plans that are allowed to cover only those items excluded from the public benefit package. While Canada bans the sale of private coverage that duplicates the public plan's benefits, it has always allowed supplemental coverage, and that hasn't sabotaged its system.

The efficiencies of a single-payer system would make universal coverage affordable and give everyone in the United States their free choice of doctors and hospitals. But that goal will remain out of reach if private insurers are allowed to continue gaming the system. Preserving the choice of insurer for some would perpetuate the affordability crisis that has bedeviled the US health care system for generations.

https://www.thenation.com/article/archive/insurance-health-care-medicare/
(See hyperlink for full text and references.) Used with permission.

The 'Public Option' on Health Care Is a Poison Pill
(Part 2 of 2: Kamala Harris' Public Option)

By David U. Himmelstein and Steffie Woolhandler
Co-Founders, PNHP ; 7 October 2019

Some Democratic candidates are pushing it as a free-choice version of Medicare for All. That's good rhetoric but bad policy.

Medicare Advantage for All

The public option approach favored by Kamala Harris would mimic the current Medicare Advantage program. Medicare Advantage plans are commercial managed care products currently offered to seniors by private insurers. The Centers for Medicare and Medicaid Services (CMS), the federal agency that administers Medicare, collects the taxes that pay for the program and passes the funds ($233 billion in 2018) along to the insurance companies. Under this approach, the public option would operate alongside the private Medicare Advantage plans and compete with them, as the traditional fully public Medicare program currently does.

In US Health Insurance, Good Guys Finish Last

Decades of experience with Medicare Advantage offer lessons about that program and how private insurers capture profits for themselves and push losses onto their public rival — strategies that allow them to win the competition while driving up everyone's costs.

A public option plan that facilitates enrollees' genuine access to health care can't compete with private insurers that avoid the expensively ill and obstruct access to care. Despite having overhead costs almost seven times that of traditional Medicare (13.7 versus 2 percent), Medicare Advantage plans have grown rapidly. They now cover more than one-third of Medicare beneficiaries, up from 13 percent in 2005. Greed has trumped efficiency, and the efforts of regulators to level the playing field have been overwhelmed by insurers' profit-driven schemes to tilt it.

Private insurers employ a dizzying array of profit-enhancing schemes that would be out of bounds for a public plan. These schemes, which

242

continually evolve in response to regulators' efforts to counter them, boil down to four strategies that are legal, in addition to occasional outright fraud.

§ **Obstructing expensive care.** Plans try to attract profitable, low-needs enrollees by assuring convenient and affordable access to routine care for minor problems. Simultaneously, they erect barriers to expensive services that threaten profits — for example, prior authorization requirements, high co-payments, narrow networks, and drug formulary restrictions that penalize the unprofitably ill.

While the fully public Medicare program contracts with any willing provider, many private insurers exclude (for example) cystic fibrosis specialists, and few Medicare Advantage plans cover care at cancer centers like Memorial Sloan Kettering.

Moreover, private insurers' drug formularies often put all of the drugs — even cheap generics — needed by those with diabetes, schizophrenia, or HIV in a high co-payment tier.

Insurers whose first reaction to a big bill is "claim denied" discourage many patients from pursuing their claims. And as discussed below, if hassling over claims drives some enrollees away, even better: The sickest will be the most hassled and therefore the most likely to switch to a competitor.

§ **Cherry-picking and lemon-dropping**, or selectively enrolling people who need little care and disenrolling the unprofitably ill. A relatively small number of very sick patients account for the vast majority of medical costs each year. A plan that dodges even a few of these high-needs patients wins, while a competing plan that welcomes all comers loses.

In the employer market, cherry-picking is easy: Private insurers offer attractive premiums to businesses with young, healthy workers and exorbitant rates to those with older, sicker employees. As a letter this summer to *The New York Times* put it, like casinos, health insurers are profitable because they know the odds of every bet they place — and the house always wins.

The CMS, in theory, requires Medicare Advantage plans to take all comers and prohibits them from forcing people out when they get sick.

243

But regulators' efforts to enforce these requirements have been overwhelmed by insurers' chicanery.

To avoid the sick, private insurers manipulate provider networks and drug formulary designs. Despite the ban on forcing enrollees out, patients needing high-cost services like dialysis or nursing home care have switched in droves from private plans to traditional, fully public Medicare. And as a last resort, Medicare Advantage plans will stop offering coverage in a county where they've accumulated too many unprofitable enrollees, akin to a casino ejecting players who are beating the house.

Finally, Medicare Advantage plans cherry-pick through targeted marketing schemes. In the past, this has meant sign-up dinners in restaurants difficult to access for people who use wheelchairs or offering free fitness center memberships, a perk that appeals mainly to the healthiest seniors.

Higher-tech approaches are just around the corner. Will "Oscar", the health insurer founded by Jared Kushner's brother (with Google's parent company as a significant investor) resist the temptation to use Google's trove of personal data to target enrollment ads toward profitable enrollees like tennis enthusiasts and avoid purchasers of plus-size clothing or people who have searched online for fertility treatments?

§ **Upcoding**, or making enrollees look sicker on paper than they really are to inflate risk-adjusted premiums. To counter cherry-picking, the CMS pays Medicare Advantage plans higher premiums for enrollees with more (and more serious) diagnoses. For instance, a Medicare Advantage plan can collect hundreds of dollars more each month from the government by labeling an enrollee's temporary sadness as "major depression" or calling trivial knee pain "degenerative arthritis." By applying serious-sounding diagnoses to minor illnesses, Medicare Advantage plans artificially inflate the premiums they collect from taxpayers by billions of dollars while adding little or nothing to their expenditures for care.

Though most upcoding stays within the letter of the law and merely stretches medical terminology, the CMS's (rare) audits of enrollees' charts indicate that Medicare Advantage plans are collecting $10 billion annually from taxpayers for entirely fabricated diagnoses.

And that's only a small fraction of their overall take from upcoding. Private insurers keep most of this pilfered money for their profits and overhead, but they use a portion to fund added benefits (for example, eyeglasses or slightly lower co-payments for routine care) that attract new enrollees and help private plans to seemingly outcompete traditional Medicare.

§ **Lobbying to get excessive payments and thwart regulators.** Congress has mandated that the CMS overpay Medicare Advantage plans by 2 percent (and even more where medical costs are lower than average). On top of that, Seema Verma, Trump's CMS administrator, has taken steps that will increase premiums significantly and award unjustified "quality bonuses," ignoring advice from the Medicare Payment Advisory Commission that payments be trimmed because the government is already overpaying the private plans. And she has ordered changes to the CMS's Medicare website to trumpet the benefits of Medicare Advantage enrollment.

In sum, a public option insurer that, like traditional Medicare, doesn't try to dodge unprofitable enrollees would be saddled with more than its share of sick, expensive patients and would become a de facto high-cost, high-risk pool. The CMS's decades-long efforts to level the playing field have been thwarted by insurers' upcoding, belying their promises of fair competition.

And insurance companies have used their political muscle to sustain and increase their competitive advantage over traditional Medicare. The result: The public plan (and the taxpayers) absorbs the losses while private insurers skim off profits, an imbalance so big that private plans can out-compete a public plan despite squandering vast sums on overhead costs, CEO salaries, and shareholder profits.

Single Payer Would Save, Public Option Won't

This year alone, private insurers will take in $252 billion more than they pay out, equivalent to 12 percent of their premiums. A single-payer system with overhead costs comparable to Medicare's (2 percent) could save about $220 billion of that money. A public option would save far less - possibly zero, if much of the new public coverage is channeled through Medicare Advantage plans, whose overhead, at 13.7 percent, is even higher than the average commercial insurer.

Moreover, a public option would save little or nothing on hospitals' and doctors' sky-high billing and administrative costs. In a single-payer system, hospitals and other health facilities could be funded via global, lump-sum budgets - similar to the way cities pay fire departments - eliminating the need to attribute costs to individual patients and collect payments from them and their insurers.

That global budget payment strategy has cut administrative costs at hospitals in Canada and Scotland to half the US level. The persistence of multiple payers would preclude such administrative streamlining, even if all of the payers are charged the same rates. (Under Maryland's mislabeled global budget system, the state's hospitals charge uniform rates but continue to bill per patient; our research indicates that their administrative costs haven't fallen at all, according to their official cost reports.)

Similarly, for physicians and other practitioners, the complexity involved in billing multiple payers, dealing with multiple drug formularies and referral networks, collecting co-payments and deductibles, and obtaining referrals and prior authorizations drives up office overhead costs and documentation burdens.

The excess overhead inherent to multi-payer systems imposes a hidden surcharge on the fees that doctors and hospitals must charge all patients - not just those covered by private insurance. <u>All told, a public option reform would sacrifice about $350 billion annually of single payer's potential savings on providers' overhead costs, over and above the $220 billion in savings it could sacrifice annually on insurers' overhead.</u>

Finally, a public option would undermine the rational health planning that is key to the long-term savings under single payer. Each dollar that a hospital invests in new buildings or equipment increases its operating costs by 20 to 25 cents in every subsequent year. At present, hospitals that garner profits (or "surpluses" for nonprofits) have the capital to expand money-making services and buy high-tech gadgets, whether they're needed or not, while neglecting vital but unprofitable services.

For instance, hospitals around the country have invested in proton-beam-radiation therapy centers that cost hundreds of millions of dollars apiece. (Oklahoma City alone now has two.) Yet there's little evidence that those machines are any better for most uses than their far cheaper alternatives.

Similarly, hospitals have rushed to open invasive cardiology and orthopedic surgery programs, often close to existing ones. These duplicative investments raise costs and probably compromise quality.

Meanwhile, primary care and mental health services have languished, and rural hospitals and other cash-strapped facilities that provide much-needed care spiral toward closure.

As in Canada and several European nations, a single-payer system could fund new hospital investments through government grants based on an explicit assessment of needs, instead of counting on private hospitals to use their profits wisely. That strategy has helped other nations direct investments to areas and services with the greatest need and to avoid funding wasteful or redundant facilities. Public option proposals would perpetuate current payment strategies that distort investment and raise long-term costs.

Because a public option would leave the current dysfunctional payment approach in place, it would sacrifice most of the savings available via single-payer reform. The bottom line is that a public option would either cost much more or deliver much less than single payer.

A final point: While allowing private insurers to compete with a public plan amounts to a poison pill, the same isn't true for supplemental private plans that are allowed to cover only those items excluded from the public benefit package. While Canada bans the sale of private coverage that duplicates the public plan's benefits, it has always allowed supplemental coverage, and that hasn't sabotaged its system.

The efficiencies of a single-payer system would make universal coverage affordable and give everyone in the United States their free choice of doctors and hospitals. But that goal will remain out of reach if private insurers are allowed to continue gaming the system.

Preserving the choice of insurer for some would perpetuate the affordability crisis that has bedeviled the US health care system for generations.

Proponents of the public option portray it as a nondisruptive, free-choice version of single payer. That may be good campaign rhetoric, but it's terrible policy.

Mr. President: Please Don't Be Swayed by Neera Tanden's Bias Against Medicare for All

The Office of Management and Budget (OMB) is the largest office within the Executive Office of the President of the United States (EOP). OMB's most prominent function is to produce the president's budget, but it also examines agency programs, policies, and procedures to see whether they comply with the president's policies and coordinates inter-agency policy initiatives.

On November 30, 2020, President-elect Joe Biden introduced Neera Tanden as his nominee for Director of the Office of Management and Budget. Immediately afterwards, Tanden deleted over 1,000 of her previous tweets, and changed her Twitter bio from "progressive" to "liberal".

On March 2, 2021, President Biden withdrew the nomination after Ms. Tanden wrote "it now seems clear that there is no path forward to gain confirmation". In May 2021, Tanden was hired to become a senior adviser to President Biden.

Tanden is a longtime ally of Hillary Clinton and has often vocally criticized both Republicans and Democrats, especially supporters of Bernie Sanders.

Much of Tanden's work relates to healthcare policy in America. In 2003, she had a central role in founding CAP: the Center for American Progress. Tanden worked on the passage of the Affordable Care Act during the Obama administration, and supports a multi-payer universal healthcare system, and opposes single-payer healthcare, including Medicare for All proposals.

In 2018, under Ms. Tanden's leadership, CAP released "Medicare Extra for All" – a proposal that preserves a role for employer coverage and for the health insurance industry.

This differs greatly from true "Medicare for All" which emphasizes that significant cost savings cannot be achieved as long as the huge profits of the insurance industry continue to be protected. As indicated by Dr. Abdul El-Sayed, co-author of "Medicare for All: A Citizen's Guide" (**https://www.commonwealthclub.org/events/archive/video/citizens-**

guide-medicare-all), in an interview with The Commonwealth Club, one hasn't thoroughly removed risk in the swimming pool if one leaves the barracudas in the pool.

Any role that Ms. Tanden might play in The Biden Administration would undermine the desire of approximately 70% of voters who support "Improved Medicare for All" as outlined in Senate Bill 1129 spearheaded by Senator Bernie Sanders and H.R.1976 spearheaded by Representative Pramila Jayapal.

https://pnhp.org/news/caps-medicare-extra-for-all-what-it-really-is/
(See hyperlink for full text and references.)

What is this "Medicare Extra for All" proposal by CAP?
Comment by Don McCanne, M.D., 22 February 2018

What is this "Medicare Extra for All" proposal by the Center for American Progress (CAP), and where does it or should it stand in the movement for health care for all?

First of all, it is not a single payer proposal. It leaves in place much of our multi-payer system, including Medicare, Medicare Advantage, employer-sponsored health plans, the individual and small group market plans, TRICARE, Veterans Affairs medical care, and FEHBP – the Federal Employees Health Benefits Program. Private insurers continue to thrive – selling us risk-bearing plans favorable to them and/or excessive administrative services. Their iniquitous tools such as excessive cost sharing and narrow provider networks will not go away. The fundamental health care infrastructure remains in place in spite of the fact that some admittedly beneficial tweaks are recommended in this proposal.

What this proposal really is is a glorified version of the public option – a Medicare-like government plan that would be used to attempt to cover those who are uninsured and could be a replacement for those who are underinsured. If you carefully review the CAP proposal you will see that it adds both costs and administrative complexity to our existing health care financing system. It forgoes much of the cost containment and administrative simplicity of a bona fide single payer system.

As one example, look at their description of the administrative efficiencies they tout in their plan. They claim that they "would take advantage of the current Medicare program's low administrative costs," but their Medicare Extra plan adds other administrative costs and yet it would represent only a small fraction of health care financing considering that most of the existing multi-payer system would remain in place. They claim that electronic submission of claims through electronic health records would provide efficiencies, yet yesterday's Quote of the Day demonstrated that those savings have not been realized and costs were actually increased when considering investments in the technology. They have not seriously addressed the profound administrative waste in our system.

A particular irony in this proposal is that they suggest replacing the private Medicare Advantage plans with private Medicare Choice plans. This reverts to the prior Medicare + Choice plans which were paid at rates of 95 percent of the costs in the traditional Medicare program, allowing them to prove that they could provide higher quality at lower costs. They couldn't, and the program began to tank until it was rescued by the Medicare Advantage program which gave the private plans a tremendously unfair advantage at taxpayer expense. The authors of Medicare Extra don't even give us a hint as to how they will entice the private insurers to jump back into their Medicare Choice plans.

A little bit of history of the Center for American Progress is enlightening. It was founded by John Podesta – Bill Clinton's Chief of Staff. It has professed to represent and advance progressive/liberal values, but it really represents the neo-liberal element that has assumed control of the Democratic Party. Their current CEO is Neera Tanden who led the forces that successfully blocked the Sanders camp from inserting a single payer plank in the Democratic Party platform, protecting Hillary Clinton who considered single payer to be a threat. The neo-liberals have been very protective of the private insurance industry and have been successful to the degree that they lured many single payer progressives into their camp in support of the Affordable Care Act – legislation designed to protect and enhance the interests of the private insurance industry. How could we have expected more out of the Center for American Progress than this highly deficient proposal with a pro-industry bias?

Already the media is jumping on this as a new, liberal, Medicare for All proposal. Even the progressive New York Times columnist David Leonhardt is calling this "A Better Single-Payer Plan." Worse, he is falling into line with the comment, "I still favor more modest health care proposals to sweeping, ambitious plans, for reasons of realpolitik." Shades of HCAN (see * below) and the erection of political barriers to single payer reform. We've said repeatedly, single payer policy is right but it's the politics that are wrong. Don't change good policy; change bad politics!

We can't leave this topic without acknowledging the one bit of good news here. Single payer Medicare for All is a vastly superior model of financing health care – a model we desperately need in this nation – and a majority of the public now realizes that. The neo-liberal Democrats realize that they cannot go into an election touting a model that many feel has fallen far short of our needs, especially when the concept of an improved Medicare for all has gained so much traction. CAP recognizes the threat and takes this challenge so seriously that they have elected to "go bolder" by dummying up a fake Medicare for All plan, calling it "Medicare Extra for All." We just have to be sure that the public is not lured by this siren song. They want the real thing.

Stay informed! Visit https://pnhp.org/news-category/quote-of-the-day/ to sign up for daily email updates.

*"Shades of HCAN"** (Referenced in above article):
https://www.healthcare-now.org/about/regarding-hcan/
(See hyperlink for full text and references.)

Regarding HCAN: Healthcare-NOW Position Regarding Health Care for America Now
Prepared by the Healthcare-NOW Board Steering Committee

On July 8, 2008, a coalition of organizations called Health Care for America Now (HCAN) announced a campaign for healthcare reform. A spokesperson for the group stated that they plan to run a multi-million dollar ad campaign and will promote health care reform that offers a mix of public funding and private insurance.

Partly because the name of the new group is so similar to our own, it is important that we point out what distinguishes the HCAN position from ours. Even more essential, the distinction is important because the policy issue is the crucial foundation of successful health care reform.

<u>The central role of private insurance companies in the HCAN plan will leave us with the same bad actors that are currently running amok in our health care.</u> We cannot place the fox in the hen house and then hope to regulate his diet.

It is in the nature of private health insurance corporations to seek to enhance their profit. The private health insurance system we have leaves 48 million Americans uninsured, causes 18,000 deaths/year, and accounts for half of the bankruptcies each year.

Liz Fowler is Back!
And She's Writing US Health Policy Again
By Kay Tillow, 7 June 2021

Liz Fowler is back! For those who followed the battles of the health care reform of 2009-2010, no name rouses more controversy than that of Elizabeth "Liz" Fowler who, as Chief Health Counsel to Senate Finance Committee Chairman Max Baucus, played a critical role in the writing of the Affordable Care Act.

Fowler, former vice president of public policy and external affairs at Wellpoint, the giant health insurance company that later became Anthem, wrote the reform policy to protect the future and the profits of the industry from which she came. Thanks to her efforts, Anthem and other for-profit insurance companies prospered from Fowler's ability to craft the Affordable Care Act to their liking. In 2020, Anthem reported over $4.5 billion in net income.

Now Liz Fowler is back, writing U. S. health care policy in line with insurance company desires. President Biden appointed her to head up the Center for Medicare and Medicaid Innovation (CMMI) within the Center for Medicare and Medicaid Services (CMS). She's back to the top spot to direct the future of health care.

Back in 2009, the insurance industry and anti-single payer policy experts promoted CMMI and wrote it into the Affordable Care Act to promote cost cutting in Medicare, Medicaid and CHIP through value-based payment models. But CMMI's work is based on the wrong-headed theory that U. S. healthcare is too expensive because of overuse. Value-based payment advocates claim that too many doctors and hospitals are giving too much care. CMMI wants to reverse the payment scheme and pay doctors and hospitals more for doing less. They contend they will be paying for quality or value rather than quantity.

Their attempts to force doctors to fill out endless forms are stressing physicians, but they have yet to find a way to accurately measure value. CMMI is working from a false premise: in the U.S., patients see their

253

doctors an average of 4 times annually while in the U. K., France, Canada, Australia, Germany and Japan, patients see their physicians from 5 to over 12 times a year. In the U.S., Americans spend an average of .6 days per year in the hospital, whereas residents of other wealthy countries spend up to three times that number. So, if Americans are seeing their doctors less and spending fewer days in the hospital, why are we still spending more than other wealthy countries on health care?

There is a battle raging over what must be done to cover everyone and rein in costs. Single payer, improved Medicare for All, advocates assert that the key is to remove profit-making insurance companies and hospitals from the system, slashing administrative waste to the point where savings can improve care for those who are covered and expand it to those who are uninsured.

Costs will be stabilized and even reduced because the profitmaking mechanisms are the source of the high costs, not the overutilization of services. Single payer advocates point to the fact that the U.S. spends on health care about double, per capita, what other wealthy countries spend. Yet the US has, on average, worse outcomes.

A plan to remove profit-making from the system is the only plan that would rein in costs. The CMMI, meanwhile, is constructed around insurance company magical thinking of health care reform: cut costs while giving less but better care.

Over the past decade, CMMI has experimented by setting up a number of alternate payment schemes designed to shift insurance risk onto hospitals and physicians. The results have not been good. Most of the CMMI experiments have been disappointing — either they don't improve care, or they worsen care, or they don't save money. Only 4 models of over 48 experiments have been adopted.

The conclusion should be that if we are to expand care and reduce costs, we should adopt a well-designed national single payer plan. But the Biden Administration has rejected that logical conclusion. Instead, the President has brought back Liz Fowler to find a way to make their pro-insurance company plan work.

The voluntary experiments of the CMMI have not proven the quality gains and cost saving that the insurance industry and its loyal experts predicted. Thus, Liz Fowler to the rescue. Fowler and others have hinted that they're looking to move from voluntary to mandatory experiments that will force greater risks onto physicians, other caregivers, and hospitals.

How much more of this nonsensical misery must the nation endure?

A decade ago, Marcia Angell, MD, former editor of the New England Journal of Medicine, explained that in a for-profit insurance system, costs and care move in the same direction. To increase care, cover more people with better care, costs are increased as well. In a for-profit system, cutting costs also cuts care. To shift the dynamics and improve care while reining in costs, one must change to a single payer, not-for-profit system. She was right.

When Senator Max Baucus refused to allow single payer advocates to participate in the hearings on the Affordable Care Act, nurses, doctors, and others stood to speak. Baucus called the police and had them arrested. But their courage to act sparked a debate and planted a banner for single payer. It's time to lift up that banner once again.

See also https://www.singlepayeraction.org/: Liz Fowler Defending Trump Program to Privatize Medicare (16 January 2022)

https://student.pnhp.org/category/blog/
(Published in The Lens: https://thelensnola.org/2019/04/18/rep-richmond-should-co-sponsor-the-medicare-for-all-act/)

Our Elected Officials Must Support Medicare for All

By Frances Gill, 24 April 2019
**"Our healthcare system is rotten to the core,
and half-measures and meager reforms won't cut it."**

In late February (2019), Seattle-area U.S. Rep. Pramila Jayapal introduced a "Medicare for All" bill in Congress that immediately attracted more than 100 Democratic co-sponsors. The legislation, if passed, would provide comprehensive healthcare coverage — medical, dental, prescriptions, long-term care, mental health, and more — to every resident in the United States, with no copays, premiums, or deductibles.

Medicare for All is a wildly popular policy. Recent polls show that 70 percent of Americans support Medicare for All, including 85 percent of Democrats and 52 percent of Republicans.

Why, then, has our Representative Cedric Richmond (LA-02) not co-sponsored his fellow Democrat's bill, one that saves working families money and guarantees healthcare security to every single person in America?

Perhaps he fears that Medicare for All is too pie-in-the-sky. Comprehensive, universal coverage? How could we afford something so extravagant? One estimate from Senator Bernie Sanders' office calculated that through a combination of progressive income taxes, capital gains and dividends taxes, and limits on tax deductions for the wealthy, we could raise $1.8 trillion over 10 years without needing to raise taxes on the middle and working class.

There are also significant savings associated with transitioning to a Medicare for All program, due to decreased administrative costs and the federal government's ability to negotiate drug prices. Consequently, even a study from a libertarian think tank, the Mercatus Center, showed that Medicare for All would ultimately save trillions of dollars.

Meanwhile, the average family of four with employer-sponsored insurance spent $28,166 on health insurance in 2018. Medicare for All would likely save the average working person thousands of dollars per year by eliminating co-pays, deductibles, and premiums.

Or perhaps Richmond doesn't want to rock the boat? Isn't the American healthcare system the envy of the world? But the reality is that we are already spending more money than any other industrialized nation — about double what other rich countries spend per capita — and still achieving worse outcomes.

The U.S. spends a fifth of our GDP on healthcare costs, yet our maternal mortality rate continues to rise, even as the global maternal mortality rate falls. Over the last few years, the rate of congenital syphilis — a completely preventable and debilitating illness — has more than doubled. In Louisiana, Black women are four times more likely to die in childbirth than white women.

Although universal healthcare coverage is not a panacea, it would at least ensure that there are no gaps in coverage during a person's lifetime, greatly increasing the likelihood that new mothers would receive timely prenatal care.

Perhaps Richmond is worried about longer wait times, or perhaps he fears that transitioning to Medicare for All will lead to rationing of care. But the reality is that we are already rationing care: patients with money or excellent insurance can get seen quickly, while the rest of us have to wait.

Perhaps Richmond thinks we simply don't need Medicare for All. After all, thanks to the expansion of Medicaid, hundreds of thousands of Louisianans gained coverage. But currently, 11.4 percent of Louisianans live without health insurance. And for those with insurance, instead of comprehensive care that's free at the point of service, as Medicare for All would be, insurance companies deliver high premiums, deductibles, copays and denials of service.

Health justice activists have been fighting for universal coverage for decades. Now, in part due to a powerful national coalition formed between National Nurses United, the Democratic Socialists of America, and several other organizations, we are closer than ever before to making this a reality.

Our local New Orleans chapter of the DSA — an organization that has almost 60,000 dues-paying members nationally and hundreds locally — has been building a campaign to demand Medicare for All. We've been canvassing our neighborhoods, tabling at public events, organizing community health fairs, and pressuring our politicians. Most importantly, we've been listening to the community's healthcare horror stories. We, the people of New Orleans, are in dire need of better healthcare, and Medicare for All is the only policy tool that can make that happen.

We've talked to people who waited weeks to see a specialist because there are so few physicians who accept Medicaid insurance. We've spoken with neighbors who paid thousands of dollars in medical bills even though they had insurance. We've met people who are afraid to go to the doctor at all — they're afraid of what they might find and what it might cost. The Medicare for All legislation put forward by Jayapal is sorely needed to correct the inadequacies and failures of our nation's healthcare system.

Other politicians have also proposed solutions, but they all fall short. Presidential candidate Beto O'Rourke, a former congressman, has spoken in support of the Medicare for America Act, but this program wouldn't provide universal coverage, and it doesn't eliminate co-pays, premiums, or deductibles. (Note how the name similarity of "Medicare for All" and "Medicare for America" allows politicians to capitalize on Medicare for All's popularity by using the #M4A hashtag.)

By retaining private insurance alongside public insurance, Medicare for America would simply perpetuate the tiered, hierarchical system we have now. A crucial aspect of the Medicare for All plan is that it brings everyone together under the same health plan, thus moving us towards a future where everyone has access to the same, high-quality care.

Other approaches, such as the "public option," which allows individuals to buy into the Medicaid or Medicare programs, have been shown to be deeply ineffective. In 2013, the Congressional Budget Office (CBO) reported that this approach would have "minimal impacts" on the number of uninsured Americans.

Our healthcare system is rotten to the core, and half-measures and meager reforms won't cut it. We need to pursue radical transformation and effect real change. Right now, we have the political opportunity to do so.

Consistently, when we are talking to our fellow constituents in Richmond's district, we hear the same refrain: of course we want this, of course we need this, how is it possible that our congressman doesn't support this?

Soon, for the first time in U.S. history, legislation on the implementation of a single-payer healthcare system will be heard before congressional committees. These hearings will be great opportunities to show Louisianans how transformative a Medicare for All program would be.

Richmond has voiced tentative support for the bill, but we need him to turn that talk into action: we need him to co-sponsor this legislation. As the former head of the Congressional Black Caucus, Richmond is a leader on Capitol Hill. We need his leadership on healthcare. Otherwise, his constituents will continue to endure substandard care, to be driven into medical bankruptcy, and to die of preventable illnesses.

If Richmond truly believes that all Louisianans, no matter their income or their age or their medical history, deserve comprehensive healthcare, he will co-sponsor the Medicare for All Act and champion it in the halls of Congress. If he chooses not to do that, we hope he'll tell us: which of his constituents does he believe should go without healthcare?

Frances Gill is a medical student and co-chair of the Health Care Committee in the New Orleans chapter of the Democratic Socialists of America. The DSA is a national organization with chapters in New Orleans and Baton Rouge. Email healthcare@dsaneworleans.org for more information.

<u>Lobbyist Documents Reveal Health Care Industry Battle Plan Against "Medicare for All"</u>

"By Lee Fang and Nick Surgey. Originally published on November 20, 2018. Reprinted with permission from *The Intercept* [https://theintercept.com/2018/11/20/medicare-for-all-healthcare-industry/], an award-winning nonprofit news organization dedicated to holding the powerful accountable through fearless, adversarial journalism."
(Underline not in original article: added by L. O'Connell)

Now that the midterms are finally over, the battle against "Medicare for All" that has been quietly waged throughout the year is poised to take center stage.

Internal strategy documents obtained by The Intercept and Documented reveal the strategy that private health care interests plan to use to influence Democratic Party messaging and stymie the momentum toward achieving universal health care coverage.

At least 48 incoming freshman lawmakers campaigned on enacting "Medicare for All" or similar efforts to expand access to Medicare. And over the last year, 123 incumbent House Democrats co-sponsored "Medicare for All" legislation — double the number who supported the same bill during the previous legislative session.

The growing popularity of "Medicare for All" in the House has made progressives optimistic that the Democratic Party will embrace ideas to expand government coverage options with minimal out-of-pocket costs for patients going into the 2020 election. But industry groups have watched the development with growing concern.

Over the summer (of 2018), <u>leading pharmaceutical, insurance, and hospital lobbyists formed the Partnership for America's Health Care Future, an ad hoc alliance of private health interests, to curb support for expanding Medicare.</u>

The campaign, according to one planning document, is designed to "change the conversation around Medicare for All," then "minimize the potential for this option in health care from becoming part of a national political party's platform in 2020."

Behind the scenes, the group attempted to sway candidates during the midterms, encouraging several of them to focus on shoring up the ACA instead of supporting single-payer health care.

The documents show that Partnership representatives spoke to the staffs of Democratic Sens. Bill Nelson of Florida and Joe Donnelly of Indiana, and received confirmation that both senators would maintain their "moderate position". When the team met with Rep.-elect Lori Trahan, D-Mass., she said that although she does not speak about the issue, she agreed that "language around single payer should be tempered." (None of the three politicians' offices provided responses to inquiries from The Intercept.)

In several competitive races, the Partnership pressed candidates to use industry-crafted talking points when speaking about health care. In one internal planning document circulated with health care lobbyists, the Partnership touted its influence over Danny O'Connor, the Columbus, Ohio-area Democrat who ran for the 12th Congressional District, claiming that O'Connor used Partnership talking points "in national news interviews." (O'Connor's campaign did not respond to a request for comment.)

Several of the candidates who agreed to embrace the Partnership's messaging and policy ideas, including Donnelly and O'Connor, came up short on Election Day. A recount ending on November 18 confirmed that Nelson received fewer votes than Republican challenger Rick Scott. But soon after Election Day results came in, the Partnership went on the offensive, informing reporters that candidates who embraced "Medicare for All" had also lost, pointing to the defeat of progressives such as Kara Eastman in Nebraska. The group also relied on research from the business-friendly Democratic think tank Third Way to argue that victorious pro-"Medicare for All" candidates couldn't attribute their success to having supported "Medicare for All" because few Democrats explicitly mentioned the policy in their campaign advertisements.

"'Medicare for All' didn't win," said Joel Kopperud, the vice president of government affairs at the Council of Insurance Agents and Brokers, one of the industry groups backing the Partnership. "I don't think that the Bernie Sanders $32 trillion solution that's going to eviscerate the insurance for 156 million Americans is really something that's going to be helpful to the party in critical states," he added in an interview with The Intercept.

Kopperud represents insurance brokers who sell employer-based health insurance coverage. He noted that his organization has a vested interest in backing the Partnership. "Medicare for All," as some envision the policy, would eventually eliminate the need for most health insurance plans — a death knell for companies represented by the CIAB.

Private health care lobbyists are confident that they can prevent any federal expansion of Medicare in Congress, given Republican control of the Senate and the White House. In the states, CIAB and other private health groups have easily defeated measures to develop single-payer proposals, such as the ColoradoCare ballot question in 2016.

But the political calculus could be changing. Recent election gains by Democrats in state government could create new opportunities for proponents of expanded government-backed health care initiatives. Gov.-elect Gavin Newsom of California campaigned on single payer and is expected to have one of the largest Democratic supermajorities in recent memory in the legislature, though California has a notoriously complex state constitution that would likely require an amendment before any significant government plan could be created.

The growing momentum for "Medicare for All" could raise expectations for the next time Democrats are in full control of power in Washington, industry groups worry. They are already pressuring conservative-leaning caucuses in the House of Representatives, such as the Blue Dogs and New Democrats Coalition, to push back against insurgent progressives' demands.

Reframing the Debate

For industry opponents of expanded government health insurance, there are two main challenges. One is combating growing public support for the idea. The other is shaping elite opinion within the Beltway.

Over the last two years, several opinion surveys show rising support for expanding Medicare. In March (2018), the Kaiser Health Tracking Poll found that 59 percent of Americans support the idea, and by August, a poll conducted by Reuters-Ipsos found an astounding 70 percent of Americans support "Medicare for All," including a majority of self-identified Republicans.

But the Partnership is quick to zero in on research that shows support for the idea drops precipitously when respondents are told that the plan would require ending employer-based coverage, tax increases, and increased government control.

The campaign has worked with advertising agencies to draw up a series of messages to convince select audiences. Several of the messages, categorized as "positive," are dedicated to educating the public on more minimal reforms that do not include expanding Medicare. Other messages, categorized as "persuasion" and "aggressive," are designed to instill fear about what could happen if "Medicare for All" passes.

In the coming weeks, the Partnership plans to ramp up a campaign designed to derail support for "Medicare for All." The group, working with leading Democratic political consultants, will place issue advertisements to target audiences, partner with Beltway think tanks to release studies to raise concerns with the plan, and work to shape the public discourse through targeted advocacy in key congressional districts.

The Partnership has tapped consulting firms with deep ties to Democratic officials. Forbes-Tate, a lobbying firm founded by former officials in President Bill Clinton's administration and conservative Democrats in Congress, is managing part of the Partnership coalition. Blue Engine Message & Media, a firm founded by former campaign aides to President Barack Obama, has handled the Partnership's interactions with the media.

In one planning document circulated over the summer, the Partnership suggested a series of messages to wean Americans away from supporting single payer. The talking points emphasize that the current system provides "world-class care," and that any move away from the Affordable Care Act would be "ripping apart our current system."

The strategy exploits familiar themes that have long been used by business groups against new government health care programs, calling for allies to say lines such as "bureaucrats in DC have no understanding of a person's medical situation and will be making decisions about your health care instead of doctors."

The Partnership plans to form a speakers bureau of former Democratic elected officials who can leverage the media to make the case that expanding Medicare is bad politics and policy. The memo names former Democratic Majority Leader Tom Daschle, now a health insurance lobbyist at the law firm Baker Donelson, as one such potential surrogate.

The memo points to early success in shaping media coverage, citing several "earned media" columns such as one published in August by former Rep. Jill Long Thompson, D-Ind., which argues that Democrats should only focus on small reforms to the Affordable Care Act, and warns against wasting political capital on pursuing a "government-controlled health insurance system." Thompson, now an associate professor at Indiana University Bloomington, did not respond to a request for comment.

Adam Gaffney, president-elect of Physicians for a National Health Program, a national coalition that advocates in favor of "Medicare for All," said he is not surprised by the messaging.

"What we're seeing is the wages of success: With single payer on the rise, it was only a matter of time before the insurance companies, big pharma, and other big-money groups came out swinging," said Gaffney, who also serves as an instructor at Harvard Medical School.

"The smear of 'socialized medicine' has been used a thousand times and has lost its bite," he added.

Influencing the 2020 Democratic Field

"We're all focused on 2020," Lauren Crawford Shaver, a partner at Forbes-Tate who is helping to manage the Partnership campaign, recently told the National Association of Health Underwriters in a podcast produced by the group.

Shaver, a former top staffer for the Hillary Clinton presidential campaign, explained to the group that she is working to peel support away from the "Medicare for All" bill sponsored by Sen. Bernie Sanders, I-Vt. The Sanders bill is currently sponsored by several rumored 2020 Democratic presidential candidates, including Sens. Elizabeth Warren, D-Mass.; Kamala Harris, D-Calif.; and Kirsten Gillibrand, D-N.Y.

"The No. 1 thing we need to focus on is that there are a lot of likely candidates that currently support the Senate bill," said Shaver. "We need to make sure we educate the public, we educate both parties, and we educate all the campaigns about both the policy and political challenges."

Shaver encouraged health care companies concerned about the growing popularity of "Medicare for All" to mobilize opposition among clients, customers, and employees. Industry groups will likely have workers or customers residing in key districts who can be tapped to influence wavering lawmakers on Capitol Hill.

The Partnership plans to "take stories of how these proposals would directly impact your clients and the constituents of the policymakers who are voting for or against these proposals," Shaver said.

The Partnership strategy echoes the health insurance industry's campaign to shape the 2008 presidential primary. At that time, the health insurance lobby group known as America's Health Insurance Plans, or AHIP, tapped the consulting firm APCO to develop an effort to label any government-run insurance option as an existential threat to Democratic political goals. The initiative emerged from a plan to minimize the impact of Michael Moore's documentary "Sicko," which was deeply critical of the American health care system.

The campaign involved planting studies with think tanks, mobilizing pundits on television, and sponsoring YouTube videos on "the horrors of government-run systems," among other publicity tactics. The APCO-crafted blitz leaned on right-wing voices such as Fox News pundit John Stossel, conservative think tanks like the American Enterprise Institute, and centrist Democratic groups such as the Democratic Leadership Council, a now-defunct group associated with the Third Way. The 2008 campaign adopted a two-pronged strategy: position private health insurance as the only positive solution to America's health care woes and "disqualify government-run health care as a politically viable solution."

Now, the same lobby groups are involved in a similar effort. AHIP, the insurance trade group behind the 2008 plan, is also a sponsor of the Partnership's 2020 campaign, along with the Federation of American Hospitals, Pharmaceutical Research and Manufacturers of America, the

Blue Cross Blue Shield Association, the Biotechnology Innovation Organization, and the American Medical Association.

Not only are the same health insurance groups financing a renewed campaign against "Medicare for All," but many of the same players who worked to undermine the public option during the ACA debate are now fighting for influence within the party. The public option was the government-run insurance plan that advocates intended to use to compete with private insurance and bring down consumer costs. In one version of the plan, the public option would pay doctors and other providers the same reimbursement rates as Medicare.

Despite a pledge by many Democratic candidates to eschew corporate PAC donations, health care lobbyists have funneled cash to many incoming lawmakers through the New Democrats PAC, the Blue Dog PAC, and other centrist committees. Unsurprisingly, the centrist New Democrats Coalition, the caucus of business-friendly centrist Democrats, has worked to depress momentum for "Medicare for All," reprising the role centrist Democrats played in killing the public option during the Obama administration. In 2009, then-Sen. Joe Lieberman, I-Conn., a founding member of the New Democrats caucus, threatened to join the Republican filibuster against health reform unless the public option was dropped from the bill.

Immediately following the midterm elections this month, the Washington Post published a column by Third Way warning that "Medicare for All" "failed the Hippocratic Oath" because opposition to the plan helped Republican candidates, thus causing "harm" to the long-term health interests of voters.

But advocates for "Medicare for All" are feeling optimistic.

"In terms of tactics, it sounds like they will just be updating the same lines they used in the 1990s to sideline reform efforts and in the ACA fight to keep single-payer health care off the table," said Eagan Kemp, a health care policy advocate with Public Citizen. "The Partnership for America's Health Care Future would be more accurately titled the 'Partnership for Profiting Off America's Health Care.'"

Private health care interests will certainly have much more money, media attention, and political resources with which to campaign. Advocates, however, are hoping Americans see past the public relations smokescreen and support health care as a human right.

"There is no brand loyalty to insurance companies, which are rightly seen as parasitic," Gaffney, the PNHP leader, said.

"Once single payer is widely understood as a program that covers everyone, that doesn't impose copays and deductibles, that has more comprehensive benefits than existing plans, and that doesn't employ restrictive insurance 'networks,' support will only grow," he added.

"By Lee Fang and Nick Surgey. Originally published on November 20, 2018. Reprinted with permission from *The Intercept* [https://theintercept.com/2018/11/20/medicare-for-all-healthcare-industry/], an award-winning nonprofit news organization dedicated to holding the powerful accountable through fearless, adversarial journalism."

Partnership for America's Health Care Future slide presentation:

Objectives

1. Change the national conversation around single payer / Medicare for All
2. Minimize the potential for this option in health care from becoming part of a national political party's platform in 2020

From: Support from left health care thought leaders (inside the Beltway)
To: Support only from the far left and minimal political support

From: Strong support but a lack of understanding around why Medicare for All (and all other proposals) actually is
To: A moderate and left of center voter base that understands what Medicare for All is and no longer supports it / supports building upon the current system and fixing what is broken

---

Our Work: Summer 2018

Beltway Narrative

Goal: Influence key thought leaders

Speakers Bureau: Amplify our message with like-minded allies

Thought Leader Engagement: Regular updates on the intersection of health care and politics

Digital Ads: Create Beltway specific digital ads targeted at the DC audience

Third Party Engagement: Collaborate with Beltway think tanks and other organizations

Regional Narrative

Goal: Create unique local messages that are state-specific and serve as a resource for candidates by providing polling, research and messaging

Candidate Briefings / Roundtables

AZ – Rep Kyrsten Sinema   WV – Senator Joe Manchin

Voter Education

Goal: Engage voters and educate them about the health care policies at hand

Pittsburgh Post-Gazette: Republicans are wrecking Obamacare

Herald Times: Fix, don't scrap Affordable Care Act protections

Sentinel and Enterprise: Improving ACA should be our top priority

The Columbus Dispatch: We should improve health care law, not throw it out

---

Quotes from the above slide of Lobbyist "Partnership for America's Health Care Future:

GOAL: Create unique local messages that are state-specific and serve as a resource for candidates by providing polling, research, and messaging.

AZ – Rep. Krysten Sinema: Field team briefed Rep. Sinema and District Director Michelle Davison. Rep. Sinema recently spoke out against Medicare for All. The field team is assisting with setting up two health care roundtables.

WV – Sen. Joe Manchin: Held a roundtable event with 15 health care advocates and provided messaging to his staff.

https://www.politico.com/news/2020/02/26/anti-medicare-for-all-south-carolina-117771   (See hyperlink for full text and references.)

Anti-Medicare for All Ad Campaign Launches in South Carolina
By Holly Otterbein and Maya King, 26 February 2020

The Partnership for America's Healthcare Future (PAHCF), a consortium of pharmaceutical, hospital and health insurance lobbyists, purchased over $200,000 in TV ads to run in Charleston and Columbia media markets Tuesday through Saturday during the Democratic debate (to) underline the message that Medicare for All, the Medicare buy-in and the public option are costly and ineffective in practice.

Wendell Potter, former head of communications at Cigna who is now president of Business for Medicare for All, said in a statement to POLITICO: "To protect the current system that puts corporate profits over patient care, the healthcare industry will launch the mother of all propaganda campaigns, and this last-ditch spending effort in South Carolina is a key part."

PACHF, whose members include Ascension, Ardent and the American Senior Alliance, has spent millions of dollars on anti-Medicare for All advertising in early primary states.

Still, Medicare for All remains a popular policy option among Democratic voters, according to early state exit polls. In Iowa, Nevada and New Hampshire, six out of 10 voters supported single payer.

https://www.ahip.org/ahip-submits-statement-for-congressional-hearing-on-medicare-for-all-legislation/ (See hyperlink for full text and references.)

America's Health Insurance Plans (AHIP) Submits Statement for Congressional Hearing on "Medicare for All" Legislation
By AHIP, 30 April 2019

On April 30, 2019, AHIP submitted a statement for a hearing in the House Rules Committee that focused on the "Medicare for All Act of 2019."

Our statement emphasizes that lowering health care costs is our most important priority, while also explaining that AHIP has developed a comprehensive set of affordability recommendations on steps that Congress and the Administration can take to provide relief from rising health care costs.

We express strong opposition to the "Medicare for All Act of 2019" and similar proposals to force government insurance systems upon Americans. We caution that such proposals do nothing to address our top challenge: a growing health care affordability crisis. We also highlight our concern that these proposals would result in higher taxes on all Americans, higher total premiums and costs for people enrolled in private coverage, longer wait times, and lower quality of care.

Our statement emphasizes that health insurance providers deliver coverage that is working for hundreds of millions of Americans — including 180 million Americans who are covered through their jobs, 22 million covered through Medicare Advantage, 55 million covered through Medicaid managed care, and 20 million who buy their own coverage. While noting that the foundation for an effective health care system already exists, we urge Congress to build on the lessons learned in these markets to improve what's working and fix what's broken, ensuring that all Americans have affordable, comprehensive health coverage that promotes timely access to high-quality care.

Head of Health Insurance Lobby Responds to Sanders: "We disclose all of our lobbying."

By Peter Sullivan for THE HILL, 21 August 2019

The head of the health insurance lobby said his industry is taking "Medicare for All" "seriously" and discloses all of its lobbying in response to a letter from Sen. Bernie Sanders (I-Vt.) pressing him for how much he would spend opposing the proposal.

"I mean we're taking it very seriously and we disclose all of our lobbying," Matt Eyles, the CEO of America's Health Insurance Plans (AHIP), said in an interview with The Hill when asked to respond to Sanders's letter. "So you can see what we're spending on lobbying. Not all of it will be on Medicare for All, there's a lot of other issues we'll be spending on, but it is an important issue to us."

Lobbying records show that AHIP spent about $5 million on lobbying in the first half of this year, though there are also additional avenues like campaign contributions and advertising spending.

Sanders, a presidential candidate who champions Medicare for All and frequently denounces the health insurance industry, wrote a letter to Eyles, as well as Steve Ubl, the CEO of the Pharmaceutical Research and Manufacturers of America, earlier this month asking how much the powerful groups would spend opposing Medicare for All.

"At a time when your profits are soaring, please tell me how many hundreds of millions of dollars the pharmaceutical industry and health insurance industry will be spending in advertising, lobbying and campaign contributions in opposition to Medicare for All," Sanders wrote.

Sanders said a better use of the money would be to "make sure that no one in the wealthiest country in the world dies or goes bankrupt because they cannot afford to purchase life-saving prescription drugs or go to a doctor."

Eyles did not punch back at Sanders personally, but said <u>his group is fighting back against Medicare for All because the proposal threatens the survival of the private health insurers he represents.</u>

Asked what his pitch is to lawmakers who are thinking of signing onto Medicare for All, Eyles pointed to the need to build on the Affordable Care Act (ACA), widely known as ObamaCare.

"Building on what we have, the infrastructure that we have, through the ACA, is the best way to expand coverage," Eyles said. "The disruption that you would have, by getting rid of private insurance, in the employer market, telling 180 million Americans that they need to give up their coverage through their employer is really not the best way to fix the problems and expand coverage in our health care system," he added.

<u>AHIP is also a member of a coalition of industry groups, the Partnership for America's Health Care Future, that is fighting Medicare for All</u>, as well as somewhat more incremental proposals like former Vice President Joe Biden's idea of giving anyone the option to buy into a government-run "public option."

Eyles argued that the insurance industry has improved its practices since a decade ago, before the Affordable Care Act, when insurers were able to engage in practices like denying coverage to people with pre-existing conditions.

"The way that this industry operates compared to the way it was a decade ago, I would say is, is fundamentally different," Eyles said.

"I mean, we are a consumer-centered, patient-centered industry that is really trying to change the way that health care is being delivered for the benefit of the American people in a way that I don't think was really recognized, you know, 10 years ago," he said. "The industry really has evolved."

MEDICARE FOR ALL: INVOKE RICO ?

How many members of Congress (in both The Senate and The House of Representatives) are receiving campaign donations from big health insurance corporations as incentive to deny "Medicare for All" (aka Universal Healthcare) to their constituents and, by extension, to all Americans?

This chapter is about the "deprivation of the right of citizens to the honest services of their elected officials".

See:
**http://www.fbi.gov/elpaso/press-releases/2010/ep090210.htm &
https://www.justice.gov/usao-wdtx/pr/four-sentenced-connection-el-paso-corruption-investigation**

In El Paso, Texas in 2010, United States Attorney John E. Murphy and Federal Bureau of Investigation Special Agent in Charge David Cuthbertson announced that a federal grand jury indicted 11 individuals in connection with the El Paso corruption investigation on RICO charges for allegedly assisting AccessHealthSource, a local health care provider, in obtaining and maintaining lucrative contracts with local and state government entities in the city of El Paso, Texas, "through bribery of and kickbacks to elected officials or himself and others, extortion under color of authority, fraudulent schemes and artifices, false pretenses, promises and representations and **deprivation of the right of citizens to the honest services of their elected local officials**". RICO stands for "Racketeer Influenced and Corrupt Organizations" Act.

On February 19, 2013, former El Paso County Commissioner Larry Medina, El Paso attorney David Escobar, and former Ysleta Independent School District (YISD) Trustees Linda Chavez and Mickey Duntley were sentenced for their roles in a corruption scheme involving healthcare service contracts with AccessHealth, Inc. (ACCESS). "The FBI, along with our law enforcement partners, will continue our pursuit of individuals and elected officials whose actions violate the public's trust and confidence," stated FBI Special Agent In Charge Mark Morgan.

https://www.fiercehealthcare.com/regulatory/health-insurer-lobbying-single-payer-democrats-campaign-contributions
(See hyperlink for full text and references.)

Health Insurers' Political Contributions
May Be Stalling the Single-payer Movement
By Leslie Small ; 1 February 2018

Though public and political support for a single-payer healthcare system seems to be growing, few can say that it's very close to becoming a policy reality.

One of the reasons for that disconnect, according to a new analysis from the Center for Responsive Politics, is the influence that the health insurance industry wields over elected officials.

To prove its case, the organization examined the contributions that health insurance companies made to leadership PACs and campaign committees of Democratic lawmakers in the House and Senate.

In the House, almost two-thirds of the Democratic caucus has cosponsored the Expanded & Improved Medicare for All Act. But House Democrats who did not cosponsor the bill received 137% more money, on average, from health insurance companies during the 2016 cycle than those who have.

A similar trend can be seen in the Senate, where more than a third of Democrats have cosponsored Sen. Bernie Sanders' Medicare for All Act. Democratic senators who did not cosponsor the bill received 146% more contributions, on average, from health insurance companies between 2011 and 2016 than those who did cosponsor it.

The analysis also found a correlation between contributions from the pharmaceutical industry and Democratic lawmakers' support of single-payer legislation. However, it noted that Sen. Cory Booker (NJ) and Rep. Joseph Crowley (NY) are outliers, as both Democrats have cosponsored single-payer proposals despite being well-funded by the pharma industry.

Other notable Democrats highlighted in the analysis include Senate Minority Leader Chuck Schumer, who led his caucus in donations from health insurance companies, and Missouri Sen. Claire McCaskill, whose top corporate donor is Centene. Schumer hasn't committed to supporting the Medicare-for-all bill, and McCaskill said last fall that she's not ready to back a single-payer system.

Though health insurers appear to be successfully discouraging a move to a single-payer system, there have been reasons to question whether their lobbying influence is as strong as it once was. Three of the country's largest insurers have left the industry's chief trade group — America's Health Insurance Plans (AHIP) — and the Trump administration has largely ignored insurers' advice against repealing the Affordable Care Act.

On the other hand, recent Medicare Advantage policy proposals have been well-received by the industry, and some insurers have benefited handsomely from the GOP's new tax law.

https://www.theglobalist.com/republican-tax-bill-trump-corruption/
(See hyperlink for full text and references.)

The Republican Crime Syndicate Takes Control
By Richard Phillips, 6 December 2017

The Republican Party has become a Racketeer Influenced Corrupt Organization (RICO). As with other criminal organizations, its purpose is to rape, pillage and plunder America.

The GOP has abandoned its core principles and has become a **Racketeer Influenced Corrupt Organization (RICO).**

This law, passed in 1970, provides for extended criminal penalties and a civil cause of action for acts performed as part of an ongoing criminal organization. Unfortunately, the RICO Act doesn't apply to political parties.

Otherwise, it would certainly be applicable as the Republican Party has ceased playing a constructive role in improving the lot of its constituents and instead has become a racket, rife with corrupt practices.

With each passing day, a new crime is perpetrated against the American people that concentrates wealth in the hands of a group of oligarchs that exert greater and greater control over how the wealth of America is distributed.

This oligarchy pays off Republican politicians with donations that underpin their political careers. Without these nefarious donations, these paid predators would be out of a job. The donations are nothing other than bribes aimed at securing the financial well-being of their recipients.

And for those who suggest there is even a semblance of moral equivalency between Republicans and Democrats, they should keep solidly in mind one important distinction: Democrats want tax cuts for the middle class, health insurance for all, a decent and protected environment, net neutrality and food for poor kids. All anyone can hope for is that voters wise up to what the GOP has been up to.

http://www.differencebetween.net/miscellaneous/politics/difference-between-lobbying-and-bribing/
(See hyperlink for full text and references.)

Difference Between Lobbying and Bribing

Lobbying, in general, refers to the act of trying to influence members of a legislative body to vote in favor of the 'lobbyist'. In some governments, 'lobbyists' have formally recognized groups, whose interests are 'lobbied' for, that may be wholly or partially funded by organizations, or even nations. On a softer side, lobbying may just involve political support offered in return for political influence, or action. Lobbying that is legalized by a government does not involve financial support.

Bribery, on the other hand, involves offering money in return for political action or influence. Often this bribery comes in cash form, without involving bank transactions, and this is one of the reasons many lobbyists have been accused of bribery. Therefore, bribery is when money contributions are made to a political group in expectation of being favored in political or legislative decisions. Priorities and decisions of legislators, governors, councilmen and the President alike, are defined by money handouts by lobbyists.

At times, there seems to be just a fine line between the two. Lobbyists have become very aggressive in pushing for their agendas, and this has led many to think that their practices have become unacceptable, as it unfairly swings the political landscape in favor of the rich and the big corporations that can use their monetary influence. Definitely, this kind of system has major drawbacks, since the concerns of the 'common man' will not matter if they are contrary to the interests of the big businesses. Some business leaders have such a grip on the avenues to power, that the gap between the businesses and the file and rank (who are the customers) is very wide.

Precisely put, bribery is when a business, individual or a group of individuals, offer cash or property in exchange for a specific influence in their favor. For instance, when a legislator tells his constituent that he will vote for certain legislation in return for a certain amount of money, then that is bribery.

Many times, proving a bribe can be as hard as it can be to distinguish between bribery (which is illegal) and lobbying (which is legal in some governments), unless informers are used. Informers will have to offer the real bribes, and tape the officials accepting the money offers. Alternatively, if there's some written agreement with the official consenting to the bribery, it could also prove the acceptance of a bribe. Otherwise, proving a connection between the two parties without tangible evidence can seem like a 'mountain to climb.'

Summary: Lobbying is trying to influence politicians to decide in your favor, while bribing means the same, except that there is an offer of money or property. Lobbying is legal (although contentious), while bribery is out rightly illegal.

NOTE: In 2021, according to OpenSecrets.org, the top three spenders trying to influence government policy were the U.S. Chamber of Commerce ($46.4 million), the National Association of Realtors ($31.0 million), **and the Pharmaceutical Research & Manufacturers of America ($22.9 million). Blue Cross/Blue Shield ($18.7 million) and the American Hospital Association ($17.6 million) were near the top of the list.** (See https://www.opensecrets.org/federal-lobbying/top-spenders?cycle=2021)

https://www.healthcare-now.org/legislation/national-timeline/
(See hyperlink for full text and links.)

HEALTHCARE-NOW!

The long history of efforts to win national healthcare in the United States is, in the words of one scholar, "a drama in too many acts." Below is a timeline of national health reform efforts in Congress, which links to hundreds of pages of legislation, Congressional analysis, and public hearings. This timeline encompasses the complete transformation of medical care in the United States, the abolition of Jim Crow in the South, and the eventual birth of a social movement for single-payer healthcare.

You can also view our sortable list of national legislation, a listing of Congressional hearings on single-payer in the 1940s and 1970s, and a listing of economic impact studies of single-payer at the state and the national levels.

Jump to a Time Period:

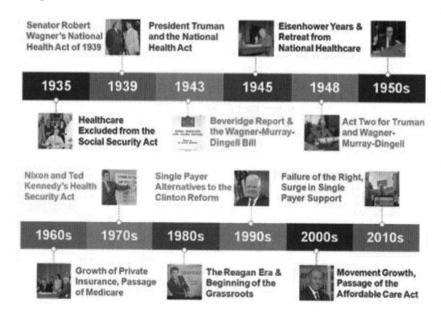

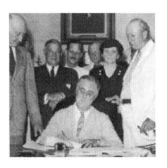

Roosevelt signs Social Security Bill

1935: Healthcare Excluded from the Social Security Act

President Roosevelt and Democratic leadership in Congress strip all mention of healthcare from the Social Security Act after opposition threatens the entire bill. The Social Security Act is passed into law on August 14, 1935.

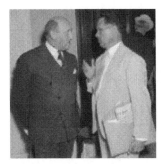

President of the AMA Lobbying Against the Wagner Bill

1939: Senator Robert Wagner's National Healthcare Act of 1939

President Roosevelt convenes a National Health Conference in July 1938, out of which comes Senator Wagner's National Health Act of 1939, which provides for federal grants-in-aid to states for voluntary expansion of healthcare coverage and public health. The bill, considered on the eve of World War II, faces fierce opposition from the American Medical Association (AMA) at Senate hearings, and fails to advance with the onset of war.

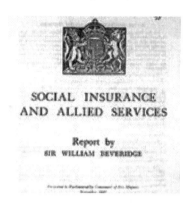

The U.K's "Beveridge Report" proposing social insurance.

1943: Beveridge Report & the Wagner-Murray-Dingell National Social Insurance Proposal

In 1942 the United Kingdom publishes the wildly popular "Beveridge Report," a government proposal to establish a welfare state, including a national health service. The author **William Beveridge tours the U.S.** in 1943, and his proposal for a broad program of social insurance is embodied in the Wagner-Murray-Dingell Bill, which proposes compulsory medical insurance for workers, as well as disability benefits, unemployment compensation, maternity benefits, and more. The bill's authors introduce it to start a conversation, but don't expect it to advance in Congress.

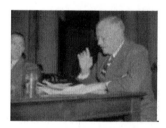

Senator Wagner testifying to a Senate subcommittee.

1945: President Truman and the Wagner-Murray-Dingell National Health Act

At the end of 1944 President Roosevelt finally instructs his administration to make a push for national health reform, but dies shortly thereafter in April 1945. Harry Truman becomes President and delivers a Special Message to Congress calling for a Comprehensive Health Program on November 19. Senators Wagner and Murray and Rep.

Dingell team up again to introduce the National Health Act, which would cover seniors, working residents, and their dependents through a national program, and provides separately via grants to states for the unemployed, mothers, and children. Major hearings are held by the Senate in 1946, which Republicans boycott. With poor prospects in the House, Sen. Murray shelves the bill for next session, but Republicans retake Congress in 1946, holding their own hearings from 1947-48 to attack Truman's healthcare plan as socialist during an election year.

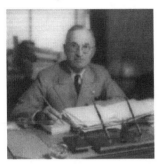

President Harry Truman at the White House.

1948: Act Two for President Truman and the Wagner-Murray-Dingell Bill

During the 1948 elections **Truman campaigns on a national healthcare platform**, and takes office with large Democratic majorities in both houses. Murray, Wagner, and Dingell revise their bill, re-filing it as the National Health Insurance and Public Health Act, which receives 15 days of public hearings by the Senate in 1949. The bill fails to gain support from Southern Democrats necessary for passage.

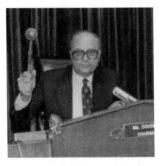

Representative John Dingell of Michigan in Congress.

1950s: The Eisenhower Years and a Retreat from National Health

Insurance

With Dwight Eisenhower serving as President from 1953 through 1961, and Republicans controlling both houses of Congress from 1955 through 1961, the prospects for a national health program diminish. However, upon the death of Rep. John Dingell Sr. in 1955, his son John Dingell wins a special election to take his seat and introduces the National Health Insurance Act in 1957 based on the legislation his father had filed in the 1940s, a bill he will introduce every session for 54 years through 2010.

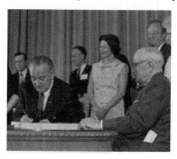

President Lyndon Johnson signing Medicare and Medicaid into law.

1960s: Growth of Private Health Insurance & Passage of Medicare and Medicaid

Employer-sponsored health insurance coverage grows rapidly through the 1950s and early 1960s, and both organized labor and Democratic leadership shift focus towards winning healthcare coverage for seniors and the low-income. In 1961 John F. Kennedy becomes President and Democrats win large majorities in both houses. The "Social Security Amendments of 1965," which include the Medicaid and Medicare programs, are signed into law on July 30th, 1965.

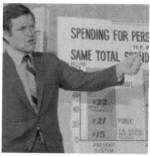

**Senator Ted Kennedy pitching his health reform
to an AFSCME meeting.**

1970s: President Nixon & Ted Kennedy's Health Security Act

During the early 1970s runaway inflation leads President Nixon to impose wage and price controls across the economy, including healthcare services. A sense of inevitability pervades Congress that national health reform of some sort will pass. The primary legislative vehicle for single payer healthcare is Senator Ted Kennedy's Health Security Act. An alternate single-payer proposal is sponsored by Republican Senator Jacob Javits. These bills, along with competing proposals from President Nixon, the American Medical Association, and the American Hospital Association, receive extensive public hearings in 1971. These include Kennedy's "Health Care Crisis in America" hearings that tour around the country, as well as additional hearings in the House and the Senate. In 1974 Sen. Kennedy introduces compromise legislation that preserves a role for health insurers as intermediaries, losing support from unions in the process, but a deal with Nixon is derailed by Watergate and his resignation from office in August. When Gerald Ford succeeds to the Presidency, Rep. Mills attempts to move an even further compromised bill through House Ways & Means, but is unable to gain support from Republicans and Southern Democrats.

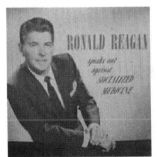

An AMA recording from 1961 featuring Reagan, attacking "socialized medicine"

1980s: The Reagan Era and the Beginning of a Grassroots Organization (PNHP)

Ronald Reagan, who in the 1960s had been recruited by the American Medical Association (AMA) to attack national healthcare as socialist, serves as President from 1981 through the end of the decade. Reagan leads an assault on organized labor and the role of government in public life. No proposals for single-payer healthcare receive significant attention during this period. However, Physicians for a National Health

Program is launched in 1986, and from 1988-1990 the bipartisan "Pepper Commission" in Congress develops a recommendation for universal healthcare that sets the stage for the next round of healthcare reform.

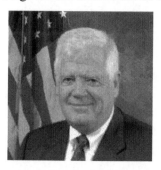

Rep. McDermott filed H.R. 1200 in the House for 24 years.

1990s: Single-Payer Alternatives to the Clinton Health Security Act

In early 1991 during the second term of George H.W. Bush, Representative Marty Russo introduces the Universal Health Care Act, which gains 72 co-sponsors - a record high for single-payer legislation in the House. Later in '91 Harris Wofford becomes the first Democrat in 23 years to win a Senate seat in Pennsylvania during a special election, closing a 44 percent polling gap by campaigning for national health insurance. Bill Clinton wins the 1992 Presidential elections promising to implement a universal healthcare plan, and while his Presidential Task Force on National Health Reform meets behind closed doors during 1993, Rep. Jim McDermott and Sen. Paul Wellstone introduce their single-payer proposal, the American Health Security Act with 90 co-sponsors in the House and 4 in the Senate. Clinton instead proposes his "Health Security Act" based on employer mandates, subsidies for the unemployed, and "managed competition," but the bill fails to advance through Committee. Democrats lose control of both houses of Congress for the next decade.

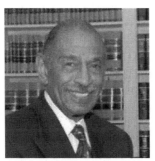

**Rep. Conyers's HR676 came to receive
unprecedented support in the House.**

2000s: Growth of the Movement and Passage of the Affordable Care Act

George W. Bush serves as President from 2001-2008, but a network of grassroots organizations fighting for single-payer healthcare forms across the country during the 1990s and early 2000s. In 2003, Rep. John Conyers introduces the Expanded and Improved Medicare for All Act, H.R. 676, and Healthcare-NOW is launched in 2004 to advocate for it. For two sessions from 2005-2008, Senator Ted Kennedy and Rep. Dingell file a new national healthcare proposal, the Medicare for All Act. However, when Barack Obama is elected President in 2008 along with Democratic majorities in both houses of Congress, Democratic leadership keeps single-payer proposals off the table while debating and passing the Affordable Care Act from 2009 to 2010.

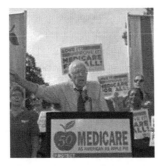

Sen. Bernie Sanders at a rally for Medicare-for-All.

2010s: Failure of the Right, Surge in Single-Payer Support

While the Affordable Care Act is not fully implemented until 2014, in 2011 Bernie Sanders introduces a Senate companion bill to the American Health Security Act, which Rep. McDermott had continued sponsoring in the House since 1993. In 2016 Donald Trump is elected President along with Republican majorities in both houses, promising to repeal the Affordable Care Act. National opposition not only prevents the GOP "repeal and replace" effort, but leads to a surge in support for single-payer healthcare. By 2017 Rep. Conyers' Expanded and Improved Medicare for All Act hits an historic high of 120 co-sponsors in the House, and Sen. Bernie Sanders introduces a new single-payer bill, the Medicare-for-All Act with 16 co-sponsors in the Senate.

Contact HEALTHCARE-NOW!

info@healthcare-now.org ; (215)732-2131

1534 Tremont Street, Boston, MA 02120

https://pnhp.org/a-brief-history-universal-health-care-efforts-in-the-us/
(See hyperlink for full text and references.) Used with permission.

A Brief History: Universal Health Care Efforts in the US

**(Transcribed from a talk given by Karen S. Palmer MPH, MS
in San Francisco at the Spring, 1999 PNHP meeting)**

Late 1800's to Medicare

The campaign for some form of universal government-funded health care has stretched for nearly a century in the US. On several occasions, advocates believed they were on the verge of success; yet each time they faced defeat. The evolution of these efforts and the reasons for their failure make for an intriguing lesson in American history, ideology, and character.

Other developed countries have had some form of social insurance (that later evolved into national insurance) for nearly as long as the US has been trying to get it. Some European countries started with compulsory sickness insurance, one of the first systems, for workers beginning in Germany in 1883; other countries including Austria, Hungary, Norway, Britain, Russia, and the Netherlands followed all the way through 1912. Other European countries, including Sweden in 1891, Denmark in 1892, France in 1910, and Switzerland in 1912, subsidized the mutual benefit societies that workers formed among themselves.

So for a very long time, other countries have had some form of universal health care or at least the beginnings of it. The primary reason for the emergence of these programs in Europe was income stabilization and protection against the wage loss of sickness rather than payment for medical expenses, which came later. Programs were not universal to start with and were originally conceived as a means of maintaining incomes and buying political allegiance of the workers.

In a seeming paradox, the British and German systems were developed by the more conservative governments in power, specifically as a defense to counter expansion of the socialist and labor parties. They used insurance against the cost of sickness as a way of "turning benevolence to power".

US circa 1883-1912, including Reformers and the Progressive Era:

What was the US doing during this period of the late 1800's to 1912?

The government took no actions to subsidize voluntary funds or make sick insurance compulsory; essentially the federal government left matters to the states and states left them to private and voluntary programs. The US did have some voluntary funds that provided for their members in the case of sickness or death, but there were no legislative or public programs during the late 19th or early 20th century.

In the Progressive Era, which occurred in the early 20th century, reformers were working to improve social conditions for the working class. However, unlike European countries, there was not powerful working class support for broad social insurance in the US. The labor and socialist parties' support for health insurance or sickness funds and benefits programs was much more fragmented than in Europe. Therefore the first proposals for health insurance in the US did not come into political debate under anti-socialist sponsorship as they had in Europe.

Theodore Roosevelt 1901 — 1909

During the Progressive Era, President Theodore Roosevelt was in power and although he supported health insurance because he believed that no country could be strong whose people were sick and poor, most of the initiative for reform took place outside of government. Roosevelt's successors were mostly conservative leaders, who postponed for about twenty years the kind of presidential leadership that might have involved the national government more extensively in the management of social welfare.

AALL Bill 1915

In 1906, the American Association of Labor Legislation (AALL) finally led the campaign for health insurance. They were a typical progressive group whose mandate was not to abolish capitalism but rather to reform it. In 1912, they created a committee on social welfare which held its first national conference in 1913. Despite its broad mandate, the committee decided to concentrate on health insurance, drafting a model bill in 1915. In a nutshell, the bill limited coverage to the working class and all others that earned less than $1200 a year, including dependents. The services of physicians, nurses, and hospitals were included, as was sick pay, maternity benefits, and a death benefit of fifty dollars to pay for funeral expenses. This death benefit becomes significant later on. Costs were to be shared between workers, employers, and the state.

AMA supported AALL Proposal

In 1914, reformers sought to involve physicians in formulating this bill, and the American Medical Association (AMA) actually supported the AALL proposal. They found prominent physicians who were not only sympathetic, but who also wanted to support and actively help in securing legislation. In fact, some physicians who were leaders in the AMA wrote to the AALL secretary: "Your plans are so entirely in line with our own that we want to be of every possible assistance." By 1916, the AMA board approved a committee to work with AALL, and at this point the AMA and AALL formed a united front on behalf of health insurance. Times have definitely changed along the way. In 1917, the AMA House of Delegates favored compulsory health insurance as proposed by the AALL, but many state medical societies opposed it. There was disagreement on the method of paying physicians and it was not long before the AMA leadership denied it had ever favored the measure.

AFL opposed AALL Proposal

Meanwhile the president of the American Federation of Labor repeatedly denounced compulsory health insurance as an unnecessary paternalistic reform that would create a system of state supervision over people's health. They apparently worried that a government-based insurance system would weaken unions by usurping their role in providing social benefits. Their central concern was maintaining union strength, which was understandable in a period before collective bargaining was legally sanctioned.

Private insurance industry opposed AALL Proposal

The commercial insurance industry also opposed the reformers' efforts in the early 20th century. There was great fear among the working class of what they called a "pauper's burial," so the backbone of insurance business was policies for working class families that paid death benefits and covered funeral expenses. But because the reformer health insurance plans also covered funeral expenses, there was a big conflict. Reformers felt that by covering death benefits, they could finance much of the health insurance costs from the money wasted by commercial insurance policies that had to have an army of insurance agents to market and collect on these policies. But since this would have pulled the rug out from under the multi-million dollar commercial life insurance industry, they opposed the national health insurance proposal.

WWI and anti-German fever

In 1917, the US entered WWI and anti-German fever rose. The government-commissioned articles denouncing "German socialist insurance" and opponents of health insurance assailed it as a "Prussian menace" inconsistent with American values. Other efforts during this time in California, namely the California Social Insurance Commission, recommended health insurance, proposed enabling legislation in 1917, and then held a referendum. New York, Ohio, Pennsylvania, and Illinois also had some efforts aimed at health insurance. But in the Red Scare, immediately after the war, when the government attempted to root out the last vestiges of radicalism, opponents of compulsory health insurance associated it with Bolshevism and buried it in an avalanche of anti-Communist rhetoric. This marked the end of the compulsory national health debate until the 1930's.

Why did the Progressives fail?

Opposition from doctors, labor, insurance companies, and business contributed to the failure of Progressives to achieve compulsory national health insurance. In addition, the inclusion of the funeral benefit was a tactical error since it threatened the gigantic structure of the commercial life insurance industry. Political naivete on the part of the reformers in failing to deal with the interest group opposition, ideology, historical experience, and the overall political context all played a key role in shaping how these groups identified and expressed their interests.

The 1920's

There was some activity in the 1920's that changed the nature of the debate when it awoke again in the 1930's. In the 1930's, the focus shifted from stabilizing income to financing and expanding access to medical care. By now, medical costs for workers were regarded as a more serious problem than wage loss from sickness. For a number of reasons, health care costs also began to rise during the 1920's, mostly because the middle class began to use hospital services and hospital costs started to increase. Medical, and especially hospital, care was now a bigger item in family budgets than wage losses.

The CCMC

Next came the Committee on the Cost of Medical Care (CCMC). Concerns over the cost and distribution of medical care led to the formation of this self-created, privately funded group. The committee was funded by 8 philanthropic organizations including the Rockefeller, Millbank, and Rosenwald foundations. They first met in 1926 and ceased meeting in 1932. The CCMC was comprised of fifty economists, physicians, public health specialists, and major interest groups. Their research determined that there was a need for more medical care for everyone, and they published these findings in 26 research volumes and 15 smaller reports over a 5-year period. The CCMC recommended that more national resources go to medical care and saw voluntary, not compulsory, health insurance as a means to covering these costs. Most CCMC members opposed compulsory health insurance, but there was no consensus on this point within the committee. The AMA treated their report as a radical document advocating socialized medicine, and the acerbic and conservative editor of JAMA called it "an incitement to revolution."

FDR's first attempt: failure to include in the Social Security Bill of 1935

Next came Franklin D. Roosevelt (FDR), whose tenure (1933-1945) can be characterized by the Great Depression, WWII, and the New Deal, including the Social Security Bill. We might have thought the Great Depression would create the perfect conditions for passing compulsory health insurance in the US, but with millions out of work, unemployment insurance took priority followed by old age benefits. FDR's Committee on Economic Security, the CES, feared that inclusion of health insurance in its bill, which was opposed by the AMA, would threaten the passage of the entire Social Security legislation. It was therefore excluded.

FDR's second attempt: Wagner Bill, National Health Act of 1939

But there was one more push for national health insurance during FDR's administration: The Wagner National Health Act of 1939. Though it never received FDR's full support, the proposal grew out of his Tactical Committee on Medical Care, established in 1937. The essential elements of the tactical committee's reports were incorporated into Senator Wagner's bill, the National Health Act of 1939, which gave general support for a national health program to be funded by federal grants to states and administered by states and localities. However, the 1938 election brought a conservative resurgence and any further innovations in social policy were extremely difficult. Most of the social policy legislation precedes 1938. Just as the AALL campaign ran into the declining forces of progressivism and then WWI, the movement for national health insurance in the 1930's ran into the declining fortunes of the New Deal and then WWII.

Henry Sigerist

About this time, Henry Sigerist was in the US. He was a very influential medical historian at Johns Hopkins University who played a major role in medical politics during the 1930's and 1940's. He passionately believed in a national health program and compulsory health insurance. Several of Sigerist's most devoted students went on to become key figures in the fields of public health, community and preventative medicine, and health care organization. Many of them, including Milton Romer and Milton Terris, were instrumental in forming the medical care section of the American Public Health Association, which then served as a national meeting ground for those committed to health care reform.

Wagner-Murray-Dingell Bills: 1943 and onward through the decade

The Wagner Bill evolved and shifted from a proposal for federal grants-in-aid to a proposal for national health insurance. First introduced in 1943, it became the very famous Wagner-Murray-Dingell Bill. The bill called for compulsory national health insurance and a payroll tax. In 1944, the Committee for the Nation's Health (which grew out of the earlier Social Security Charter Committee) was a group of representatives of organized labor, progressive farmers, and liberal physicians who were the foremost lobbying group for the Wagner-Murray-Dingell Bill. Prominent members of the committee included Senators Murray and Dingell, the head of the Physician's Forum, and Henry Sigerist. Opposition to this bill was enormous and the antagonists launched a scathing red baiting attack on the committee saying that one of its key policy analysts, I.S. Falk, was a conduit between the International Labor Organization (ILO) in Switzerland and the United States government. The ILO was red-baited as "an awesome political machine bent on world domination." They even went so far as to suggest that the United States Social Security board functioned as an ILO subsidiary. Although the Wagner-Murray-Dingell Bill generated extensive national debates, with the intensified opposition, the bill was never passed by Congress despite its reintroduction every session for 14 years! Had it passed, the Act would have established compulsory national health insurance funded by payroll taxes.

Truman's Support

After FDR died, Truman became president (1945-1953), and his tenure is characterized by the Cold War and Communism. The health care issue finally moved into the center arena of national politics and received the unreserved support of an American president. Though he served during some of the most virulent anti-Communist attacks and the early years of the Cold War, Truman fully supported national health insurance. But the opposition had acquired new strength. Compulsory health insurance became entangled in the Cold War and its opponents were able to make "socialized medicine" a symbolic issue in the growing crusade against Communist influence in America.

Truman's plan for national health insurance in 1945 was different than FDR's plan in 1938 because Truman was strongly committed to a single universal comprehensive health insurance plan. Whereas FDR's 1938 program had a separate proposal for medical care of the needy, it was Truman who proposed a single egalitarian system that included all classes of society, not just the working class. He emphasized that this was not "socialized medicine." He also dropped the funeral benefit that contributed to the defeat of national insurance in the Progressive Era. Congress had mixed reactions to Truman's proposal. The chairman of the House Committee was an anti-union conservative and refused to hold hearings. Senior Republican Senator Taft declared, "I consider it socialism. It is to my mind the most socialistic measure this Congress has ever had before it." Taft suggested that compulsory health insurance, like the Full Unemployment Act, came right out of the Soviet constitution and walked out of the hearings. The AMA, the American Hospital Association, the American Bar Association, and most of the nation's press had no mixed feelings; they hated the plan. The AMA claimed it would make doctors slaves, even though Truman emphasized that doctors would be able to choose their method of payment.

In 1946, the Republicans took control of Congress and had no interest in enacting national health insurance. They charged that it was part of a large socialist scheme. Truman responded by focusing even more attention on a national health bill in the 1948 election. After Truman's surprise victory in 1948, the AMA thought Armageddon had come. They assessed their members an extra $25 each to resist national health insurance, and in 1945 they spent $1.5 million on lobbying efforts which at the time was the most expensive lobbying effort in American history. They had one pamphlet that said, "Would socialized medicine lead to socialization of other phases of life? Lenin thought so. He declared socialized medicine is the keystone to the arch of the socialist state."

The AMA and its supporters were again very successful in linking socialism with national health insurance, and as anti-Communist sentiment rose in the late 1940's and the Korean War began, national health insurance became vanishingly improbable. Truman's plan died in a congressional committee. Compromises were proposed but none were successful. Instead of a single health insurance system for the entire population, America would have a system of private insurance for those who could afford it and public welfare services for the poor. Discouraged by yet another defeat, the advocates of health insurance now turned toward a more modest proposal they hoped the country would adopt: hospital insurance for the aged and the beginnings of Medicare.

After WWII, other private insurance systems expanded and provided enough protection for groups that held influence in America to prevent any great agitation for national health insurance in the 1950's and early 1960's. Union-negotiated health care benefits also served to cushion workers from the impact of health care costs and undermined the movement for a government program.

Why did these efforts for universal national health insurance fail again?

For many of the same reasons they failed before: interest group influence (code words for class), ideological differences, anti-communism, anti-socialism, fragmentation of public policy, the entrepreneurial character of American medicine, a tradition of American voluntarism, removing the middle class from the coalition of advocates for change through the alternative of Blue Cross private insurance plans, and the association of public programs with charity, dependence, personal failure and the almshouses of years gone by.

For the next several years, not much happened in terms of national health insurance initiatives. The nation focused more on unions as a vehicle for health insurance, the Hill-Burton Act of 1946 related to hospital expansion, medical research and vaccines, the creation of national institutes of health, and advances in psychiatry.

Johnson and Medicare/Medicaid

Finally, Rhode Island congressman Aime Forand introduced a new proposal in 1958 to cover hospital costs for the aged on social security. Predictably, the AMA undertook a massive campaign to portray a government insurance plan as a threat to the patient-doctor relationship. But by concentrating on the aged, the terms of the debate began to change for the first time. There was major grass roots support from seniors and the pressures assumed the proportions of a crusade. In the entire history of the national health insurance campaign, this was the first time that a ground swell of grass roots support forced an issue onto the national agenda.

The AMA countered by introducing an "eldercare plan," which was voluntary insurance with broader benefits and physician services. In response, the government expanded its proposed legislation to cover physician services, and what came of it were Medicare and Medicaid. The necessary political compromises and private concessions to the doctors (reimbursements of their customary, reasonable, and prevailing fees), to the hospitals (cost plus reimbursement), and to the Republicans created a 3-part plan, including the Democratic proposal for comprehensive health insurance ("Part A"), the revised Republican program of government subsidized voluntary physician insurance ("Part B"), and Medicaid. Finally, in 1965, Johnson signed it into law as part of his Great Society Legislation, capping 20 years of congressional debate.

What does history teach us? What is the movement reacting to?

1.   Henry Sigerist reflected in his own diary in 1943 that he "wanted to use history to solve the problems of modern medicine." I think this is, perhaps, a most important lesson. Damning her own naivete, Hillary Clinton acknowledged in 1994 that "I did not appreciate how sophisticated the opposition would be in conveying messages that were effectively political even though substantively wrong." Maybe Hillary should have had this history lesson first.

2.   The institutional representatives of society do not always represent those that they claim to represent, just as the AMA does not represent all doctors. This lack of representation presents an opportunity for attracting more people to the cause. The AMA has always played an oppositional role and it would be prudent to build an alternative to the AMA for the 60% of physicians who are not members.

3.   Just because President Bill Clinton failed doesn't mean it's over. There have been periods of acquiescence in this debate before. Those who oppose it cannot kill this movement. Openings will occur again. We all need to be on the lookout for those openings and also need to create openings where we see opportunities. For example, the focus on health care costs of the 1980's presented a division in the ruling class and the debate moved into the center again. As hockey great Wayne Gretzky said, "Success is not a matter of skating to where the puck is, it is a matter of skating to where the puck will be."

4.   Whether we like it or not, we are going to have to deal with the persistence of the narrow vision of middle class politics. <u>Vincente Navarro says that the majority opinion of national health insurance has everything to do with repression and coercion by the capitalist corporate dominant class.</u> He argues that the conflict and struggles that continuously take place around the issue of health care unfold within the parameters of class and that coercion and repression are forces that determine policy. I think when we talk about interest groups in this country, it is really a code for class.

5.   Red-baiting is a red herring and has been used throughout history to evoke fear and may continue to be used in these post Cold War times by those who wish to inflame this debate.

6.   Grass roots initiatives contributed in part to the passage of Medicare, and they can work again. Ted Marmor says that "pressure groups that can prevail in quiet politics are far weaker in contexts of mass attention — as the AMA regretfully learned during the Medicare battle." Marmor offers these lessons from the past: "Compulsory health insurance, whatever the details, is an ideological controversial matter that involves enormous financial and professional stakes. Such legislation does not emerge quietly or with broad partisan support. <u>Legislative success requires active presidential leadership, the commitment of an</u>

Administration's political capital, and the exercise of all manner of persuasion and arm-twisting."

7.   One Canadian lesson — the movement toward universal health care in Canada started in 1916 (depending on when you start counting), and took until 1962 for passage of both hospital and doctor care in a single province. It took another decade for the rest of the country to catch on. That is about 50 years all together. It wasn't like we sat down over afternoon tea and crumpets and said please pass the health care bill so we can sign it and get on with the day. We fought, we threatened, the doctors went on strike, refused patients, people held rallies and signed petitions for and against it, burned effigies of government leaders, hissed, jeered, and booed at the doctors or the Premier depending on whose side they were on. In a nutshell, we weren't the stereotypical nice polite Canadians. Although there was plenty of resistance, now you could more easily take away Christmas than health care, despite the rhetoric that you may hear to the contrary.

8.   Finally, there is always hope for flexibility and change. In researching this talk, I went through a number of historical documents and one of my favorite quotes that speaks to hope and change come from a 1939 issue of Time Magazine with Henry Sigerist on the cover. The article said about Sigerist: "Students enjoy his lively classes, for Sigerist does not mind expounding his dynamic conception of medical history in hand-to-hand argument. A student once took issue with him and when Dr. Sigerist asked him to quote his authority, the student shouted, "You yourself said so!" "When?" asked Dr. Sigerist. "Three years ago," answered the student. "Ah," said Dr. Sigerist, "three years is a long time. I've changed my mind since then." I guess for me this speaks to the changing tides of opinion and that everything is in flux and open to renegotiation.

Acknowledgements:

Special thanks to medical historians and PNHP colleagues Corinne Sutter-Brown and Ted Brown for background information, critical analysis, and editing.

About the Speaker:

Karen S. Palmer MPH, MS, is an adjunct professor at the Faculty of Health Sciences in Simon Fraser University in Burnaby, British

Columbia. For 25+ years, Karen's passion has been comparative health care funding and delivery systems, policies, and reforms (mostly US, Europe, and Canada), underpinned by a belief that health care is a human right.

References:

Much of this talk was paraphrased/annotated directly from the sources below, in particular the work of Paul Starr:

1. Bauman, Harold, "Verging on National Health Insurance since 1910" in Changing to National Health Care: Ethical and Policy Issues (Vol. 4, Ethics in a Changing World) edited by Heufner, Robert P. and Margaret # P. Battin, University of Utah Press, 1992.

2. "Boost President's Plan", Washington Post, p. A23, February 7, 1992.

3. Brown, Ted. "Isaac Max Rubinow", (a biographical sketch), American Journal of Public Health, Vol. 87, No. 11, pp. 1863-1864, 1997

4. Danielson, David A., and Arthur Mazer. "The Massachusetts Referendum for a National Health Program", Journal of Public Health Policy, Summer 1986.

5. Derickson, Alan. "The House of Falk: The Paranoid Style in American House Politics", American Journal of Public Health", Vol. 87, No. 11, pp. 1836 – 1843, 1997.

6. Falk, I.S. "Proposals for National Health Insurance in the USA: Origins and Evolution and Some Perspectives for the Future', Milbank Memorial Fund Quarterly, Health and Society, pp. 161-191, Spring 1977.

7. Gordon, Colin. "Why No National Health Insurance in the US? The Limits of Social Provision in War and Peace, 1941-1948", Journal of Policy History, Vol. 9, No. 3, pp. 277-310, 1997.

8. "History in a Tea Wagon", Time Magazine, No. 5, pp. 51-53, January 30, 1939.

9. Marmor, Ted. "The History of Health Care Reform", Roll Call, pp. 21,40, July 19, 1993.

10. Navarro, Vicente. "Medical History as a Justification Rather than Explanation: Critique of Starr's The Social Transformation of American Medicine" International Journal of Health Services, Vol. 14, No. 4, pp. 511-528, 1984.

11. Navarro, Vicente. "Why Some Countries Have National Health Insurance, Others Have National Health Service, and the United States has Neither", International Journal of Health Services, Vol. 19, No. 3, pp. 383-404, 1989.

12. Rothman, David J. "A Century of Failure: Health Care Reform in America", Journal of Health Politics, Policy and Law", Vol. 18, No. 2, Summer 1993.

13. Rubinow, Isaac Max. "Labor Insurance", American Journal of Public Health, Vol. 87, No. 11, pp. 1862 – 1863, 1997 (Originally published in Journal of Political Economy, Vol. 12, pp. 362-281, 1904).

14. Starr, Paul. The Social Transformation of American Medicine: The rise of a sovereign profession and the making of a vast industry. Basic Books, 1982.

15. Starr, Paul. "Transformation in Defeat: The Changing Objectives of National Health Insurance, 1915-1980", American Journal of Public Health, Vol. 72, No. 1, pp. 78-88, 1982.

16. Terris, Milton. "Crisis and Change in America's Health System", American Journal of Public Health, Vol. 63, No. 4, April 1973.

17. "Toward a National Medical Care System: II. The Historical Background", Editorial, Journal of Public Health Policy, Autumn 1986.

18. Trafford, Abigail, and Christine Russel, "Opening Night for Clinton's Plan", Washington Post Health Magazine, pp. 12, 13, 15, September 21, 1993.

CONGRESSIONAL PROGRESSIVE CAUCUS MEMBERS (see hyperlink): https://progressives.house.gov/caucus-members/

CONGRESSIONAL PROGRESSIVE CAUCUS HEALTHCARE for ALL

https://progressivecaucusactionfund.org/issues/healthcare

(See hyperlink for full text and references.)

Healthcare is a human right, but nearly 40 million Americans have no health insurance and millions more are struggling with crushing medical debt or making impossible choices between needed care and making ends meet. No one should have to turn to a "go fund me" to pay for surgery, or ration insulin to be able to pay the rent.

We need Medicare for All now including access to health, vision, dental, mental health and long-term care, affordable medicines, solutions for families drowning in medical debt. Medicare for All means every doctor and every hospital is in network. Medicare for All means every person has access to high quality healthcare with no copays, no hours wasted begging insurance companies for care, and no devastating medical debt.

CONGRESSIONAL PROGRESSIVE CAUCUS Universal Health Care Statement

https://progressives.house.gov/universal-health-care

The United States is the only developed nation in the world that fails to provide Universal Health Care to its people. The result: despite spending more per capita on health care than anywhere else, America has far worse health outcomes -- higher infant and maternal mortality, lower life expectancy, higher rates of suicide and higher rates of chronic disease. More than 27 million Americans were uninsured in 2018, and medical debt is the leading cause of bankruptcy in the United States.

Health care is a human right -- and the failure of the United States to fulfill this basic need for millions is a stain on our country. At the Progressive Caucus, we're fighting to pass the Medicare For All Act to guarantee health care to all people living in the United States. It's past time to remove the profit motive from health care and ensure that every person has access to the treatment and care that they need.

At the Progressive Caucus, we also recognize that the greed of Big Pharma is a public health crisis with life-threatening implications for millions of families. Nearly one in four Americans report struggling to afford a prescription drug. This is a national public health crisis caused by the greed of Big Pharma. Congress must act to rein in the price-gouging in the pharmaceutical market, require the direct negotiation of drug prices between pharmaceutical companies and the federal government, ensure robust competition in the marketplace, and institute critical safeguards to prevent any lifesaving drugs from being removed from the market.

Lastly, at the Progressive Caucus we believe that reproductive freedoms are a critical part of any universal health care system. We must permanently end the discriminatory Hyde Amendment, which prevents countless low-income women and women of color from accessing their constitutional right to reproductive health care. And given the unprecedented attacks on Roe v. Wade, Congress must act to codify Roe and make it clear that women's reproductive freedoms are not up for debate.

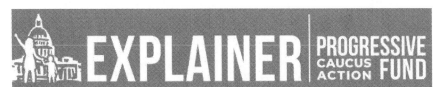

https://static1.squarespace.com/static/53cab2c3e4b0207d2957d0d2/t/605b72
e1d6fc1a50a52c01d0/1616605921216/House+Support+for+Medicare+for+A
ll+Growing.pdf   (See hyperlink for full text and references.)

House Support for Medicare for All Growing But Still Needs to Catch Up with Voters

www.progressivecaucusactionfund.org
Last updated 22 March 2021

Support for Medicare for All in the House of Representatives has grown in recent years. On March 17, 2021, Reps. Pramila Jayapal and Debbie

Dingell introduced the Medicare for All Act of 2021 with a record 112 original cosponsors. The Medicare for All Act of 2019 (H.R. 1384 – now H.R. 1976) ended the 116th Congress with a total of 118 cosponsors and four congressional hearings.

However, Members of Congress are still far behind the general public. While only one in four House Members have cosponsored the Medicare or All Act, voters consistently favor Medicare for All in public polling. This gap between Members and their constituents shows up in all the key committees that may consider Medicare for All in the House.

Support for Medicare for All is strong across the country. A national exit poll from the 2020 general election found that 72 percent of Americans are in favor of switching to a government-run healthcare plan like Medicare for All. A Kaiser Family Foundation tracking poll found that Medicare or All consistently had majority support from June 2017 to January 2020. The COVID-19 pandemic has increased support for Medicare for All. A Morning Consult poll found that "more than two in five U.S. adults say the outbreak has increased their likelihood of supporting universal health care proposals where the government would provide all Americans with health insurance," including one in four Republicans and 34 percent of independents.

KEY HOUSE COMMITTEES

Healthcare jurisdiction is divided up between many committees in the House. As a result, the Medicare for All Act of 2019 was referred to six House committees: Energy and Commerce, Ways and Means, Education and Labor, Rules, Oversight and Reform, and Armed Services. Four House committees held hearings on the bill: Budget, Energy and Commerce, Ways and Means, and Rules. Information on those committees and additional committees of interest is provided below.

Energy & Commerce Committee:

• Subcommittee on Health: The Subcommittee on Health is the primary committee of jurisdiction for the Medicare for All Act. It has broad jurisdiction over public health, health providers, Medicaid, the Indian Health Service and other matters relevant to Medicare for All.

• Hearing: The Energy & Commerce Subcommittee on Health held a hearing - Proposals to Achieve Universal Health Care Coverage - on

December 10, 2019 on the Medicare for All Act of 2019 as well as eight other bills. Witnesses included:

➢ Rep. Pramila Jayapal

➢ President Jean Ross, National Nurses United

➢ Douglas Holtz-Eakin, President, American Action Forum (Republican witness)

➢ Scott W. Atlas, David and Joan Traitel Senior Fellow, Hoover Institution, Stanford University (Republican witness)

Ways & Means Committee:

● Subcommittee on Health: Beyond the Ways and Means Committee's general jurisdiction over taxes and revenue, the Health Subcommittee's jurisdiction includes Medicare, drug pricing, and existing subsidies for private health insurance.

● Hearing: The Ways and Means Subcommittee on Health held a hearing - Pathways to Universal Health Coverage - on June 12, 2019 on ways to strengthen the Affordable Care Act, the addition of a lower-cost public option, Medicare and Medicaid buy-ins, Medicare for America, and Medicare for All. Witnesses included:

➢ Rebecca Wood, Patient advocate and mother who lives outside of Boston, Massachusetts

➢ Tricia Neuman, Senior Vice President and Director of the Program on Medicare Policy, Henry J. Kaiser Family Foundation

➢ Donald M. Berwick, President Emeritus and Senior Fellow, Institute for Healthcare Improvement and Former Administrator, Centers for Medicare & Medicaid Services

➢ Pam MacEwan, Chief Executive Officer, Washington Health Benefit Exchange

➢ Chiquita Brooks-LaSure, Managing Director, Manatt Health

➢ Grace-Marie Turner, President of the Galen Institute (Republican witness)

Education & Labor Committee: The Education and Labor Committee has jurisdiction over employee benefits, including health benefits.

Rules Committee: In addition to considering rules to bring major legislation to the House floor, the Rules Committee also has original jurisdiction for legislation that affects the rules of the House. Given the congressional hearings required by the Medicare for All Act, it could come before the House Rules Committee as an original jurisdiction matter in addition to a standard Rules Committee meeting.

- Hearing: The Rules Committee held a hearing on Medicare for All on April 30, 2019. Witnesses included:

➤ Dr. Dean Baker, Senior Economist, Center for Economic and Policy Research

➤ Dr. Sara Collins, Vice President for Health Care Coverage and Access, Commonwealth Fund

➤ Dr. Doris Browne, Immediate Past-President, National Medical Association

➤ Dr. Farzon Nahvi, Emergency Room Physician

➤ Mr. Ady Barkan, Founder, Be A Hero Organization

➤ Ms. Grace-Marie Turner, President of Galen Institute (Republican witness)

➤ Dr. Charles Blahous, J. Fish and Lillian F. Smith Chair and Senior Research Strategist, Mercatus Center (Republican witness)

Oversight & Reform Committee: In addition to being the main investigative committee in the House, the Committee on Oversight and Reform has jurisdiction over federal workers and general jurisdiction over government operations and efficiency.

Armed Services Committee: The House Armed Services Committee, specifically the Subcommittee on Military Personnel, has jurisdiction over Medicare for All to the extent it affects military personnel and their families.

Budget Committee: While the Medicare for All Act of 2019 was not referred to the House Committee on the Budget, the Budget Committee would have to hold a markup if Medicare for All advanced through the budget reconciliation process.

- Hearing: The Budget Committee held a hearing, "Key Design Components and Considerations for Establishing a Single-Payer Health Care System," on May 22, 2019 with the focus on Medicare for All. Witnesses included:

  ➢ Mark Hadley, Deputy Director, Congressional Budget Office

  ➢ Dr. Jessica Banthin; Deputy Assistant Director for Health, Retirement, and Long-Term Analysis; Congressional Budget Office

  ➢ Dr. Jeffrey Kling, Associate Director for Economic Analysis, Congressional Budget Office

Small Business Committee: The Medicare for All Act of 2019 was not referred to the Small Business Committee. Nevertheless, the committee frequently holds hearings on healthcare issues in relation to small businesses.

Leadership of Key House Committees in the 117th Congress Committee and subcommittee chairs set the agenda, deciding on hearings and markups. Support among committee leaders is essential to advancing Medicare for All through the House. Chairs of seven of the eight key committees (and one key subcommittee) have cosponsored the Medicare for All Act. However, the Chairs of the Ways & Means Committee and Health Subcommittee of the Energy & Commerce Committee have not yet cosponsored.

(See charts using hyperlink above and as follows:
https://static1.squarespace.com/static/53cab2c3e4b0207d2957d0d2/t/
605b72e1d6fc1a50a52c01d0/1616605921216/House+Support+for+Me
dicare+for+All+Growing.pdf)

CONCLUSION:

Congressional support is less than half of what it should be relative to broad support among the general public. Only 26 percent of House members have cosponsored the Medicare for All Act. Slightly more than half of House Democrats have cosponsored, and no House Republicans have.

The House Oversight & Reform Committee, House Education & Labor Committee, and House Rules Committee register the highest levels of support for Medicare for All among key committees, with about 40 percent of their committee members supporting the bill. On the Oversight & Reform Committee, three-quarters of Democrats support Medicare for All. In addition, more than one-third of House Budget Committee members (and 62 percent of Democratic members) support Medicare for All.

While Medicare for All has majority support among Americans, it lacks proportional support among members on the two most important committees of jurisdiction: the Energy & Commerce and Ways & Means Committees. Not only do all Republicans on those committees fail to support Medicare for All, half of Democrats on those committees have not cosponsored the bill yet. (In fact, they cosponsor Medicare for All at a slightly lower rate than House Democrats overall.) This suggests a major schism between those members of those committees and the people they represent. The case to committee members should be convincing whether they care more about public health or family budgets: a Lancet study found that implementing Medicare for All would save lives and money (over $450 billion annually).

Unfortunately, the Small Business Committee shows the least support for Medicare for All of the key committees - with only three members cosponsoring. This is out of step with the needs of small businesses. Prior to the pandemic, small business owners already struggled with healthcare costs and the pandemic has exacerbated the situation. A Medicare for All system would alleviate many of the financial burdens small businesses face by eliminating healthcare costs.

Americans recognize that Medicare for All is more vital than ever as the country recovers from the COVID-19 pandemic. Members of Congress, particularly those on key House committees, need to catch up.

ORGANIZATIONS THAT PROMOTE UNIVERSAL HEALTHCARE

HEALTHCARE-NOW!

Executive Director: Benjamin Day

WEBSITE: www.healthcare-now.org

Each January, HEALTHCARE-NOW! AND LABOR FOR SINGLE-PAYER host a "Single-Payer Strategy Conference". This is an amazing gathering of advocates from around the country who come together to listen to speakers, participate in group sessions and share methods of advocating for universal healthcare. You can see agendas for their various events by searching Google for "Single-Payer Strategy Conference": 2017 in NYC, 2018 in Minneapolis, 2019 in Portland, and 2020 and 2021 virtually due to COVID. Watch for future Conferences and plan to attend!

LABOR FOR SINGLE-PAYER

WEBSITE: https://www.laborforsinglepayer.org/

Contact: organizers@laborforsinglepayer.org

Major unions support Single Payer:

PNHP: PHYSICIANS FOR A NATIONAL HEALTH PROGRAM

President: Susan Rogers, MD, FACP

WEBSITE: https://pnhp.org/

STUDENTS FOR A NATIONAL HEALTH PROGRAM

Students for a National Health Program is the student arm of Physicians for a National Health Program (PNHP). The SNaHP 2021 Summit (virtual) was held on 4/24/2021. The summit is a gathering of medical and health professional students from institutions all over the country who support single-payer national health insurance. See **https://student.pnhp.org/about/** for SNaHP local chapters (by state) all across the country.

NATIONAL NURSES UNITED

Executive Director: Bonnie Castillo, RN

Presidents: Deborah Burger, Zenei Triunfo-Cortez, Jean Ross

WEBSITE: **https://www.nationalnursesunited.org/**

DUH: Demand Universal Healthcare

Donna Ellington, DUH Social Media

https://www.facebook.com/groups/858099384918591/

National Improved Medicare for All

Executive Director: Donna Ellington

https://www.facebook.com/groups/182119008587323

HEALTH OVER PROFIT FOR EVERYONE = HOPE

National Coordinator: Margaret Flowers

WEBSITE: **http://healthoverprofit.org/**

Margaret Flowers: "MEDICARE ADVANTAGE DANGERS: Medicare Advantage plans are private health insurance plans available to people who are eligible for Medicare. While the name sounds positive, Medicare Advantage plans are privatizing Medicare (sending dollars that could be used for care to investor's bank accounts), preventing seniors who need care from getting it and taking us down a wrong path."

TARBELL.ORG - Tarbell's mission is to provide objective

investigative reporting on hard hitting topics effecting Americans; specifically related to healthcare, the environment, defense, and culture.

NETWORK

Executive Director: Mary Novak

WEBSITE: https://networklobby.org/issues/healthcare/

Catholic Social Justice tells us it is our moral responsibility to guarantee access to health care for all, regardless of social or economic status, race, or ability to pay. Our government must expand health care affordability and access, eliminate disparities in health outcomes based on race and economic status, and curb the exploitative behavior of the pharmaceutical industry. We have seen too many family members, friends, and neighbors die from lack of care and unaffordable medicines in our country.

https://www.americanswhotellthetruth.org/portraits/dr-rev-william-barber-ii

Dr. Rev. William Barber II: Minister, Organizer
Our concern is the moral fabric of our society. It's about a deep vision of society that says we must look at two guiding stars. The first is our state and national Constitutions, with their insistence on the common good, the good of the whole, and establishing equal justice under the law. And the second guiding star comes from the best of all our moral and ethical traditions, loving your neighbor and doing justice. It is from these two perspectives that public policy ought to be developed. We should ask are policies constitutionally consistent, morally defensible, and economically sane.

https://en.wikipedia.org/wiki/Poor_People%27s_Campaign: A National Call for a Moral Revival

"Poor People's Campaign: A National Call for a Moral Revival is an American anti-poverty campaign led by William Barber II and Liz Theoharis. According to Jelani Cobb, writing in The New Yorker, the movement demands "federal and state living-wage laws, equity in education, an end to mass incarceration, **a single-payer health-care** system, and the protection of the right to vote." The aim of the campaign centers on connecting movements that seem to be interconnected, such as racism, sexism, anti-Native American policies, ableism and classism.

https://wholewashington.org/

IN THE ABSENCE OF NATIONWIDE UNIVERSAL HEALTHCARE SOME STATES ARE CRAFTING THEIR OWN

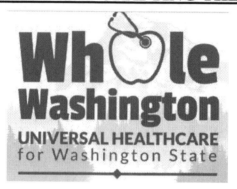

We want everyone to have high-quality, comprehensive healthcare.

By 'everyone' we mean every single resident of Washington State. Our healthcare should not be tied to our employment, our spouse, our age, or our ability to pay.

By 'comprehensive' we mean inpatient, outpatient, vision, dental, mental healthcare services, and more.

We want the care our doctor recommends, not what an insurance company decides or is willing to pay.

We want to change the way we pay.

Instead of paying profit-motivated insurance companies, we want fair and dedicated taxes to fund a trust that covers our healthcare expenses.

We want the elimination of deductibles, co-pays, unaffordable prescriptions, and other unpredictable out-of-pocket costs, and no more medical bankruptcies or crowdfunding campaigns, ever.

We want to pay nothing at the time services are rendered. We want to walk out of the hospital or doctor's office with no bills looming ahead of us.

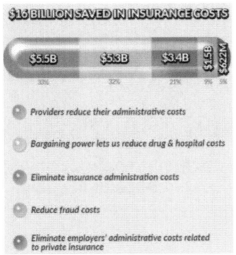

We want freedom.

We want to go to the doctor of our choice. No networks, referrals, or prior authorizations.

We want freedom from worry. If we're sick or injured, we want to focus on healing, not financial ruin. If we're healthy, we want the preventive care to stay that way.

We don't want to be locked into jobs or relationships out of fear of losing health insurance. We want the freedom to pursue our dreams.

We believe our health is our wealth.
It's time to invest in our most valuable resource: us!

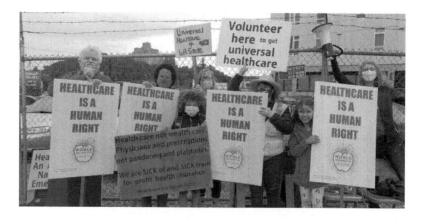

**Hundreds of additional organizations
are listed in the final chapter.**

SONGS

"We're Nursing As Fast As We Can"
https://www.youtube.com/watch?v=UQfzAdBhObk

"Medicare For All"
https://www.youtube.com/watch?v=NsgHm-ZMYvQ
https://wicklinefamilyandfriends.bandcamp.com/track/medicare-for-all-single-payer-2

DOCUMENTARIES & FILMS

By far, these are not the only documentaries and feature films about the U.S. healthcare system, but they're the ones we know best and which you can watch for free or for a minor cost on the Internet or Netflix. Gather your friends or form a "Medicare for All" Advocate Group to view these films and documentaries together.

THE MOVIE THAT STARTED IT ALL:

SICKO by Michael Moore

https://www.youtube.com/watch?v=_XWgw3Ea4WU

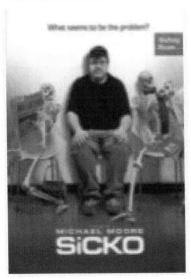

Rating: PG-13

Released: 2007

2 hours

FULL FEATURED MOVIES & VIDEOS:

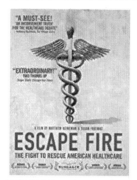

ESCAPE FIRE: The Fight to Rescue American Healthcare
http://www.escapefiremovie.com/trailer

FIXIT - HEALTHCARE AT THE TIPPING POINT:
https://www.youtube.com/watch?v=KS-olhBvEkc

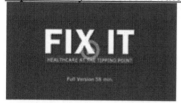

BIG PHARMA - MARKET FAILURE:
https://www.youtube.com/watch?v=W6c3yhBGGMU

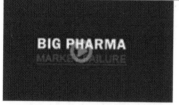

BIG MONEY AGENDA – DEMOCRACY ON THE BRINK:
https://fixithealthcare.com/watch-the-movie/big-money-agenda/

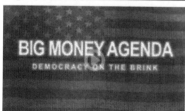

Medicare for All Short Videos:

Bernie Sanders & Medicare For All -
https://www.youtube.com/watch?v=olRR_wNTd9A&t=237s

"Bernie's Bill" – The Humanist Report, Episode 111 (Mike Figueredo: START at 52:40 – STOP at 1:17:25). Ah, yes: "The Senate just overwhelmingly approved a $700 billion military spending bill. You don't need to explain spending on our military industrial complex and killing people, but you must justify spending to provide healthcare to Americans."

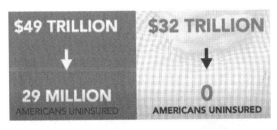

| In the youtube video, Sanders says, "Let me thank the Koch brothers, of all people, for sponsoring a study that shows that Medicare for All would save the American people $2 trillion over a 10-year period." **https://www.youtube.com/watch?v=pyC 4grL-Uag** | 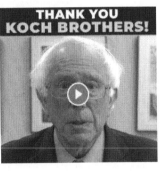 |

Healthcare: is it a right or a luxury? | Tarik Sammour

https://www.youtube.com/watch?v=jCVmY1iOJQs

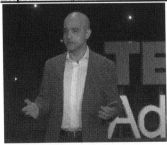 01/25/2018

DEMAND UNIVERSAL HEALTHCARE (DUH!)

https://www.commonwealthclub.org/events/archive/video/citizens-guide-medicare-all (See their book: Citizen's Guide to Medicare for All)

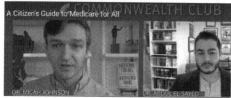 02/22/2021

https://www.youtube.com/watch?v=hQV4SZic0lE

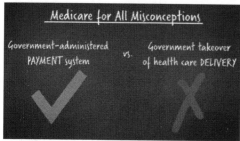 03/11/2019

https://www.youtube.com/watch?v=IyGYXEKRQ7c

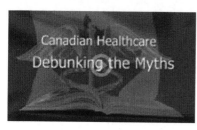 12/06/2018

https://www.youtube.com/watch?v=1DLHLHpeA-E

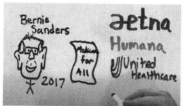 12/30/2019

https://www.youtube.com/watch?v=dvP1IaI8m44

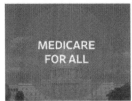 07/23/2019

https://www.youtube.com/watch?v=PuqYC-1abVM

 03/25/2019

https://vimeo.com/314654894

Medicare for All: How do we pay for it?

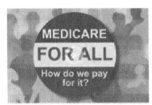 2019

https://www.laborcampaign.org/resources

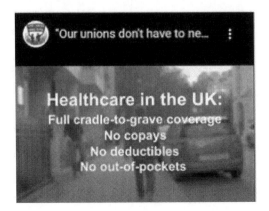

"THE HEALTHCARE MOVIE" &
"NOW IS THE TIME: Healthcare for Everybody"
By Filmmakers Terry Sterrenberg & Laurie Simons

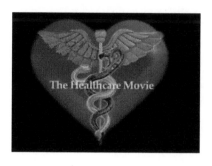
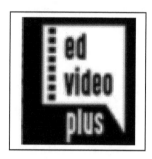

This documentary provides the real story of how the health care systems in Canada and the United States evolved to be so completely different, when at one point they were essentially the same. An intense political struggle led to the universal medical care system in Canada. Meanwhile, for almost a century, negative PR campaigns have been prevalent in the U.S. to dissuade the public from supporting national health care. https://edvideoplus.net/the-healthcare-movie/

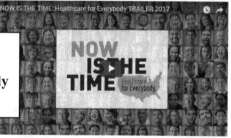

NOW IS THE TIME:

Healthcare for Everybody

TRAILER 2017

www.nowisthetimemovie.com - The United States pays almost twice as much for healthcare as any other industrialized nation, yet it still does not provide care for all its citizens. Polls show that 58% of Americans favor a national publicly funded healthcare program. This documentary delves into what single payer healthcare is, how it saves money, and what we can do to make it happen. https://www.youtube.com/watch?v=SMiZ1co0S0M

DRIVE for UNIVERSAL HEALTHCARE

Our 2013 trip thru the Northeast to the Midwest advocating for Universal, single-payer healthcare for all. Sue Saltmarsh, Donna Ellington, Terry Sterrenberg, Laurie Simons, and Bob Sisler speak about the need for Universal, Single-Payer Healthcare in easy to understand language.

https://www.youtube.com/watch?v=hObcysTDEcE

HEALTHCARE JUSTICE MARCH

https://www.youtube.com/channel/UCzAyfuoKs0kc_3fiUQd2PXQ/videos

Dr. Louis Klein, a psychiatrist, and member of SPAN--Ohio, at the Healthcare Justice Rally on August 1, 2015.

https://www.youtube.com/watch?v=YtHYMokr940

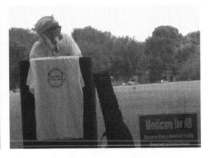

Sue Saltmarsh of DUH - Drive for Universal Healthcare on Universal Health Care vs The ACA

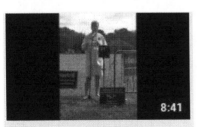

Sue Saltmarsh speaks at the Healthcare Justice March o...

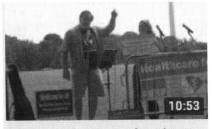

Margaret Flowers and Kevin Zeese of Popular Resistanc...

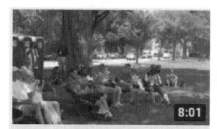

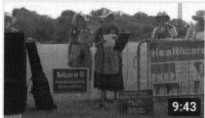

Dr. Bill Honigman sings
Silence is Consent....

The Raging Grannies at
Healthcare Justice Rally on...

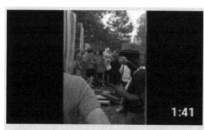

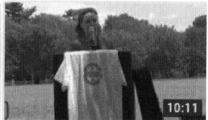

Bernie Sanders - Partial from
Medicare turns 50 event IM...

Michaeleen Crowell, Chief of
Staff for Bernie Sanders...

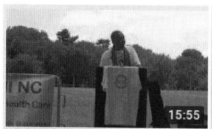

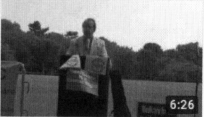

Pastor Thomas Dixon of
Charleston, SC at the...

Pastor Neal Jones speaking
at the Healthcare Justice...

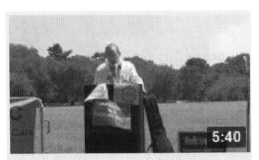

Dr Zarr, President of PNHP
DSCN0675

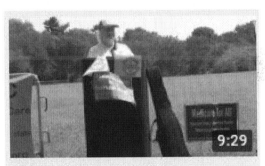

Donna Ellington, at the
Healthcare Justice Rally on ...

https://www.facebook.com/groups/182119008587323

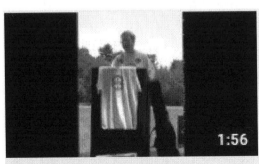

Sue closes the Healthcare
Justice March - 8/1/15

BOOKS – MEDICARE FOR ALL

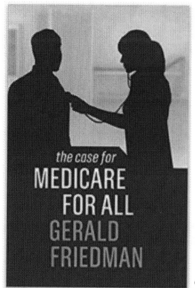

This bold and brilliantly argued book is essential reading for anyone who wants to see Congress and the White House act to provide America with a 21st century healthcare system. Largely privately funded with relatively little public regulation, the United States healthcare system is both expensive and inefficient, providing poor care to large parts of the population. For decades, Americans have wrestled with how to fix their broken healthcare system. In this razor-sharp contribution to the healthcare debate, leading economist and former adviser to Bernie Sanders Gerald Friedman recommends that we build on what works: a Medicare system that already efficiently provides healthcare for millions of Americans. Rejecting the discredited idea that healthcare should be treated like any other commodity, Friedman shows that healthcare is distinctive and can be best provided only through a universal program of social insurance. Deftly exposing the absurdities of the opponents of reform, Friedman shows in detail how the solution to our health care crisis is staring us in the face: enroll everyone in Medicare to improve the health of all Americans. (https://www.abebooks.com/first-edition/Case-Medicare-Paperback-Gerald-Friedman-Polity/30558616408/bd)

322

https://www.forewordreviews.com/reviews/medicare-for-all/
Abdul El-Sayed & **Micah Johnson**
Bernie Sanders (Contributor) & **Pramila Jayapal** (Contributor)

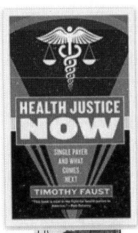

Healthcare policy is notoriously complex, but what Americans want is simple: good healthcare that's easy to use and doesn't break the bank. Polls show that a majority of Americans want the government to provide universal health coverage to all Americans. Discussing both problems with American health care and potential solutions, Abdul El-Sayed and Micah Johnson's *Medicare for All* acknowledges that "health insurance doesn't make health care affordable, and it doesn't protect you from financial ruin," and so proposes that Medicare be made available to everyone.

https://pnhp.org/news/timothy-faust-health-justice-now-a-must-read/
(full text) and https://www.youtube.com/watch?v=x0ikEx-qXtg

"What single-payer can do, I believe, is serve as a ladder we can climb, all together, into a better world. A properly designed single-payer program is one titanic step toward making people safe in their own homes, in their own bodies. It is a reprieve from our continual fucking-over by the structure and stricture of private insurance. And it is a method of finally demanding accountability from a state that permits (or even encourages) the sins that cause mass suffering—and the medical inequities they produce." – Timothy Faust

Which Country
Has the
World's Best
Health Care?

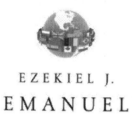

E Z E K I E L   J.
EMANUEL

WHICH COUNTRY HAS THE WORLD'S BEST HEALTH CARE?

HARDCOVER | PURCHASE

The preeminent doctor and bioethicist Ezekiel Emanuel is repeatedly asked one question: Which country has the best healthcare? He set off to find an answer. The US spends more than any other nation, nearly $4 trillion, on healthcare. Yet, for all that expense, the US is not ranked #1 – not even close. In **Which Country Has the World's Best Healthcare?** Ezekiel Emanuel profiles 11 of the world's healthcare systems in pursuit of the best or at least where excellence can be found.

Using a unique comparative structure, the book allows healthcare professionals, patients, and policymakers alike to know which systems perform well, and why, and which face endemic problems. From Taiwan to Germany, Australia to Switzerland, the most inventive healthcare providers tackle a global set of challenges in pursuit of the best healthcare in the world.

For the answer and all the facts, you'll have to read Dr. Emanuel's book.

Here is a glimpse, showing his conclusions on 22 Dimensions of Performance as compared to Australia, Canada, China, France, Germany, Netherlands, Norway, Switzerland, Taiwan and The United Kingdom:

The United States among the Best-Performing Countries:

- Comprehensiveness of benefits
- Innovation in payment
- Excellent chronic-care coordination (all selective areas)
- Excellent mental health care (all selective areas)
- Innovation in care delivery
- Access to innovative drugs

The United States among the Notably Poor-Performing Countries:

- Universal Coverage
- Simplicity and ease of obtaining coverage
- Affordability at point of service
- Progressive financing
- Specially subsidized groups - low income, children, and chronically ill
- Effective limits on total health care spending
- Simplicity in paying by patients
- Simplicity in payment to physicians and hospitals
- Choice of physicians and hospitals
- Simplicity of getting services
- Low drug prices
- Rigorous and objective mechanism to price drugs

N/A Dimension (The United States):

- Dedicated mechanism for financing long-term care
- Alignment of payment incentives
- Excellent Primary care
- Waiting times

https://fivebooks.com/best-books/austin-frakt-healthcare-reform/
(See hyperlink for full text and references.)

THE BEST BOOKS on HEALTHCARE REFORM

Recommended by Austin Frakt, a health economist and the creator of the blog The Incidental Economist. Interview by Sophie Roell

If you were starting from scratch, no one would design a healthcare system like America's. The health economist tells us how it evolved and what needs to change. He picks the best books on US healthcare reform.

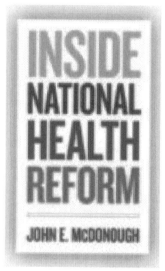
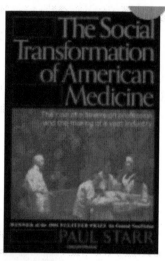
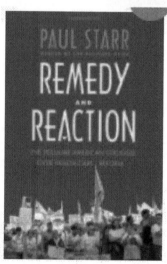

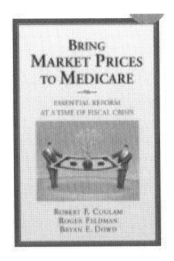
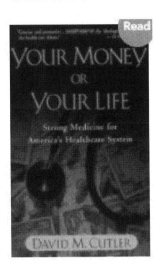

Leaving aside the insurance issue, why is the absolute price of American healthcare so high? The price of going to the doctor in the U.S., or buying drugs, can on occasion be 10 times what it is in Europe.

It's particularly surprising when in every other area – from clothing to electronic goods to gas – American consumers are incredibly cost conscious and prices are almost invariably lower than elsewhere.

There are many reasons why US health spending is so high – and why we allow it to be high. One of the main lines of Paul Starr's book ***The Social Transformation of American Medicine*** is that physicians have, over many decades, amassed considerable power over the policies that have been enacted, and they've shaped them to their benefit economically. So a lot of money flows to healthcare providers, physicians and hospitals, and also to suppliers of drugs and medical equipment. Those organisations are relatively powerful and they've been able to keep it going.

Also, Americans mostly don't see the prices. Because of insurance, they don't directly feel how expensive it is when they enter the system in any way – whether it's a visit to a physician or a visit to a hospital. Worse than that, they mostly don't even see the price of insurance directly. The vast majority of Americans have employer-based health insurance and much of the premium is paid by the employer. It doesn't show up on their pay stub, and it doesn't appear, to them, to come out of their own pocket – even though actually it does, through lower wages. When you think you're getting something for free or pretty cheaply – whether it's the insurance or the healthcare itself – you're not that motivated to shake things up.

That's for people who work. Then for retirees, almost all of them are on Medicare, so they're getting considerable benefit through a public programme. They don't see why that should change either. So things just keep marching along. We haven't been able to put in place sustainable cost controls, either publicly or privately, largely because it's politically difficult to do that.

You do see articles about spiraling insurance premiums and healthcare costs. Are attitudes changing, with people becoming more aware that this is unsustainable?

Healthcare is like every other issue in the American political discourse – it has its moments. It can rise to the surface if other things aren't in the way. If the economy is bad, that's always going to dominate what people are thinking about. Or other issues can dominate, depending on the news and where the crisis of the day is. But every once in a while, the spending on healthcare and the problems in healthcare markets do come up. They start to weigh heavily on people's minds, and when that coincides with a political opportunity to do something then reform can happen.

That coincidence tends not to happen often. Maybe once every 15 to 20 years we get a genuine opportunity to do something substantial in health, and it doesn't always succeed. That's how Medicare happened in 1965. It had been considered, worked on and thought about for more than a decade in various forms. Other comprehensive health reforms have failed over the decades including, famously, the Clinton plan of the early 1990s. That was a time when there was a lot of attention paid to healthcare. People thought we should do something, and it seemed politically feasible. But it just wasn't managed in a way that succeeded, because the politics are so hard. It's like threading a needle. You have to do *everything* right to get something passed, even if it's imperfect. Finally, in 2010, it was remarkable how well everything came together. It was very messy, but that's the nature of it. It was the finest of margins, every vote in the Senate counted. They needed 60. They got 60.

I've seen charts showing that increased spending in the US doesn't

translate into higher life expectancy. Is that because the uninsured bring down the average lifespan?

There are studies out there showing that lack of insurance leads to higher mortality, but the estimates are not precise. It's exceedingly hard to empirically relate insurance to mortality, because many health-related issues that lead to lower life expectancy take years to develop. In America, by the time you're 65 you're insured on Medicare. If you've reached that age, you're likely to live quite a bit longer. What is the effect on mortality, after age 65, of being uninsured for some number of years when you're younger? That's very hard to tell.

Why we have lower life expectancy is a good question. Insurance does play a role, but it's not the only thing that matters. What is true is that we spend dramatically more than any other country – twice as much as the next highest-spending country – and we have not just higher mortality but a whole range of quality measures that are worse than elsewhere. Sometimes much worse. So what one can confidently say is that we're spending a lot but not showing a lot for it. That doesn't mean that if we spend less, or just cut the budget, then we won't lose something. It's likely that we are getting something for all that spending – we're just not getting it very efficiently.

One barrier to change is that rich and educated people, including members of Congress, believe that the US has the best doctors and hospitals in the world – and that if they move to more socialised medicine, as in Europe, then they will lose that.

It's definitely a concern among the elite and health policy wonks. The way it plays out more broadly is that there's immense status quo bias. That's true everywhere. People tend to be comfortable with what they know. Everybody wants to believe that what they have and where they live is fantastic. People are very reluctant to give up the idea that the US is number one.

And you *can* receive the very best care in the world in this country. There is a reason why princes from Saudi Arabia fly into the US for treatment. But only a very tiny fraction of the population has access to the very best healthcare in the US. They don't want to give it up, and I don't want them to give it up either. But there are many people who don't have access to the best care. In fact, there are many people who don't even have access to basic healthcare. We're not talking about state-of-the-art, triple-transplant surgery. We're talking about routine preventative care, screenings, office visits and immunisations. The disparity is large between what the very best and the bottom quintile are able to obtain.

But _is_ it true that the US is the best country in the world for top-end healthcare? Are there studies proving that if I'm treated for cancer at a top US cancer hospital, then my survival rate is higher than in other systems?

There are certain cancers we rate very highly on. Breast cancer is one of them – our survival rate for breast cancer is very good. But when you read anything claiming that the US has the best care in the world, they are cherry picking three or four specific diseases where we have very good survival rates. It could be because the care on those diseases is good. It could also just be that if you run enough statistics, then by random variation we're going to be number one on a few things, even if we are middle of the pack or worse on 99 other things. It's not a good way of judging the overall quality of healthcare.

Given the average age of members of Congress, they must have either been sick themselves or had a relative who has been, and so know what it's like to deal with the healthcare system and insurance companies. Or do they have some sort of gold-plated insurance that means they're shielded from the worst of it?

Actually, I am an employee of the US federal government so I have the same health benefits that congressmen do. It's pretty much standard employee health benefits. For people who have decent jobs – as I do and as congressmen do – routine healthcare is not a big deal. But I've heard that it comes as a shock to people like us whenever they engage intensively with the healthcare system, for example if they or a family member becomes incredibly ill and is in hospital for a long time.

That's when some of them finally say, "Boy, I was at a good hospital and still. Ugh. It was really unpleasant and I kept being asked the same questions. They didn't seem to know that I'd already had that test. Thank God I had my wife with me during all this so she could make sure they didn't amputate the wrong leg." The stories are just shocking. There's a story just recently that a large proportion of physicians don't follow guidelines in washing their hands. It's atrocious.

Let's talk about the Obama administration's attempt to reform the system. The first book you've picked is _Inside National Health Reform_, which explains the 2010 law (The ACA) and also the political jockeying that made it what it is.

This is really two books in one. John McDonough is an insider. He was an adviser to Senator [Ted] Kennedy's HELP committee, which was one of the two big committees in the Senate that wrote the health reform law. He was in a lot of meetings, talked to a lot of people, and tells wonderful stories about negotiations over the minutiae of the health law. It's suspenseful and interesting to see how law, and this law in particular, is really made. There's a lot about the politics but it also explains the policy rationale – why it was structured this way, why one side thought this and the other side thought something else.

That's the first half of the book, and it's not a hard read. The second half goes through the law in summary fashion, through each title and then each sub-section. It explains what they're about and why, and how much money they cost or save, in plain language. That in itself, I will admit, is pretty tedious. I've read the law and summaries of it, and it's not fun. You only do it if you are looking for something. However, he intersperses long passages explaining more of the politics and policy rationale. Those chunks are easy to pick out by eye, so you can just flip through the summary of the law and go straight to the narrative. It's just as intriguing as the first half of the book.

This book is important because most people have no idea how laws are really made in the US, and what politics really means. Not the politics of campaigns but the politics of making a law, especially one as complicated and controversial as the health reform law. In the end, the message is that the health reform law we got in 2010 was the only one we could have got in 2010, or pretty close to the only one. The range of what was politically feasible was incredibly narrow. It had to satisfy so many political constraints that it almost didn't happen. It was either that law or no law.

So while not perfect, it's the best that could be done given the politics?

No law is perfect. No law will satisfy everybody. My view is that the correct interpretation of what we have is not the national health reform we all deserve and want, but a good first step towards an evolutionary reform. There will need to be more. We can build on what we have. But the status quo was not and is not acceptable, and this makes some important changes.

What is the best thing about the law, in terms of moving in the right direction?

The reforms to the health insurance market were absolutely crucial and, abstracting from the law itself, relatively uncontroversial. Across the political spectrum, it would be hard to find many people who would say, "Actually, it's a good thing that private insurers can keep people off insurance. They should be able to keep people off, they should be able to throw people off, and it should be very expensive." In reforming the way that market functions, the law logically requires some other things that are controversial, but that principle alone is one of the best aspects.

What will it mean in practice? For people who are already insured through their employer, presumably it won't have much impact.

It will not have a substantial impact on most people who are currently insured. It is possible, depending on where you work, what your employer does and what your future holds, that you will be impacted. If you lose your health insurance for whatever reason, for example, there will be better options for you beginning in 2014. And there are some aspects of the law that will change features of your health insurance – some things you may like, some things you may not – but in relatively minor ways.

Let's go onto Paul Starr's book _The Social Transformation of American Medicine_. This explains historically why the American health system is the way it is.

This is a very long, detailed book, and it's not all that easy for someone who is not deeply into health policy and healthcare to relate it to today. Its purpose is to describe the broad sweep of the history of healthcare in America, through to about 1980. It was published in 1982 so it's not even that current. But it's necessary reading for anybody who fancies themselves as a health policy wonk or expert, or a health historian, or anybody who works in healthcare. I found it fascinating, and I didn't even know about it until relatively recently. I've put it on this list to remind people of its existence, because it should be more widely known and read.

So 30 years after it was written you still think it is relevant. What is it about the book that's so interesting?

The parallels. He traces the development of institutions, many of which remain in positions of power as they did in the past, and have been able to amass more power. There have been some changes over the century, but many things have stayed the same. He tells stories about the politics of reform and prior reform efforts – of which there were a lot, even before 1980. You could lift so many passages from that book and people would say "Oh, you're talking about 2009" and you'd say "No, that was 1917 or 1937". It would be great to impress upon people that these issues of healthcare reform that we fight about so passionately today are the same issues people have been fighting about in the US for 100 years. That's the reason to read this book.

We have spent decades on these issues, and perhaps up to half of us are *still* not convinced that we've taken a reasonable step in the latest reform. Just thinking about that is stunning – the number of years we've gone with the level of uninsurance we have in this country, and the rate of increase in healthcare costs. They've been escalating faster than any other country since about 1980. Unfortunately, Starr's book ends right when the US healthcare trajectory, in terms of spending, diverges from the rest of industrialised countries. Look at the graphs and it's in about 1980 that the US starts taking off, and everybody else stays at a lower level. And we're still diverging.

One key difference with other countries is that in the U.S., employers provide health insurance. Why is that so embraced here?

This is partly what my next choice, Paul Starr's most recent book *__Remedy and Reaction__*, is really about. It's describing what he and others call the U.S. health policy trap. That trap is that we've evolved to a point where most people and most voters are insured, either through an employer or Medicare. Therefore, they and the institutions that they benefit are resistant to change. It's very hard to move the system to something that would be more sensible. Right now, the reason people cling to employer-based care is because it's what they know. On one level, it works. Yes it's expensive and inefficient, but it's what they know, it seems to work for them. That's why it's hard to change.

Do healthcare economists think it's a good thing?

No. It's widely recognised that a more rational system would sever the connection between health insurance and employment. To the extent that the debate is over policy, it's about how to get there and under what terms. To the extent that the debate is over politics, it's just too easy to use the spectre of change to frighten people.

Why is it so inefficient?

It creates too many distortions in the labour market. A lot of people will take and hold onto jobs for the health insurance, not because the job makes sense in terms of the work or even in terms of wages. There are many people who don't retire because of health insurance. There are even studies that show that there is lower creation of small businesses and less entrepreneurship because of health insurance. It's an unnecessary constraint on the labour market and on job creation, and it just doesn't need to be that way.

I get the sense that if you started from scratch, you would not create a system like American healthcare.

No, and it's not just me. I would defy anybody to come up with it. If you could go to a world where you are unaware of the American system and then design a system, there is no way you would come up with anything like what we have here. It's just preposterous. It doesn't make sense on so many levels. The risk pools are chopped up, there are many inefficiencies and strange subsidisations. Nobody would do it that way. One couldn't even imagine that it would be possible. You can't make this stuff up.

Tell me more about _Remedy and Reaction_. It just came out, and takes us pretty much up to the present.

Yes. It's mostly focused on the last several decades, and relatively more attention is paid as we get closer to the present, including the most recent healthcare reform effort. Quite a lot of it is on the Clinton effort as well. It's really about more modern development of health policy in the U.S. and the policy rationale for the 2010 health reform law. It includes much of the politics that were in McDonough's book but not the stories, because Paul Starr wasn't sitting in on those kinds of meetings. If you want to read one book and learn something about the policy and the politics of health reform, this is a fine choice. It has all the arguments and all the nuances.

What in particular makes you recommend it?

As you know, I've been paying a lot of attention to this. There's almost no issue about health reform policy and politics that I haven't read about and seen debated. What really impressed me is how on every single issue that I'm familiar with, he said all the things that I knew and was expecting, and then he'd say one more thing that I hadn't quite assimilated yet, or I hadn't recognised. It was a nuance or an insight that went one step beyond and blew me away. There was always a little bit more from him that I hadn't seen anyone else put on paper. Paul Starr just puts it all together better and more completely than I've seen anywhere else.

Your fourth book is _Bring Market Prices to Medicare_. I know from your blog that you believe we should take the authors' advice on this, and that it would reduce Medicare expenditure by 8% – some $50bn (£32bn) a year. Can you explain?

One of the perennial debates about Medicare is how much we should support the participation of private plans, and how much we should make it a public-only programme. It started as just a public health insurance programme. All the bills were paid directly by the federal government, it was a uniform national benefit and there was no choice: You're on Medicare, everyone is in the same programme, it's one big risk pool. Then, starting in the 1970s but increasingly in the late 90s and 2000s, private plans have participated. You can enroll in what is now called Medicare Advantage Plan, through which you get all your Medicare benefits and maybe more. You pay them a premium, they get a subsidy from the government and it's like a private plan arm of Medicare. Also, the Medicare prescription drug programme, which includes drug-only private insurance, is entirely through private plans. Medicare does not have a public prescription drug programme.

Every year in Congress, and also elsewhere, we debate: How much should these private plans be subsidised? Is it a good deal? Do they save money? Are they treating beneficiaries well? Are they just cream-skimming, i.e. choosing the healthiest beneficiaries and making a lot of profit off taxpayers? Conversely, is traditional Medicare – the public option – serving beneficiaries well? Is it slow to innovate? Is it inflexible? Is it wasting money? Is it not managing care well? One approach that would resolve the question of how much we should pay these private plans is to have them compete, along with traditional Medicare, for the rate of subsidy that they're given. This kind of competition is akin to the sort that each of us would put a contractor through if we were remodeling our kitchen or having our house repainted. You would solicit bids from qualified painters or construction companies, and you would weigh the price of the bids against quality. You would probably ultimately pick a bid based largely on price.

Medicare Advantage and traditional Medicare could do the same, but they don't. You could have these plans compete, bid for how much of a subsidy they would need to provide the Medicare benefit, and then Medicare would say, "OK, we're going to pick the lowest subsidy rate and give all plans that same amount. They can all participate, but if beneficiaries want to choose a more expensive plan then they have to pay the difference." That's what this book is about. It gives a lot of detail on Medicare pertaining to some of the things that we debate regularly. It gets into questions like: What really is the Medicare benefit? What is the social contract? Does the Medicare benefit have to include a public option that's available to everyone at the same price? Or can it be a different price in different areas, depending on how plans bid and compete? Do plans have to provide access to all willing providers or can they establish provider networks, as private plans do and traditional Medicare doesn't?

Is this competitive bidding going to happen? From the way you describe it, it sounds like a no-brainer.

It's a political battle. Plans don't want to compete. They're very happy with the relatively lavish payments they receive now.

Is the book comprehensive on Medicare?

No, it's not the place to go on Medicare generally. For that, John Oberlander's ***The Political Life of Medicare*** is a good book. That would be the place to go on the history of Medicare and why it was shaped the way it was – the political bargaining leading up to it, and its history since. But it was published in 2003, so it doesn't get into the Prescription

Drug Programme which was passed in 2003 and enacted in 2006.

Let's move onto the last book, by another highly regarded healthcare economist, David Cutler of Harvard. Why have you chosen _Your Money or Your Life_?

I suggested this book because it raises some very important points about healthcare spending in the US. We spend a lot, and it's generally believed there is a lot of waste. There are a lot of things we could cut, or ways we could save on spending that wouldn't harm health. Looking internationally suggests that this must be true. But even so, Cutler's argument is that we do receive great value from our spending on healthcare. He argues that even if you look at just a few health conditions – heart conditions, mental health, low-birth-weight infants – and work out the value that we've received from improvements in healthcare, quality of life and prolonged life, it is greater than what we spend. He says we get high value for all this money. That doesn't mean we shouldn't spend less and still get that high value, it just means that we're still making, on average, investments that are worth it.

Are you recommending this book because that's not an argument you often hear?

If one is in favour of cutting health spending because there's so much waste and so forth, then the next easy place to go – which is often where we do go – is to make very crude cuts across the board. To just cut Medicare, for example. That runs the risk of throwing out the baby with the bathwater. The book suggests that we do need to get smarter about how we make our health system more efficient. You can cut spending in a way that could be harmful to health or, in principle, you can cut it in a way that isn't. We know ways to cut that aren't going to harm health, we know some things that we shouldn't be paying for. But we don't know as much as we ought to.

For our international readers, can you outline how bad things are in the U.S. for people who cannot afford health insurance? You hear horror stories, but there is also protection such as Medicaid for those with a very low income.

Things are very bad if you don't have insurance. If you become ill, then not only will you suffer from that illness but you will also suffer from bill collectors. They don't care – it's not their job to care how badly you may be doing. They will harass you and repossess what they can. Eventually you'll have nothing. You will be bankrupt. This does happen to people in the US. The reason it happens is that the safety net has a lot of holes in it.

You mention Medicaid, which is supposed to be the programme for the poor. Ultimately, if things are bad enough, if you spend all your money and have no job or income, then you might be able to go on Medicaid. But actually, it doesn't even cover all the poor. You have to be poor *and* you have to fall into one of a number of qualifying categories, like being pregnant, elderly, blind or disabled. Beyond those federally mandated categories, individual states have the discretion to cover more. Many of them don't. Or if they do, they only cover them if your income is extremely low, a fraction of the poverty level.

So it is possible in the US to be horribly poor and not have access to any health insurance programme. You're at the mercy of charity care. And there is charity care. You can also walk into an emergency room and if it's an emergency they will treat you. But that is no way to have a healthy, satisfying life.

People always tell me this, that if you're really in trouble you can always walk into an emergency room and you will be treated. But the bill collectors will come after you if you don't pay that bill, presumably?

Yes. They will try to collect payment but eventually, if you can't pay, they can't take what you don't have. Many states have uncompensated care pools, so they'll try and collect that or just write it off. Sometimes hospitals don't get reimbursement for the care they provide.

Is there also a lot of difference depending on where you live?

There's a lot of variation. In urban areas, there will tend to be better access and support for such things, because of population density and infrastructure. In rural areas, obviously there's a lot less. And even though you may have access, it is constrained; you may not have access to many specialists, and you're at the mercy of whatever quality those programmes are. There are many studies showing that your access is greatly restricted, and you're not getting regular preventative care.

And some doctors just don't accept Medicaid even if you have it.

Oh yes. Many doctors don't take Medicaid. It's not in any way a requirement and reimbursements are low.

I always thought Medicaid covered all low-income people.

That's widely misunderstood, and is one thing that the health reform law will change. As of 2014, anyone with income within 133% of the poverty level is eligible for Medicaid, independent of anything else.

Support Five Books
Five Books interviews are expensive to produce. If you've enjoyed this interview, please support us by donating a small amount.

Five Books aims to keep its book recommendations and interviews up to date. If you are the interviewee and would like to update your choice of books (or even just what you say about them) please email us at editor@fivebooks.com *(Donate: **https://fivebooks.com/support-us/**)*

Read the full text of these bills:

S. 1129 (pending reintroduction) - Bernie Sanders & Co-sponsors:
https://www.congress.gov/bill/116th-congress/senate-bill/1129/text
&
H.R. 1976 (17 March 2021) - Pramila Jayapal & Co-sponsors:
https://www.congress.gov/bill/117th-congress/house-bill/1976/text

MEDICARE for ALL BILLS

in THE SENATE & THE HOUSE of REPRESENTATIVES

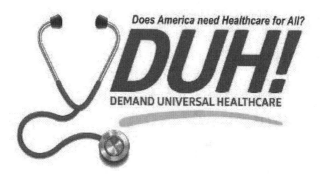

Follow Demand Universal Healthcare - DUH on Facebook!

https://www.facebook.com/groups/858099384918591/

Visit our new website – www.peopleenergizingpolitics.org/

Sue Saltmarsh (1956 - 2021), Founder of DUH, said: The general public - especially young people who are the ones who will push "Medicare for ALL" - wants to know:

1. How much will I have to pay?

2. What's covered and what's not?

3. What about undocumented immigrants?

4. What about abortion?

5. Will there still be co-pays, deductibles, networks?

6. What about long wait times?

What is true universal, or single-payer, healthcare?

- No premiums. No deductibles. No co-pays or co-insurance. No medical debt.

- 100% of your costs would be paid by government revenues. Under the Affordable Care Act (ACA) only 70% is covered by silver exchange plans.

- ALL necessary testing, care, and treatment would be covered, including mental health, dental, vision and hearing aids.

- Your access to healthcare would never depend on your ability to pay.

Is it free?

- No – everyone who works would pay into the system. As with Medicare/Medicaid, there would be a Healthcare trust that would be funded through payroll deductions. The original proposed funding of H.R. 676 (now H.R. 1976) would increase payroll tax for most people to 4.75% of their income. Proposed 1/3 (.003) of 1% tax on stock sales – Wall Streeters have to pay some too!

- We don't know what HR 1976 will end up being, but estimates are 5% for most people, 8% and up for those earning more than $250,000 per year.

- Too much? What do you pay for health insurance now, including premiums & deductibles & co-pays & unspecified income taxes (& monthly deductions from your Social Security, Seniors)?

Is it good for business?

- Yes – employers would pay a set payroll tax, no longer facing rising premiums.

- No more paying for medical costs under worker's comp.

- Labor and management would no longer have to fight over healthcare benefits, including pensions.

- If employers didn't have to pay exorbitant healthcare costs, they could hire more people.

- Consumers will have more money to spend to purchase products and services, increasing business profitability and making our economy stronger.

If I'm healthy, why should I have to pay higher taxes for someone else's healthcare?

- Your taxes help pay for police/fire protection, public education, infrastructure, and our military even though you may never be the victim of a crime, have a home that burns down, have children in school, drive on roads, or personally need military intervention. Why not guarantee healthcare?

- Healthcare is a basic need for everyone. Providing it for each other makes our country healthier, stronger, and more united.

- Right now you are paying via taxes for the healthcare of those who are uninsured, underinsured, and have no access to care except the ER. Why not pay less and get more for everyone?

Wouldn't the government be able to interfere in my healthcare decisions?

- Insurance companies interfere already and spend up to 30% on administrative costs. Their vested interest is in profit and happy investors. The government spends around 3% administering Medicare / Medicaid. The government's interest is like ours – improving America's health and lowering the cost of healthcare.

- Under a true universal system, no provider or facility would be "outside the network."

- There will be no more fighting with insurance companies when you should be fighting your illness.

- Decisions will be made by you and your doctor, not by bureaucrats with no medical training.

How would a National Improved Medicare for All (NIMA) healthcare plan work for businesses?

Currently, businesses that offer health insurance to their employees pay at least 10% of operating costs (most pay more) for covering their employees. The ACA's convoluted requirements for different sized businesses based on number of employees have caused some employers to cut down on or not be able to hire full-time workers in order to save money on ever-rising premiums.

- Though we can't yet know specific numbers for HR 1976, under HR 676 in the past, cost was proposed to be around a 4.75% payroll tax, significantly less than the current system, with no rising premiums.

- Medical costs associated with worker's comp would be covered.

- All employees, part-time or full-time, would receive all medically necessary care and treatment they needed, including in- and outpatient care, primary care, surgery, testing, lab work, physical and occupational therapy, dental, vision, long term care, mental health and addiction recovery, and dental and vision care.

- There would be no administrative work to be done as far as claims, eligibility, or purchasing different kinds of policies.

- Neither the employer nor the employees would ever see a medical bill. Patients would go to the doctor(s) *they* choose, receive the services they need, the doctor and/or the hospital would send the bill to the government, and the government would pay.

- Medical bankruptcy would no longer exist and businesses would no longer have to choose between hiring a full-time worker and paying an insurance premium they can't afford, cutting benefits, buying a cheaper, inadequate plan, or shifting more cost to employees who also can't afford it.

Isn't this socialized medicine?

No. In a socialized plan like the one in the UK, the government not only pays the bill, but (similar to our VA system) they also employ the providers, and own the hospitals, facilities, and labs. Under "Medicare for All", doctors and other providers are either solo practitioners or members of a private practice group, as they are now. Hospitals, imaging facilities, labs, etc. are privately owned and operated. The government pays the bill and that's it.

I don't want some federal bureaucrat deciding what treatment I can and cannot have – no death panels!

Private insurance companies driven only by profit motive now limit care based on cost. They hand down death sentences every day by denying medically necessary, doctor-preferred treatment in favor of whatever's cheaper. This leads to more than 45,000 unnecessary deaths per year. The government has no profit motive. The top concern is keeping us healthy, thus lowering costs, which is why NIMA (New & Improved Medicare for All) promotes primary and preventive care, as well as the best appropriate treatment.

What if employers move their business to another state?

Medicare for All ("a card in your wallet") is completely portable for both business owners and their employees. No matter where in the U.S. you move, your insurance goes with you. And if some employees choose to go back to school, or start a business of their own, they will not lose their healthcare. It will stay the same no matter what. Once they leave the job, their employer won't pay a tax for them anymore.

Medicare for All is simple, cost-effective, and offers the greatest benefit to our society. It makes sense and cents! The participation of the People, relentless in our demand, is what it will take to make it a reality!

https://spanwv.org/
(See hyperlink for full text and references.)

How Would National Improved Medicare for All / Single-Payer Work?

Lynn Moses Yellott, Author. The SPANWV website was designed and built by Terry Thorson, BlueStars Design, with additional design input by the late Ann Louise Coulter of Shepherdstown WV.
Members of Single-Payer Action Network WV include healthcare providers and non-medical people in the Eastern Panhandle of West Virginia

- A single-payer healthcare system would provide comprehensive healthcare for everyone from birth to death.

- If you change jobs, lose your job, start a business, or get divorced—your benefits would stay the same.

- You would be able to keep your doctors/practitioners because there would be no networks to be in or out of.

- You would not need to delay or avoid seeing a doctor because of out-of-pocket expenses.

- Healthcare would be publicly funded in the same way we pool our taxes to pay for police, fire protection, education, roads, public parks, and the military — regardless of how much we use these public services. Everyone would be in one risk pool.

- You would no longer pay premiums, co-payments, or deductibles to private health insurance companies that put profit over medical needs. (Private insurance would only be for non-medically-necessary care, such as cosmetic surgery.)

- Our healthcare dollars would be spent on health**care**, decided by you and your doctor, not on health insurance with its wasteful and unnecessary administrative costs, the goal of which is denial of care.

- Two different (but somewhat similar) bills in the U.S. Congress would establish Medicare for All: H.R. 1976, the Medicare For All Act of 2021 in the House, and S. 1129, the Medicare for All Act of 2019 in the Senate.

NOTE: Proposed Funding For HR 1976 Program*

Maintain current federal and state funding for existing healthcare programs; employer payroll tax of 4.5%, an employee payroll tax of 3.3%, in addition to the already existing 1.45% for Medicare; establish a 5% health tax on the top 5% of income earners; 10% tax on top 1% of wage earners, 1/3rd of 1% stock transaction tax, closing corporate tax loop-holes; repeal the Bush tax cut for the highest income earners.

*This proposal is put forward by single-payer advocates as one example of a funding system, though HR 1976 doesn't propose a funding program.

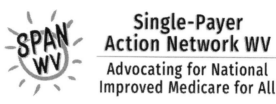

**Single-Payer
Action Network WV**

Advocating for National
Improved Medicare for All

🌐 spanwv.org
✉ MedicareForAll@spanwv.org
🐦 @SPAN_WV
f @SPANWV — Single-Payer Action Network WV

https://www.nbcnews.com/politics/2020-election/if-roe-v-wade-struck-down-would-sanders-medicare-all-n1024566
(See hyperlink for full text and references.)

If Roe v. Wade is Struck Down, Would Sanders' "Medicare for All" Still Guarantee the Right to an Abortion?

By Adam Edelman, 28 June 2019

MIAMI — Vermont Sen. Bernie Sanders, responding to a hypothetical question during Thursday night's Democratic debate, seemed to suggest that his "Medicare for All" health care plan would guarantee all women the right to an abortion even if Roe v. Wade is struck down.

Policy experts told NBC News Friday that this is wrong. It would not be possible for Sanders' health care plan — as it is written now — to ensure the right to abortion in states that decide to outlaw the procedure in a world where that landmark Supreme Court decision doesn't exist.

But, they said, the issue is a complicated one. Here's why.

MSNBC's Rachel Maddow, one of the debate's moderators, asked Sanders: "What is your plan if Roe v. Wade is struck down while you're president?"

Sanders, after talking about appointing progressive judges to the high court, eventually responded by saying, "Medicare for All guarantees every woman in this country the right to have an abortion if she wants it."

His response raised an enormous theoretical question: Assuming Roe v.

346

Wade is overturned, and Sanders' iteration of Medicare for All is in place, could women covered by the health care system still obtain an abortion in states that decide to outlaw the procedure?

Experts told NBC News that the answer would essentially be no, though there's more to the story.

If the Supreme Court were to strike down Roe v. Wade, the 1973 decision that effectively legalized abortion nationwide, states could make abortion illegal. In other words, they could deny the legal right to receive this procedure within their individual state borders.

Under Sanders' version of Medicare for All, women would have insurance that pays for the procedure. But experts on the issue told NBC News that it wouldn't matter. "Medicare for All" simply guarantees the insurance — not the procedure.

"Medicare for All could pay for abortions, but that's different than whether or not a person could get one," said Lawrence Gostin, a professor of global health law at the Georgetown University Law Center.

"It only solves the issue of payment, not the issue of access," he added.

Gostin added that, in the scenario Sanders was responding to, "a person who lives in a state where abortion is outlawed could travel to a state that still allows it," and use the insurance there.

"Which isn't really different than how things are now," he said, referring to the idea that some women are already traveling hundreds of miles to visit an abortion clinic due to restrictive laws in their home states.

Michelle Mello, a professor of law and health research and policy at Stanford University's School of Law and School of Medicine, agreed.

"The mere fact that a woman has insurance coverage available for abortion will not open a pathway for her to receive an abortion in a jurisdiction that has chosen to make it illegal," she told NBC News in an email.

"In order for Sanders' claim to make sense, the Medicare for All legislation would need to include a provision that prevents states from regulating abortion" or "asserting that Congress intends to pre-empt state law in that area," Mello added.

"I don't know whether Sanders envisions including such a provision, and

347

I can't imagine it would have a shot in a Republican-controlled Senate," she said.

A spokesman for the Sanders' campaign, when asked to elaborate on Sanders' statement from the debate, explained to NBC News that the Supreme Court striking down Roe "could mean any number of any different things because the court would be re-writing precedent" and pointed to efforts to codify Roe v. Wade into law as a more viable way to preserve abortion rights.

"If the right to abortion was annihilated, period, the solution would be codifying Roe into federal law," the spokesman said, pointing out that Sanders has supported such efforts since 1993.

Sanders is a co-sponsor of the The Women's Health Protection Act, which would codify Roe v. Wade into federal law. His Senate colleagues and fellow 2020 candidates, Sens. Elizabeth Warren of Massachusetts, Kirsten Gillibrand of New York, Cory Booker of New Jersey, Amy Klobuchar of Minnesota, Kamala Harris of California and Michael Bennet of Colorado, have also signed on to the bill.

NOTE to Reader: All through the COVID pandemic and vaccine campaign, we have been hearing people say "My body, my choice!". Hmmm…. Now where have we heard that phrase for the past few decades?

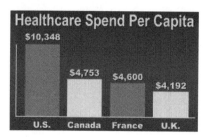

See hundreds more national, state and local organizations listed in our last chapter. Follow, join, donate, advocate, speak up!

https://www.youtube.com/watch?v=hQV4SZic0lE
Donald Berwick, MD – President Emeritus & Senior Fellow, IHI

Medicare for All

Pros	Cons
• Lower administrative costs	• "Big government"
• Publicly accountable	• Political turnover
• Transparency	• Cost savings unknown
• More say about what's covered	• Will Medicare have too much power?

UNITED STATES of AMERICA

UNIVERSAL HEALTH CARE CARD

(aka "MEDICARE for ALL" CARD)

for

You – Yes – You !

The recipient of this card is entitled to go to any qualified doctor, specialist, hospital or clinic

and receive any prescribed medication or treatment for

physical, mental, vision, dental, hearing health care   (except cosmetic)

https://pnhp.org/system/assets/uploads/2021/03/HouseBill2021_Chart.pdf
(See hyperlink for full text and references.)

Commercial Insurance vs. Medicare for All Act of 2021

pnhp.org/HouseBill ; Created March 2021

The health insurance industry (and their friends in Congress) say that commercial insurance products — including ACA marketplace, workplace, and privatized "Medicare Advantage" plans — are the best way to cover uninsured Americans. But how do these plans compare to Medicare for All?

Does it provide secure coverage for everybody in the U.S.?

- Commercial Insurance: NO. Coverage depends on your job, marriage, or income, and can be lost at any time. More than 30 million Americans are uninsured, and 40 million have high-deductible plans they can't afford to use.

- Medicare for All Act: YES. It covers everybody in the nation, regardless of age, employment, income, or immigration status. Coverage is guaranteed for life.

Does it cover health services for all parts of the body?

- Commercial Insurance: NO. Most plans do not adequately cover the full range of needed health services, forcing families to either skip care or pay for it on their own.

- Medicare for All Act: YES. It covers all medically necessary services, including hospital and doctor visits; dental, vision, hearing, mental health, and reproductive care; long-term care; ambulatory services; and prescription drugs.

Does it include free choice of doctor and hospital?

- Commercial Insurance: NO. Patients cannot see doctors or hospitals outside of the insurers' "network."

- Medicare for All Act: YES. Patients are free to choose practically any hospital or provider in the nation.

Does it reduce health costs for most families?

- Commercial Insurance: NO. Insurers pass on costs via premiums, copays, and deductibles that discourage patients from seeking care.

- Medicare for All Act: YES. Care is provided free at the point of service; families will never see a medical bill again.

Does it reduce national health spending?

- Commercial Insurance: NO. Insurers have no incentive to reduce health spending since they pass increased costs onto patients, employers, and taxpayers.

- Medicare for All Act: YES. By eliminating insurance profiteering, reducing providers' administrative costs, and negotiating drug prices, it will save at least $700 billion a year.

Does it improve health quality?

- Commercial Insurance: NO. People of color are less likely to be insured; copays and deductibles create financial barriers to care, exacerbating disparities.

- Medicare for All Act: YES. It eliminates all financial barriers to care and invests in health services and facilities for underserved urban and rural communities.

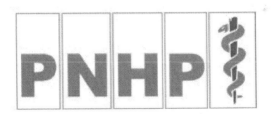

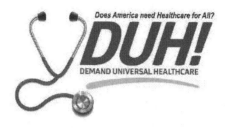

Socialized? Universal? What's the difference?
By Sue Saltmarsh (1956-2021), Founder of DUH!
https://www.facebook.com/groups/858099384918591/

Many people are confused by the ways healthcare systems are defined in today's world. In the United States, it used to be the worst thing to call something "socialized," as in Socialism, which Joe McCarthy would tell you is a step away from (gasp!) *COMMUNISM*. Socialism is defined as an economic and political system where the workers own the means of production (i.e. farms, factories, tools, and raw materials.)

Now, thanks to Bernie's courage in self-identifying as a Democratic Socialist, along with the millions of people, especially young ones, who don't think it's such a bad idea for people living in a society together to have each other's backs, the knee jerk alarm that fearmongers like McCarthy inspired is quickly becoming a thing of the past. But for Baby Boomers who may still have doubts, here is a comparison of socialized healthcare and the kind of universal system we want in this country.

SOCIALIZED HEALTHCARE
Government owns hospitals & other facilities
Providers are employees of the government
Prescription drugs may not be covered
Wait times for non-urgent issues vary by country
Government pays the bills
All necessary medical care is covered
No premiums, deductibles, co-pays
Everyone is covered from birth to death
Healthcare decisions are made by the doctor and patient

UNIVERSAL HEALTHCARE
Hospitals & other facilities are privately owned
Providers are employed privately

Prescription drugs are covered
Wait times for non-urgent issues vary by state, city, rural, etc.
Government pays the bills
All necessary medical care is covered
No premiums, deductibles, co-pays
Everyone is covered from birth to death
Healthcare decisions are made by the doctor and patient

As you can see, most differences are about whether or not the government *owns* facilities and *employs* providers. The panic about waiting for treatment for a year when you're having a heart attack is ridiculous. I waited 10 months for a hip replacement, I wait months to see the specialists I need. As far as I know, the only ones who can see a doctor the day something goes wrong are our *pets*.

There *will* be doctor shortages while a universal single-payer system is implemented and works out the kinks, but there will still be ERs – only now, you won't have to worry about meeting your deductible or paying a co-pay. **NO ONE WILL GO WITHOUT CARE!**

So stop buying into opposition propaganda – the only thing to fear about universal, single-payer, National Improved Medicare for All, is that we won't get it before we die!

https://www.commondreams.org/views/2021/03/20/all-health-public-health?utm   (See hyperlink for full text and references.)

Tinashe Goronga is at EqualHealth. Follow him on Twitter: **@tisaneg**

Dana Brown is co-director of theory, research, and policy at The Democracy Collaborative and is director of The Next System Project at the Collaborative.

Siddhartha Mehta is a member of the COVID-19 Response Collective at Progressive International. Follow him on Twitter: **@SJ_Mehta**

All Health Is Public Health

The pandemic has blown up the myth that our health is largely a product of individual choices and personal responsibilities.
Published March 20, 2021 by *Common Dreams.org*

Tinashe Goronga, Dana Brown, Siddhartha Mehta

For decades, we have been sold a myth of private health. It is a myth that our health is largely a product of individual choices and personal responsibilities. It is a myth that our healthcare is a service that private corporations can provide, and for which we must pay to survive.

But the COVID-19 pandemic has blown up this myth.

Our personal health cannot be separated from the health of our neighbors or our planet. Nor can it be separated from the structural factors and policy decisions that have determined our health outcomes long before we are born.

The right to health, in the context of these interconnections, is a universal right. Your life is worth no more and no less than that of your next-door neighbor because the fates of the two are so intimately entwined.

Today, the universal right to health is not held back by scarcity of resources or a lack of technology. On the contrary, the wealth of this world — invested well — could end the pandemic before the year's end.

Instead, we are held back by another myth: that there exists a trade-off between public health and the health of the economy. The assumption of this trade-off dictates that all public policy is subordinate to the great god of economic growth — even if it costs us our lives. The concept of private health grows out of this second myth, which makes a commodity of our bodies, and a market for essential healthcare services.

Indeed, public health systems around the world are structured carefully to serve a profit motive. Unsurprisingly, their outcomes are inequitable and insufficient, leaving poor and marginalized communities with no recourse to private health provision.

Drawing on the evidence of health impacts of the coronavirus pandemic and the impact of policy responses, the racial, gender and class dimension in the impact of the virus is undeniable. The raw reality of systemic fragility of both public health and economic systems in the North in dealing with the social crisis has also been brought to the fore. Those countries that have been successful — such as Vietnam, Cuba and New Zealand — viewed public health as economic wealth.

Once again, we return to the basic premise. Health, in all its dimensions, is a public good. How can we deliver a world that reflects this simple premise?

The first step is decolonization. Countries in the Global South cannot deliver on the promise of public health when they are curtailed by neocolonial conditionalities that come along with philanthropic funding and multilateral lending. This top-down approach strips countries of their sovereignty over how to fund health services, privatizes health infrastructure and cripples social policy provisions.

Most of these countries assured universal health services as a matter of course in the 1960s and 1970s. Then came structural adjustment. The imposition of the Washington Consensus in the course of the 1980s and 1990s led to a radical reframing of the health sector as a profitable site of privatization and deregulation. The introduction of user fees and prioritization of imported, high tech-fixes forced millions of poor people to the margins, as "private health" became the norm. Provision in the

355

form of "minimum packages" took priority over comprehensive primary and community health.

Public health, then, requires public ownership — a form of ownership that can deliver transparency and foster citizen participation in the delivery of healthcare services. Public sector clinics, homecare companies, and biomedical enterprises should be built to assure the production and distribution of essential medicines and medical technologies as well as healthcare services.

Free from the structural constraints of shareholder primacy and profit maximization, these enterprises will be able to prioritize preventative and curative technologies, fill gaps in existing treatments, and provide products at or below cost where necessary to meet public health needs.

Moreover, they can return revenue to public balance sheets, reduce inefficiencies, and create surge capacity for emergencies. Having a robust public sector infrastructure for the development, manufacture, and distribution of essential goods like medicines, personal protective equipment, and other medical instruments breaks the corporate monopoly over our supply of medical goods, reducing regulatory capture and increasing public power to demand equitable and universal access to critical health goods and services.

Health as a public good offers positive externalities for the economy and society. Even if we just follow the logic of narrow economic growth, a dollar investment in health in developing countries is estimated to result in between $2 and $4 in economic returns over time. And those dollars are best spent when communities and nations have the autonomy to prioritize their own needs and invest in long-term institution-building that will serve their communities for years to come.

Countries like Cuba and Vietnam have demonstrated that, even with modest budgets, developing a sovereign healthcare system that prioritizes primary and preventative care together with robust public health infrastructure can deliver first-rate population health outcomes. Investing in public healthcare systems has been shown to contribute to better outcomes than investing in privatized healthcare systems. Freeing the healthcare sector from market imperatives would allow for the re-centering of primary and preventative care, planning for equitable access, and robust community health outreach — not traditionally the profit-making parts of healthcare delivery. Additionally, targeted workforce development programs can be created to meet community needs while providing stable, public sector jobs that are themselves an upstream investment in community health.

Reclaiming autonomy of the public sector by sovereign nations requires a shift from the current donor-driven vertical disease control programs most funded in prioritizing the needs of the community. Vertical interventions to eradicate single diseases are often costly and have been imposed on low and middle-income countries at the expense of horizontal enhancements of public health infrastructure that would serve whole populations over the long term and make local health systems more resilient. They also contribute to internal brain drain with skilled people leaving the public sector to work for higher pay in international and nongovernmental organizations.

Reversal of structural adjustment conditions and untying loans, donor grants and external funding from conditionalities is essential in reclaiming sovereignty in the national public health decision space. Complete restructuring of the global health governance mechanisms to ensure democratic representation in decision-making by every participating country, whether they are net donors or net recipients, is vital.

Global health governance mechanisms must have measures in place to ensure that external influence exerted over countries is subordinate to national sovereignty, and that the activities of global health organizations without a democratic mandate are overseen and their impact held to account by national governments.

Representation of the most marginalized and communities most impacted by colonialism and structural adjustment on governance of global health and financial institutions is important for their priorities and perspectives to be included on the agenda and in development priorities. In addition, more community empowerment, participation, and co-planning in the process of deprivatization of healthcare services can aid in the democratization of healthcare and provide increased opportunities for transparency, citizen accountability, and oversight.

Hand-in-hand with the reclaiming of the healthcare sector for the public good should be the reclamation of essential services like water and power. Investments in public power and water — coupled with divestments from fossil fuels — would build both climate resilience and more equitable access to the basic infrastructure of public health.

Amongst the greatest challenges to public health in many countries around the world are still infectious diseases like tuberculosis, malaria, and lower respiratory infections, all of which correlate highly to social determinants like access to clean water and good living conditions, air quality, and sanitation. Any strategy to reclaim public health for the public good must center social determinants and seek to increase public power across sectors of the economy responsible for the basic conditions of human life and the stability of our environment.

The COVID-19 pandemic has opened a window of opportunity to revisit and reevaluate the many myths that held up a broken system of global health. And in doing so, it has offered us the chance to deliver a truly global public health system: equitable, inclusive and people-centered.

A withering critique of capitalism is not enough. It is time to reimagine a world where human life and environmental sustainability are the first priority, and where that universal right to health is the basis for all public policy.

A system premised on this universal right — and powered by global solidarity — is not only possible. For our species to survive, it is necessary.

https://www.epi.org/publication/medicare-for-all-would-help-the-labor-market/ Used with permission. (See hyperlink for references & full text.)

Fundamental Health Reform like 'Medicare for All' Would Help the Labor Market

Economic Policy Institute (EPI) Report by Josh Bivens, 5 March 2020

Job loss claims are misleading, and substantial boosts to job quality are often overlooked.

Fundamental health reform like "Medicare for All" would be a hugely ambitious policy undertaking with profound effects on the economy and the economic security of households in America. But despite oft-repeated claims of large-scale job losses, a national program that would guarantee health insurance for every American would *not* profoundly affect the total number of jobs in the U.S. economy. In fact, such reform could boost wages and jobs and lead to more efficient labor markets that better match jobs and workers. Specifically, it could:

- **Boost wages and salaries** by allowing employers to redirect money they are spending on health care costs to their workers' wages.

- **Increase job quality** by ensuring that every job now comes bundled with a guarantee of health care - with the boost to job quality even greater among women workers, who are less likely to have employer-sponsored health care.

- **Lessen the stress and economic shock of losing a job or moving between jobs** by eliminating the loss of health care that now accompanies job losses and transitions.

- **Support self-employment and small business development** - which is currently super-low in the U.S. relative to other rich countries - by eliminating the daunting loss of/cost of health care from startup costs.

- **Inject new dynamism and adaptability into the overall economy** by reducing "job lock" - with workers going where their skills and preferences best fit the job, not just to workplaces (usually large ones) that have affordable health plans.

- **Produce a net increase in jobs as public spending boosts aggregate demand**, with job losses in health insurance and billing administration being outweighed by job gains in provision of health care, including the expansion of long-term care.

While the overall effect of fundamental health reform on the labor market would be unambiguously positive, this does not mean policymakers should ignore the distress caused by job transitions forced by this reform. Specifically, policy support should be provided to help displaced health insurance and billing administration workers move into new positions.

But we should not let critics of Medicare for All inflate the scale of this transition challenge or falsely present the number of jobs displaced in individual sectors as the *net* effect of reform on labor markets. The number of health insurance and billing administration workers who would need to transition implies an increase in the rate of overall job market churn that is relatively small: Job losses for these workers would be equivalent to one-twelfth the size of economy-wide layoffs in 2018.

Background: The need for fundamental health reform

A fundamental reform like Medicare for All (M4A) would make coverage universal. Further, by providing a counterweight to (or outright eliminating) the substantial market power that keeps prices high and that is currently wielded by many key players in the health care sector (e.g., insurance companies, drug companies, specialty physicians, and device makers), such a reform could also have great success in containing health care cost growth. This could in turn provide relief from many of the ways that rising health costs squeeze family incomes.

An underappreciated benefit of such a reform is that it would also lead to a much better functioning labor market in many areas. Job quality would increase, job switching would become less stressful, better "matches" between workers and employers would boost productivity, and small businesses would be much easier to launch.

Despite the fact that M4A could deliver these large benefits to efficient labor market functioning, the policy often comes under fire from critics making highly exaggerated claims about the potential job loss that could occur under such a reform. The grain of truth in some of the claims is that, like any productivity improvement, the adoption of a reform like M4A would require the redeployment of workers from one sector (the health insurance and medical billing complex) to other sectors (mostly the delivery of health care). But there is little in the M4A-induced redeployment of workers that would greatly stress the American labor market over and above the uncertainty and churn that characterizes this labor market every year. Smart policy could make this redeployment eminently manageable for those workers who would be required to make the transition.

This brief highlights some labor market implications of M4A and critically examines claims that large job losses in the health insurance and billing administration sectors would make M4A an undesirable policy.

Health reform as labor market policy: Key effects for workers

Fundamental reforms like M4A could greatly aid labor market outcomes for U.S. workers. The most obvious benefits would be higher wages and salaries, increased availability of good jobs, reduced stress during spells of job loss, better "matches" between workers and employers, and greater opportunity to start small businesses.

Higher cash wages and salaries

Medicare for All could increase wages and salaries for U.S. workers by reducing employers' costs for health insurance — freeing up fiscal space to invest in wages instead. The share of total annual compensation paid to American employees in the form of health insurance premiums rather than wages and salaries rose from 1.1% in 1960 to 4.2% in 1979 to 8.4% in 2018[5].

If this post-1960 increase had been only half as large — and employers had spent the health cost savings on wages and salaries — the take-home wages of American workers would have been almost $400 billion higher in 2018[6]. Given that the share of total compensation spoken for by health insurance premiums is starting from a high base today, any reform that managed to slow the excess growth of health spending going forward would go a long way in making space for faster growth of cash compensation[7].

Increased availability of 'good jobs'

Medicare for All could increase job quality substantially by making all jobs "good" jobs in terms of health insurance coverage and by increasing the potential for higher wages. While the definition of a "good job" is always going to be a bit imprecise, the vast majority of U.S. workers would say that a good job is one that pays decent wages and that also provides the health insurance coverage and retirement income benefits that most of today's workers can only reliably access through employment. Nearly half of jobs fail this test on account of health care coverage alone: In 2016, 46.9% of workers held jobs in which their employer made no contributions to the workers' health care; for workers in the middle fifth of the wage distribution, 42.9% held jobs in which the employer made no contribution to their health care (EPI 2017).

By making health coverage universal and delinking from employment, M4A would make it far easier for employers to offer good jobs in this regard, as *every* job would now be accompanied by guaranteed health care coverage. Further, as noted above, wages and salaries would have substantial room to grow if health care costs were taken off of the backs of employers.

Schmitt and Jones (2013) estimate the share of good jobs — jobs that clear a specified wage floor[8] and provide health and retirement coverage — in overall employment each year between 1979 and 2011. They then look at various policy changes that would boost this share. They find that providing universal health coverage would boost the probability that any given job in the economy is a good job by almost 20% — and that's even before any potential boost to the share of jobs that are good jobs coming from cash wage increases provided as employers shed health care costs[9]. The boost to job quality from making health coverage universal would be even greater for women workers, as women are currently less likely to receive employer-sponsored health insurance benefits from their own employers[10].

Less damaging spells of joblessness

Medicare for All could make job losses and transitions less stressful by delinking employment and access to health insurance, emulating the universal access to health care offered by our rich country peers. The U.S. is unique among the rich countries of the world in how much it ties crucial social benefits — like health insurance and retirement income — to specific jobs.

Hacker (2002) has referred to this arrangement as the "divided welfare state," with some Americans having relatively full access to health and retirement security while others have access to virtually none, all based on the specific jobs they have. This makes some jobs in the U.S. economy especially valuable, and hence especially damaging to lose. Manufacturing workers without a college degree, for example, likely incur enormous income and social benefits losses in the event of job loss stemming from either automation or trade.

The ability of universal, public social benefits to make individual job losses less damaging has been long recognized by social scientists (see, for example, Estevez-Abe, Iversen, and Soskice 2001).

Smooth job transitions contribute to economic dynamism by helping ensure that vacancies are filled quickly by appropriate workers and that unemployed workers can quickly find new jobs that make good use of their skills. Smooth job transitions will also be an important component of meeting crucial policy goals such as mitigating greenhouse gas emissions with wholesale changes in how energy is created.

Policies that make job transitions easier and inspire less resistance from workers should be encouraged. Fundamental health reform that, like M4A, guarantees access to insurance regardless of one's current job status is a key part of making such transitions easier.

Better labor market matches between workers and employers

Medicare for All could decrease inefficient "job lock" and boost small business creation and voluntary self-employment. Making health insurance universal and delinked from employment widens the range of economic options for workers and leads to better matches between workers' skills and interests and their jobs. The boost to small business creation and self-employment would be particularly useful, as the United States is a laggard in both relative to advanced economy peers.

Substantial evidence indicates that our current system of employer-sponsored insurance (ESI) creates significant "job lock" — a condition in which workers who don't want to lose their current ESI stay in their current jobs rather than make transitions that would better meet their needs.

Making employment decisions based on access to ESI rather than on other criteria — such as work–life balance, cash wages, and commuting distance — can lead to employment "matches" that are less productive and that decrease overall worker welfare relative to job choices that are not constrained by the availability of health insurance.

More small-business formation

Despite policymakers' frequent claims that they seek to support small businesses in the U.S. economy, the United States has a notably small share of small-business employment relative to our rich country peers. In 2018, for example, the U.S. was dead-last among the members of the Organisation for Economic Co-operation and Development (OECD) in its share of self-employment, at just 6.3% of employment. Countries that are frequently portrayed in U.S. business reporting as being choked by regulation — like Spain, France, and Germany — have far higher shares of self-employment, at 16.0%, 11.7%, and 9.9%, respectively (OECD 2020).

Besides a low share of self-employment, the U.S. also had significantly lower shares of overall employment in small businesses, across nearly all industrial sectors. The latest OECD data show that the U.S. share of employment in enterprises with fewer than 50 employees is lower than in any other country except for Russia (OECD 2018, Figure 7).

In an earlier overview of trends in employment by firm size, Schmitt and Lane (2009) highlight how health care policy plays two key roles in potentially explaining cross-country trends. First, because health care is nearly universally provided in other rich countries, workers choosing to start their own businesses in those countries do not face a cost confronting would-be entrepreneurs in the U.S.: the loss of ESI (employer-sponsored insurance). Second, small businesses in the U.S. are at a distinct disadvantage in recruiting employees because the cost of providing health care coverage is significantly higher for small companies[11].

Employment effects of fundamental health reform: gains in health care, losses in insurance and billing — with likely economywide net job gains from rising economic demand

Like all positive productivity gains, Medicare for All would be more likely to increase the total number of jobs in the U.S. economy, even as health reform leads to the redeployment of workers from some sectors and into others.

Despite the many labor market benefits of fundamental health reform like M4A, many critics have claimed that such reform would lead to a loss of jobs. This claim is misleading. One small grain of truth to it is that the universal provision of health insurance would allow people who would strongly prefer *not* to work (or not to work full time), but who have remained in their current jobs in order to retain health insurance, to be free to quit. This type of voluntary reduction in labor supply following a health reform would be strongly welfare-improving.

For example, the ACA was clearly associated with a large increase in parents with young children transitioning to part-time work (see Jørgensen and Baker 2014). To the degree this occurred because these parents no longer needed to work full time to obtain ESI, and they preferred spending more time with their children for reasons of work-life balance, it should be seen as a clear win for the policy.

Generally, people expressing concern about job loss stemming from a policy are concerned about involuntary job loss that leads to a higher level of unemployment in the economy. Unemployment is almost entirely a function of the level of aggregate demand: spending by households, businesses, and governments[12].

The effect of fundamental health reform on the level of aggregate demand depends in turn on the balance of increased public spending and the means of financing this spending. All else equal, more public spending will boost aggregate demand and create jobs, while higher taxes will reduce aggregate demand and restrain job growth.

Further, the progressivity of taxes used to finance fundamental health reform will also condition its effect on aggregate demand. The more progressive the taxes that finance health reform, the less they will drag on job growth. Increased public spending combined with progressive tax increases would almost certainly boost the level of aggregate demand and lead to lower unemployment, all else equal.

While the overall number of jobs and the level of unemployment in the economy is largely a macroeconomic issue determined by aggregate demand, claims that fundamental health reform like M4A will lead to job loss sometimes sound plausible because it is easy to envision the *specific jobs* that might be displaced: jobs in the health insurance and billing administration sectors. But these job displacements would be balanced by likely job gains in other sectors — most particularly in health care delivery. The health insurance coverage expansions of M4A will boost demand for health care goods and services, and workers will need to be hired to meet this demand.

Job losses in the health insurance and billing administration sectors

A recent analysis of the economic effects of M4A (Pollin et al. 2018) includes the projection that up to 1.8 million jobs in the health insurance and billing administration sector (the divisions of hospitals and doctors' offices dedicated to administrative processing of bills and payments) could be made redundant. These potential 1.8 million lost jobs are frequently presented as if they constitute the net employment effect of M4A[13]. This is a deeply flawed misrepresentation of Pollin and his colleagues' work. In fact, their estimates are a gross (not net) measure of job displacement or "churn" — the regular process of workers starting and leaving jobs during the course of their work lives. Relative to the scale of other gross measures of job churn, the churn associated with M4A is not large.

It is true that one source of cost savings from the introduction of M4A is the reduced demand for insurance and billing administration. In turn, this reduced demand would shift employment out of these sectors. This could certainly cause challenges and economic distress for the workers within these sectors who are directly affected. But for some perspective, it is worth noting that 21.5 million workers were laid off in 2018 (BLS 2020b). If the 1.8 million workers that Pollin et al. (2018) identify as potentially being displaced by M4A were forced to transition over the four-year phase-in commonly identified with M4A plans, this would increase the national rate of layoffs by about 2%.

It is also worth noting that even within just the finance and insurance sectors, there have been 1.7 million layoffs in the past four years (BLS 2020b). This is not a shock: Our economy generates a huge amount of job churn every year. This churn is the hallmark of growth in productivity — getting more economic output with fewer inputs. While productivity growth can indeed put downward pressure on jobs in the sector experiencing it directly, Autor and Salomons (2018) demonstrate that productivity gains within a given sector strongly *boost* job growth in *other* sectors, as the savings to households and businesses stemming from enhanced productivity increase purchasing power that supports demand for these other sectors' outputs.

If workers in the insurance or billing administration sectors were particularly hard-pressed for reemployment prospects because of geographic isolation or low average levels of educational credentials, their displacement might pose particular concern to policymakers. But employment in the health insurance and billing administration sectors is not particularly geographically concentrated[14], and Pollin et al. (2018) show that 56.5% of workers in these sectors have a four-year college degree or more education, a far greater share than the overall labor force.

Substantial likely job gains in the health care sector

While it may seem counterintuitive, fundamental health reform like M4A is almost guaranteed to substantially *expand* employment in the health care sector overall, even taking reduced billing administration employment into account.

Often people hear that fundamental reform is aimed at cost containment and then imagine that part of this cost containment will take the form of fewer jobs providing health care, but this is not necessarily the case. As noted before, the U.S. is an outlier in terms of how much it *spends* on health care, but its health care workforce as a share of the total workforce is not out of line with shares in other countries. For example, in 2017 the health care workforce in the U.S. was equal to 13.4% of the overall workforce, while the share averaged 12.9% in the 20 other richest OECD countries[15]. Additionally, seven of these other countries had health care workforce shares equal to or higher than the U.S.'s 13.4%[16].

Pollin et al. (2018) estimate that expanded access to health care could increase demand for health services by up to $300 billion annually. Given the current level of health spending and employment, this would translate into increased demand for 2.3 million full-time-equivalent workers in providing healthcare[17]. Obviously all of the workers displaced from the health insurance and billing administration sectors could not necessarily transition into these jobs seamlessly, but well over 10% of workers in the health insurance sector, for example, are actually in health care occupations (e.g., they are doctors or nurses)[18].

Further, several M4A plans have provisions to pay for long-term care services. Reinhard et al. (2019) have estimated that in 2018, Americans provided roughly 34 billion hours in unpaid long-term care. If this care was divided up among full-time paid workers, it would require 17 million new positions. Of course, not all of this currently unpaid care would be converted into paid positions in the job market. But if even 10% of unpaid care translated into new jobs, it would create enough new demand for workers to essentially offset the displacement of workers in the health insurance and billing administration sectors.

The upshot: M4A creates a small amount of manageable churn but increases the overall demand for labor and boosts job quality

The job challenge relating to a fundamental health reform is managing a relatively small increase in job churn during an initial phase-in period. Most Medicare for All plans explicitly recognize and account for the costs of providing these workers the elements of a just transition. As noted previously, this sort of just transition is far easier when health care is universally provided.

Besides this challenge, the effect of fundamental reform like M4A on the labor market would be nearly uniformly positive. The effect of a fundamental reform like M4A on aggregate demand is almost certainly positive and will therefore boost the demand for labor. The number of jobs spurred by increased demand for new health care spending (including long-term care) will certainly be larger than the number displaced by realizing efficiencies in the health insurance and billing administration sectors.

Finally, the introduction of fundamental health reform like M4A — particularly reform that substantially delinks health care provision from specific jobs — would greatly aid how the labor market functions for typical working Americans. Take-home cash pay would increase, job quality would improve, labor market transitions could be eased for employers and made less damaging to workers, and a greater range of job opportunities could be considered by workers. The increased flexibility to leave jobs should lead to more productive "matches" between workers and employers, and small businesses and self-employment could increase.

Fundamental health reform would benefit typical American families in all sorts of ways. Importantly, contrary to claims that such reform might be bad for jobs, this reform could substantially improve how labor markets function for these families.

Josh Bivens joined the Economic Policy Institute in 2002 and is currently EPI's director of research. His primary areas of research include macroeconomics, social insurance, and globalization. He has authored or co-authored three books (including *The State of Working America, 12th Edition*) while working at EPI, has edited another, and has written numerous research papers, including many for academic journals. He appears often in media outlets to offer economic commentary and has testified several times before the U.S. Congress. He earned his Ph.D. from The New School for Social Research.

https://youtu.be/FEzGZOGuDOA
with Josh Bevins of EPI (Economic Policy Institute, March 2020)

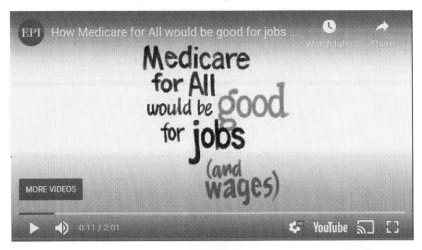

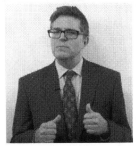

The Congressional Budget Office (CBO)

The Congressional Budget Office (CBO) is a federal agency within the legislative branch of the United States government that provides budget and economic information to Congress. It is a nonpartisan agency that estimates how much proposed and existing legislation will cost American taxpayers.

In December of 2020, the CBO undertook an analysis of "Medicare for All": https://www.cbo.gov/system/files/2020-12/56811-Single-Payer.pdf

The bottom line of the CBO analysis — that universal coverage can be affordably achieved even as benefits are expanded and cost sharing all but eliminated — should reinvigorate debate over such reform.

https://www.healthaffairs.org/do/10.1377/hblog20210210.190243/full/
(See hyperlink for full text and references.)

Congressional Budget Office Scores Medicare-For-All: Universal Coverage For Less Spending
By Adam Gaffney, David Himmelstein and Steffie Woolhandler,
16 February 2021

For the first time in a quarter century, the Congressional Budget Office (CBO) has undertaken an economic analysis of single-payer health care reform, also known as Medicare for All. The more than 200-page working paper, released last month, includes a rich explanation of methodology together with cost projections for 2030 and will no doubt serve as an important reference for years to come.

The report makes many sound assumptions but also some questionable ones that are overly pessimistic. Yet, overall, its bottom-line estimates should reassure those concerned about the economic feasibility of single payer: The CBO projects that such reform would achieve universal coverage, bolster provider revenues for clinical services, and eliminate almost all copayments and deductibles — even as overall health care spending fell.

The CBO models costs under five different variants of single payer. The first four envision universal coverage of all services other than long-term care, while the fifth incorporates a large expansion of long-term services and supports (LTSS) for people with disabilities of all ages.

Overall, the CBO report provides one of the most detailed explorations to date of the economics of single-payer financing. As we have noted, it makes many sound assumptions, particularly about payer- and provider-side administrative savings. At the same time, it adopts some unfavorable assumptions about the structure of single-payer reform (including some that conflict with key provisions of the Medicare for All bills in Congress), projects excessive windfalls for some providers, and asserts clinically nescient (*lacking knowledge, ignorant*) portrayals of "unmet demand." Nonetheless, the bottom line of the CBO analysis — that universal coverage can be affordably achieved even as benefits are expanded and cost sharing all but eliminated — should reinvigorate debate over such reform.

Authors' Note: The authors have served as leaders of Physicians for a National Health Program, a nonprofit organization that supports single-payer health care reform.

Related articles:

https://pnhp.org/news/congressional-budget-office-scores-medicare-for-all-universal-coverage-for-less-spending/

Congressional Budget Office Scores Medicare-For-All: Universal Coverage For Less Spending
**By Adam Gaffney, M.D., M.P.H. ; David Himmelstein, M.D. ;
and Steffie Woolhandler, M.D., M.P.H.
Health Affairs Blog, 16 February 2021**

https://www.vox.com/policy-and-politics/2019/3/8/18251707/medicare-for-all-bill-senate-filibuster-budget-reconciliation-byrd-rule

The Senate's Rules Will Make It Really Hard to Pass Medicare-for-All
By Dylan Scott (@dylanscott ; dylanscott@vox.com), 8 March 2019

https://www.cbo.gov/publication/56898
(See hyperlink for full text and references.)

How CBO Analyzes Proposals for a Single-Payer Health Care System
Posted by CBO Director Phill Swagel, 10 December 2020

HEY JOE – PLEASE STUDY THE COST STUDIES !

Medicare for All is Less Expensive than The Public Option!!!

https://khn.org/news/does-medicare-for-all-cost-more-than-the-entire-budget-biden-says-so-but-numbers-say-no/
(See hyperlink for full text and references.)

Would 'Medicare For All' Cost More Than U.S. Budget? Biden Says So. Math Says No.

KHN & POLITIFACT HEALTHCHECK
By Shefali Luthra (ShefaliL@kff.orf), 14 February 2020

It turns out, based on the numbers and interviews with independent experts, Biden's comparison of Medicare for All's price to total federal spending misses the mark because the calculation is flawed.

Sanders has said publicly that economists estimate Medicare for All would cost somewhere between **$30 trillion** and **$40 trillion** over 10 years. Research by the nonpartisan Urban Institute, a Washington, D.C., think tank, puts the figure in the **$32 trillion** to **$34 trillion** range.

What you would need to do is add up the Congressional Budget Office's projected budget outlays from 2020 to 2029, and compare the sum to the Medicare for All spending figure.

Marc Goldwein, senior vice president and senior policy director at the Committee for a Responsible Federal Budget, looked at the numbers another way: Including interest, he found, the federal budget would consume about $55 trillion between now and 2030. Again, that's more than what Medicare for All would cost during the same period. No matter how you slice Biden's math, his numbers are off.

HR 1976 (formerly HR 676) would Save $400 Billion
The U.S. could save enough on administrative costs with a single-payer system to cover the uninsured.

PNHP (Physicians for a National Health Program) Co-founders Drs. Steffie Woolhandler and David Himmelstein published this definitive study of the administrative costs of the U.S. health system in the August 21, 2003 edition of the New England Journal of Medicine. After analyzing the costs of insurers, employers, doctors, hospitals, nursing homes and home-care agencies in both the U.S. and Canada, they found that administration consumes 31.0 percent of U.S. health spending, double the proportion of Canada (16.7 percent). Average overhead among private U.S. insurers was 11.7 percent, compared with 1.3 percent for Canada's single-payer system and 3.6 percent for Medicare. Streamlined to Canadian levels, enough administrative waste could be saved to provide comprehensive health insurance to all Americans. You can read the study at http://www.pnhp.org/publications/nejmadmin.pdf.

Make No Mistake: Medicare for All Would Cut Taxes for Most Americans
By Emmanuel Saez and Gabriel Zucman; 25 October 2019
Emmanuel Saez and Gabriel Zucman are economics professors at the University of California, Berkeley, and the authors of The Triumph of Injustice: How the Rich Dodge Taxes and How to Make Them Pay, from which this essay is adapted.

Not only would universal healthcare reduce taxes for most people, it would also lead to the biggest take-home pay raise in a generation for most workers.

The debate about healthcare has been at the center of the Democratic primaries, yet it is hard to make sense of the conversation. For some, public universal health insurance – such as Bernie Sanders's Medicare for All bill – would involve massive tax increases for the middle class. For others, it's the opposite: Medicare for All would cut costs for most

Americans. Who is right?

The starting point of any intelligent conversation about health in America must be that it's a cost for all of us – and a massive one. The United States spends close to 20% of its national income on health. Elderly Americans and low-income families are covered by public insurance programs (Medicare and Medicaid, respectively), funded by tax dollars (payroll taxes and general government revenue). The rest of the population must obtain coverage by a private company, which they typically get via their employers. Insurance, in that case, is funded by non-tax payments: health insurance premiums.

Although they are not officially called taxes, insurance premiums paid by employers are just like taxes – but taxes paid to private insurers instead of paid to the government. Like payroll taxes, they reduce your wage. Like taxes, they are mandatory, or quasi-mandatory. Since the passage of the Affordable Care Act in 2010, it has become compulsory to be insured, and employers with more than 50 full-time workers are required to enroll their workers in a health insurance plan.

A frequent objection to calling health insurance premiums a tax is that people have some choice. Can't the poor, the argument goes, enroll in cheap health plans? If you start calling health insurance premiums a tax, then shouldn't we also call spending on food and clothes a tax?

This argument, however, is wrong, because cheap healthcare does not exist. There are cheap meals, there are cheap clothes, but there is no cheap way to treat your heart attack, to cure your cancer, or to give birth. Cheap health insurance means no healthcare when you need it. All wealthy nations, even those that try hard to control costs, spend 10% of their national income on health – the equivalent of $7,500 a year per adult in the United States. The view that healthcare services are like haircuts or restaurant meals – services for which there is a product tailored to any budget – is a myth. Healthcare is like education: everybody needs it, regardless of their budget, but it's expensive. That's why all advanced economies, except the United States, fund it through taxation.

The main difference between the insurance premiums currently paid by American workers and the taxes paid by workers in other countries is that taxes are based on ability to pay. The income tax has a rate that rises

374

with income. Payroll taxes are proportional to income, at least up to a limit. Insurance premiums, by contrast, are not based on ability to pay. They are a fixed amount per covered worker and only depend on age and the number of family members covered. Insurance premiums are the most regressive possible type of tax: a poll tax. The secretary pays the same amount as the executive.

Many people believe that the United States has a progressive tax system: you pay more, as a fraction of your income, as you earn more. In fact, if you allocate the total official tax take of the United States across the population, the US tax system looks like a giant flat tax that becomes regressive at the very top. And if you add mandatory private health insurance premiums to the official tax take, the US tax system turns out to be highly regressive. Once private health insurance is factored in, the average tax rate rises from a bit less than 30% at the bottom of the income distribution to reach close to 40% for the middle class, before collapsing to 23% for billionaires.

The health insurance poll tax hammers the working class and the middle class. At the bottom of the distribution, it's not as onerous as sales and payroll taxes. But that's because many low-income Americans rely on a family member to cover them, enroll into Medicaid, or go uninsured. For the middle-class, the burden is enormous. Take a secretary earning $50,000 a year, who has employer-sponsored health insurance at a total cost of $15,000. In reality her labor compensation is $65,000 (that's what her employer pays in exchange of her work), but the secretary only gets $50,000. The executive earning $1,000,000 also pays the same $15,000 for his healthcare. This is a terrible funding mechanism.

Funding healthcare via insurance premiums would be acceptable if this private poll tax was small. When the system of private health insurance developed initially, the cost of employer-sponsored health insurance was moderate, the equivalent of 0.5% of national income in the 1950s. Today, however, it is huge: 6% of national income, almost as much as payroll Social Security taxes. The Affordable Care Act increased the pool of Americans eligible for Medicaid and subsidized the purchase of private insurance for low-income people not covered by their employer. But it provided no relief for workers who fund their healthcare through a huge and growing poll tax.

This situation is not sustainable. Most countries have understood this a long time ago. Health and retirement benefits started, like in the United States, as negotiated arrangements between employees (represented by their unions) and employers. But the task of funding health and retirement was then gradually entrusted to the government. Private premiums morphed into regular taxes, based on ability to pay. In the United States, this transformation has not happened yet for healthcare – leading to the crises we are in now.

This is the context needed to understand the current debate at the heart of the presidential elections. Proposals such as Medicare for All would replace the current privatized poll tax by taxes based on ability to pay. Some believe that it would result in a big tax increase for America's middle class. But the data show that it would, in fact, lead to large income gains for the vast majority of workers.

Take again the case of a secretary earning $50,000 in wage and currently contributing $15,000 through her employer to an insurance company. With universal health insurance, her wage would rise to $65,000 – her full labor compensation. With an income tax of 6% – which, if applied to a base large enough, would be enough to fund universal health insurance – she would have to pay about $4,000 more in tax. But the net gain would be enormous: $11,000. Instead of taking home $50,000, the secretary would take home $61,000.

On **https://taxjusticenow.org/#/**, any interested reader can simulate the effect of replacing private health insurance premiums by taxes – progressive income taxes, wealth taxes, consumption taxes, or broad taxes on consumption or all of national income. This simulator that we developed is open-source, user-friendly, and based on a systematic exploitation of all available statistics about who earns what and pays what in taxes and health insurance in America.

As one illustration, it's possible to see how the tax plans of the leading Democratic primary candidates would affect tax rates for each group of the population. For instance, Bernie Sanders's tax proposals would be enough to replace all existing private insurance premiums, while leaving 2.6% of national income to cover the uninsured and spend on other programs. Under such a plan, the 9 bottom deciles of the income distribution would gain income on average, as would the bottom of the top 10%. With smart new taxes—such as broad income taxes exempting low wages and retirees—it is possible to make the vast majority of the population win from a transition to universal health insurance.

Supporters of Medicare for All are right. Funding universal health insurance through taxes would lead to a large tax *cut* for the vast majority of workers. It would abolish the huge poll tax they currently shoulder, and the data show that for most workers, it would lead to the biggest take-home pay raise in a generation.

https://www.thelancet.com/journals/lancet/article/PIIS0140-6736(19)33019-3/fulltext   (See Hyperlink for full text and references.)

Improving The Prognosis of Health Care in The USA
15 February 2020
by Prof Alison P. Galvani, PhD, Alyssa S. Parpia, MPH, Eric M. Foster,
Burton H. Singer, PhD, Meagan C. Fitzpatrick, PhD

SUMMARY (read full text in the link provided above):

Although health care expenditure per capita is higher in the USA than in any other country, more than 37 million Americans do not have health insurance, and 41 million more have inadequate access to care. Efforts are ongoing to repeal the Affordable Care Act which would exacerbate health-care inequities. By contrast, a universal system, such as that proposed in the Medicare for All Act, has the potential to transform the availability and efficiency of American health-care services. Taking into account both the costs of coverage expansion and the savings that would be achieved through the Medicare for All Act, we calculate that a single-payer, universal health-care system is likely to lead to a 13% savings in national health-care expenditure, equivalent to more than US$450 billion annually (based on the value of the US$ in 2017). The entire system could be funded with less financial outlay than is incurred by employers and households paying for health-care premiums combined with existing government allocations. This shift to single-payer health care would provide the greatest relief to lower-income households. Furthermore, we estimate that ensuring health-care access for all Americans would save more than 68,000 lives and 1.73 million life-years every year compared with the status quo.

https://www.salon.com/2020/02/22/multiple-studies-show-medicare-for-all-would-be-cheaper-than-public-option-pushed-by-moderates/
(See hyperlink for full text and references.)

Multiple Studies show Medicare for All would be Cheaper than Public Option pushed by Moderates

By Igor Derysh, Staff Writer for SALON ; 22 February 2020
This article first appeared in Salon.com, at http://www.Salon.com.
An online version remains in the Salon archives. Reprinted with permission.
Yale and Harvard researchers: Medicare for All reduces costs, while public option makes health care more expensive.

Two new studies found that the Medicare for All plan proposed by candidates like Sen. Bernie Sanders, I-Vt., and Sen. Elizabeth Warren, D-Mass., would cost less than the public option proposed by former Vice President Joe Biden and other moderates in the Democratic primary.

"Sanders' 'Medicare for All' plan "would cost more than the entire federal budget that we spend now," Biden claimed during a debate earlier this month, which PolitiFact rated as false (https://khn.org/news/does-medicare-for-all-cost-more-than-the-entire-budget-biden-says-so-but-numbers-say-no/).

Biden has repeatedly demanded to know how Sanders plans to pay for the proposal. Sanders has repeatedly said it would be paid for by tax increases that would cost far less than the premiums, deductibles, copayments and other costs that Americans already pay. The United States spends more than $10,000 per year for every man, woman and child's health care, far more than any other nation.

Biden is right that Sanders' plan would add trillions to the federal budget. A widely-shared study funded by a think tank backed by the Koch brothers estimated that the plan would cost $32 trillion over the next decade. But the Department of Health and Human Services estimates that the country would spend more than $34 trillion under the current profit-driven system.

Two new studies further showed that the Medicare for All plan is not only cheaper than the status quo but also costs less than the public option moderates have claimed is more fiscally sound.

(https://www.thelancet.com/journals/lancet/article/PIIS0140-6736(19)33019-3/fulltext): A study published in The Lancet on 2/15/2020 by researchers at Yale University, the University of Florida and the University of Maryland estimated that Medicare for All would save $450 billion per year — about $2,400 in annual savings per family — and would prevent more than 68,000 unnecessary deaths each year.

"Our study is actually conservative because it doesn't factor in the lives saved among underinsured Americans — which includes anyone who nominally has insurance but has postponed or foregone care because they couldn't afford the copays and deductibles," Yale researcher Alison Galvani told Newsweek.

Medicare for All would allow the government to negotiate prices for care, as most Western nations with single-payer systems already do, and reduce overhead costs.

Biden's (public option) proposal would actually increase costs, Galvani said. "Without the savings to overhead, pharmaceutical costs, hospital/clinical fees, and fraud detection, 'Medicare for All Who Want It' could annually cost $175 billion dollars more than status quo," Galvani told Newsweek. "That's over $600 billion more than Medicare for All."

Another study published in the Annals of Internal Medicine (https://www.acpjournals.org/doi/10.7326/M19-2818) by researchers at Harvard University, Hunter College and the University of Ottawa similarly estimated that switching to a single-payer system like Medicare for All could save up to $600 billion per year on administrative costs alone.

The study found that the average American pays $2,597 per year on administrative costs — overhead for insurers and hospitals, salaries, huge executive compensation packages and growing profits — while Canadians pay $551 per year.

Though Canada had costs similar to the United States and worse health outcomes before it adopted its single-payer system in 1962, Canada now has better health outcomes than the United States and only spends 17% of its health care spending on administrative costs, compared to 34% in the U.S.

"Americans spend twice as much per person as Canadians on health care. But instead of buying better care, that extra spending buys us sky-high profits and useless paperwork," lead author Dr. David Himmelstein, who teaches at Harvard and Hunter College, said in a statement. "Before their single-payer reform, Canadians died younger than Americans, and their infant mortality rate was higher than ours. Now Canadians live three years longer and their infant mortality rate is 22% lower than ours. Under Medicare for All, Americans could cut out the red tape and afford a Rolls Royce version of Canada's system."

Himmelstein told Time that the savings in administrative costs alone would be enough to eliminate "all copayments and deductibles" and still "have money left over."

But while Medicare for All would reduce these costs by eliminating private profit-seeking insurers, the public option alternative would add costs while leaving the bloated administrative costs in place.

"Medicare for All could save more than $600 billion each year on bureaucracy, and repurpose that money to cover America's 30 million uninsured and eliminate copayments and deductibles for everyone," said researcher Dr. Steffie Woolhandler, who also teaches at Harvard and Hunter. "Reforms like a public option that leave private insurers in place can't deliver big administrative savings. As a result, public option reform would cost much more and cover much less than Medicare for All."

Other studies have led to similar conclusions. A review of 22 single-payer studies published in PLOS Medicine (*) found that 19 of them "predicted net savings ... in the first year of program operation and 20 ... predicted savings over several years; anticipated growth rates would result in long-term net savings for all plans." https://journals.plos.org/plosmedicine/article?id=10.1371/journal.pmed.1003013 (*PLOS Medicine). Studies have also widely disputed other claims made by opponents of Medicare for All.

While critics have claimed that the proposal would lead to "rationing" of health care, a recent Federal Reserve survey found that roughly a quarter of "adults skipped necessary medical care in 2018 because they were unable to afford the cost." Millions of Americans have been forced to ration their insulin or avoid calling an ambulance in emergencies due to sky-high costs, including those who have insurance.

Critics also argue that wait times for care are longer in countries with single-payer systems, but a 2017 survey found that wait times have already increased in the United States by 30% since 2014 under the current system.

Critics have claimed that Medicare for All would lead to people abusing the free health care system. But a study published in the Journal of General Internal Medicine in November showed that use did not generally increase in countries that moved to single-payer systems.

All these studies make various assumptions about costs and figures associated with what a single-payer system would look like in America. "Experts answer those questions differently, which is reflected in their final cost estimates. And though we can't predict the future, we do have plenty of data on what's happening in the American health-care system right now," wrote Washington Post data journalist Christopher Ingraham. "Relative to people in other wealthy nations, Americans are less likely to be in good health and more likely to die of preventable causes. Our babies and mothers are more likely to die after child birth, and our lives are shorter overall."

But a public option is not the solution, Drs. Himmelstein and Woolhandler wrote in an op-ed "The 'Public Option' on Health Care Is a Poison Pill" in The Nation (October 21, 2019): ....
(https://www.thenation.com/article/archive/insurance-health-care-medicare/).

"The case for a public option rests on faulty economic logic and naive assumptions about how private insurance actually works," they wrote. "Tens of millions would remain uninsured or with coverage so skimpy, they still couldn't afford care. ... Moreover, a public option would save little or nothing on hospitals' and doctors' sky-high billing and administrative costs."

"Because a public option would leave the current dysfunctional payment approach in place, it would sacrifice most of the savings available via single-payer reform," they added. "The bottom line is that a public option would either cost much more or deliver much less than single-payer."

Igor Derysh is a staff writer at Salon. His work has also appeared in the Los Angeles Times, Chicago Tribune, Boston Herald and Baltimore Sun. Tips/Email: iderysh@salon.com & Twitter: @IgorDerysh

https://thehill.com/blogs/congress-blog/healthcare/484301-22-studies-agree-
medicare-for-all-saves-money   (See hyperlink for full text and references.)

22 STUDIES AGREE: 'MEDICARE FOR ALL' SAVES MONEY

By Diane Archer, Opinion Contributor THE HILL, 02/24/2020
The views expressed by Contributors are their own
and not the view of THE HILL

The evidence abounds: A "Medicare for All" single-payer system would guarantee comprehensive coverage to everyone in America and save money.

Christopher Cai and colleagues at three University of California campuses examined 22 studies on the projected cost impact for single-payer health insurance in the United States and reported their findings in a recent paper in PLOS Medicine. Every single study predicted that it would yield net savings over several years. In fact, it's the only way to rein in health care spending significantly in the U.S.

All of the studies, regardless of ideological orientation, showed that long-term cost savings were likely. Even the Mercatus Center, a right-wing think tank, recently found about $2 trillion in net savings over 10 years from a single-payer Medicare for All system. Most importantly, everyone in America would have high-quality health care coverage.

Medicare for All is far less costly than our current system largely because it reduces administrative costs. With one public plan negotiating rates with health care providers, billing becomes quite simple. We do away with three-quarters of the estimated $812 billion the U.S. now spends on health care administration.

Administrative costs are so high because thousands of insurance companies individually negotiate benefit rules and rates with thousands of hospitals and doctors. On top of that, they rely on different billing procedures — and this puts a costly burden on providers.

Administrative savings from Medicare for All would be about $600 billion a year. Savings on prescription drugs would be between $200 billion and $300 billion a year, if we paid about the same price as other wealthy countries pay for their drugs. A Medicare for All system would save still more with implementation of global health care spending budgets.

Even more savings are possible in a Medicare for All system because, like every other wealthy country, we would have a uniform electronic health records system. Such a system generates additional savings because system problems would be easier to detect and correct. A uniform claims data system helps reduce health care spending for fraudulent services. In 2018, total U.S. health care costs were $3.6 trillion, representing 17.7 percent of GDP.

Savings are in part a function of the benefits Medicare for All covers. The Mercatus report and others projected savings, even with the elimination of deductibles and out-of-pocket costs. Under both Sen. Bernie Sanders's (I-VT) Medicare for All bill and Rep. Pramila Jayapal's (D-WA) Medicare for All bill, patients would not pay deductibles or coinsurance when they receive medical care. Their bills also provide for vision, hearing and dental care, as well as long-term services and supports, such as home care and nursing home care.

No matter how you design a single-payer public health insurance system, it would have lower overall health care costs, so long as for-profit private health insurers no longer exist to drive up health care costs.

And, if you're thinking that having the federal government guarantee coverage to all Americans is a big deal, it's actually not. The government (aka taxpayers) already pays for about two-thirds of health care costs. Among other things, it pays for Medicare, Medicaid, VA, TRICARE and a wide range of state and local health care programs, along with private insurance for government employees and tax subsidies for private insurance.

Whether you call it single-payer or Medicare for All (or Universal Healthcare), it isn't some socialist pipe dream. It's a sensible, efficient, and effective way to guarantee excellent health insurance to everyone.

Diane Archer is a senior adviser at Social Security Works and president of Just Care (https://justcareusa.org/).

https://journals.plos.org/plosmedicine/article?id=10.1371/journal.pmed.100
3013   (See hyperlink for full text and references.)

PLOS MEDICINE
Projected Costs of Single-payer Healthcare Financing in the United States: A Systematic Review of Economic Analyses

Christopher Cai , Jackson Runte, Isabel Ostrer, Kacey Berry, Ninez Ponce,
Michael Rodriguez, Stefano Bertozzi, Justin S. White, James G. Kahn
Published: 15 January 2020

Abstract

Background

The United States is the only high-income nation without universal, government-funded or -mandated health insurance employing a unified payment system. The US multi-payer system leaves residents uninsured or underinsured, despite overall healthcare costs far above other nations. Single-payer (often referred to as Medicare for All), a proposed policy solution since 1990, is receiving renewed press attention and popular support. Our review seeks to assess the projected cost impact of a single-payer approach.

Methods and findings

We conducted our literature search between June 1 and December 31, 2018, without start date restriction for included studies. We surveyed an expert panel and searched PubMed, Google, Google Scholar, and preexisting lists for formal economic studies of the projected costs of single-payer plans for the US or for individual states. Reviewer pairs extracted data on methods and findings using a template. We quantified changes in total costs standardized to percentage of contemporaneous healthcare spending. Additionally, we quantified cost changes by subtype, such as costs due to increased healthcare utilization and savings due to simplified payment administration, lower drug costs, and other factors. We further examined how modeling assumptions affected results.

Our search yielded economic analyses of the cost of 22 single-payer plans over the past 30 years. Exclusions were due to inadequate technical data or assuming a substantial ongoing role for private insurers. We found that 19 (86%) of the analyses predicted net savings (median net result was a savings of 3.46% of total costs) in the first year of program operation and 20 (91%) predicted savings over several years; anticipated growth rates would result in long-term net savings for all plans. The largest source of savings was simplified payment administration (median 8.8%), and the best predictors of net savings were the magnitude of utilization increase, and savings on administration and drug costs (R^2 of 0.035, 0.43, and 0.62, respectively). Only drug cost savings remained significant in multivariate analysis. Included studies were heterogeneous in methods, which precluded us from conducting a formal meta-analysis.

Conclusions

In this systematic review, we found a high degree of analytic consensus for the fiscal feasibility of a single-payer approach in the US. Actual costs will depend on plan features and implementation. Future research should refine estimates of the effects of coverage expansion on utilization, evaluate provider administrative costs in varied existing single-payer systems, analyze implementation options, and evaluate US-based single-payer programs, as available.

Author Summary

Why was this study done?

- As the US healthcare debate continues, there is growing interest in "single-payer" also known as "Medicare for All." Single-payer uses a simplified public funding approach to provide everyone with high-quality health insurance.
- Public support for provision of universal health coverage through a plan like Medicare for All is as high as 70%, but falls when costs are emphasized.
- Economic models help assess the financial viability of single-payer. Yet, models vary widely in their assumptions and methods, and can be hard to compare.

What did the researchers do and find?

- We found and compared cost analyses of 22 single-payer plans for the US or individual states.

- Nineteen (86%) of the analyses estimated that health expenditures would fall in the first year, and all suggested the potential for long-term cost savings.
- The largest savings were predicted to come from simplified billing and lower drug costs.
- Studies funded by organizations across the political spectrum estimated savings for single-payer.

What do these findings mean?

- There is near-consensus in these analyses that single-payer would reduce health expenditures while providing high-quality insurance to all US residents.
- To achieve net savings, single-payer plans rely on simplified billing and negotiated drug price reductions, as well as global budgets to control spending growth over time.
- Replacing private insurers with a public system of insurance is expected to achieve lower net healthcare costs.

Studies Identified

We reviewed 90 studies and included primary analyses of 22 single-payer plans from 18 studies, published between 1991 and 2018, including 8 national and 14 state-level plans (Massachusetts, California, Maryland, Vermont, Minnesota, Pennsylvania, New York, and Oregon).

Included Studies (alphabetical)

1. Blahous C (2018). The Costs of a National Single-Payer Healthcare System. Arlington (VA): Mercatus Center, George Mason University; 2018 Jul [cited 2019 Dec 18]. .... Available from: https://www.mercatus.org/system/files/blahous-costs-medicare-mercatus-working-paper-v1_1.pdf

2. Congressional Budget Office (1993). Single-Payer and All-Payer Health Insurance Systems Using Medicare Payment Rates. (accessed 12/24/2019) ..... Available at https://www.cbo.gov/publication/16595

3. Friedman, Gerald (2013). Financing the Maryland Health Security Act. (accessed 12/24/2019) .... Available at https://www.healthcare-now.org/wp-content/uploads/2017/08/Maryland-Friedman-2013.pdf

4. Friedman, Gerald (2013). Funding HR 676: The Expanded and Improved Medicare for All Act: How we can afford a national single-payer health plan. (accessed 12/24/2019) .... Available at https://www.healthcare-now.org/single-payer-studies/gerald-friedman-2013/

5. Friedman, Gerald (2013). The Pennsylvania Health Care Plan Impact and Implementation. Available at https://www.healthcare-now.org/wp-content/uploads/2017/08/Pennsylvania-Friedman-2013.pdf (accessed 12/24/2019)

6. Friedman, Gerald (2015). Economic Analysis of the New York Health Act. (accessed 12/24/2019) .... Available at http://www.infoshare.org/main/Economic_Analysis_New_York_Health_Act_-_GFriedman_-_April_2015.pdf

7. Government Accounting Office (1991). Canadian Health Insurance: Lessons for the United States. (Accessed 12/24/2019) Available at https://www.gao.gov/products/T-HRD-91-35

8. Grumbach, K., Bodenheimer, T., Himmelstein, D. U., & Woolhandler, S. (1991). Liberal benefits, conservative spending: the Physicians for a National Health Program proposal. JAMA, 265 (19), 2549-2554. (Accessed 12/24/2019) .... Available at https://jamanetwork.com/journals/jama/article-abstract/385948

9. Hsiao, W., Kappel, S., & Gruber, J. (2011). Act 128: Health system reform design. achieving affordable universal health care in Vermont. Final Report to the Vermont Legislature (February 19, 2011). (Accessed 12/24/19) .... Available at https://hcr.vermont.gov/sites/hcr/files/FINAL_REPORT_Hsiao_Final_Report_17_February%202011_3.pdf

10. Lewin Group (2000). Analysis of the Costs and Impact of Universal Health Care Models for the State of Maryland: The Single-Payer and Multi-Payer Models. (Accessed 12/24/2019) .... Available at https://www.healthcare-now.org/wp-content/uploads/2017/08/Maryland-Lewin-Group-2000.pdf

11. Lewin Group (2002). Cost and Coverage Analysis of Nine Proposals to Expand Health Insurance Coverage in California. Prepared for The California Health and Human Services Agency. March 31, 2002.

(accessed 12/24/2019) .... Available at https://www.healthcare-now.org/wp-content/uploads/2017/08/California-Lewin-2002.pdf

12. Lewin Group (2012). Cost and Economic Impact Analysis of a Single-Payer Plan in Minnesota. (Accessed 12/24/2019) Available at https://www.healthcare-now.org/single-payer-studies/minnesota-lewin-group-2012/

13. Liu, Jodi L., Exploring Single-Payer Alternatives for Health Care Reform. Santa Monica, CA: RAND Corporation, 2016. .... https://www.rand.org/pubs/rgs_dissertations/RGSD375.html

14. Liu, Jodi L., Chapin White, Sarah A. Nowak, Asa Wilks, Jamie Ryan, and Christine Eibner, An Assessment of the New York Health Act: A Single-Payer Option for New York State. Santa Monica, CA: RAND Corporation, 2018. .... https://www.rand.org/pubs/research_reports/RR2424.html

15. Pollin, R., Heintz, J., Arno, P., & Wicks-Lim, J. (2017). Economic analysis of the Healthy California single-payer health care proposal (SB-562). Political Economy Research Institute, University of Massachusetts. (Accessed 12/24/2019) .... Available at https://www.peri.umass.edu/publication/item/996-economic-analysis-of-the-healthy-california-single-payer-health-care-proposal-sb-562

16. Pollin, R., Heintz, J., Arno, P., Wicks-Lim, J., & Ash, M. (2018). Economic Analysis of Medicare for All. Political Economy Research Institute, University of Massachusetts: Amherst, MA, USA (Accessed 12/24/2019) .... Available at https://www.peri.umass.edu/publication/item/1127-economic-analysis-of-medicare-for-all

17. Solutions for Progress (2000). Massachusetts Can Afford Health Care for All.. Available at https://www.bu.edu/sph/files/2012/07/UHC-1-Nov-00-FINAL.pdf

18. White, Chapin, Christine Eibner, Jodi L. Liu, Carter C. Price, Nora Leibowitz, Gretchen Morley, Jeanene Smith, Tina Edlund, and Jack Meyer, A Comprehensive Assessment of Four Options for Financing Health Care Delivery in Oregon. Santa Monica, CA: RAND Corporation, 2017. https://www.rand.org/pubs/research_reports/RR1662.html

https://jacobinmag.com/2020/04/coronavirus-medicare-for-all-m4a-single-payer-health-insurance   (See hyperlink for full text and references.)

There's Never Been a Better Time for Us to End Private Health Insurance Than Right Now

By Tim Higginbotham, April 2020
(Tim Higginbotham is an organizer with Democratic Socialists of America's Medicare for All campaign. He lives in Anchorage, Alaska.)

The coronavirus crisis will lead to health insurance premium increases by up to 40 percent next year. We can't afford that. Instead of seeing premiums skyrocket or bailing out private health companies, we need to seize this moment to abolish private insurance and create a single, national insurance plan.

The US health care system is going to be overwhelmed by the coronavirus pandemic for months to come. But when the spread of the virus finally does subside, many of its impacts will be here to stay. With millions of Americans likely to need expensive hospital stays this year, our nationwide health care costs are expected to increase by as much as $251 billion, according to a new analysis. As a result, US health insurance premiums could rise by up to 40 percent in 2021, exacerbating a crisis of ever-increasing costs that already leave Americans paying far more for care than the people of any other country.

What this means is that we're about to hit a fork in the road with the private insurance industry. The coronavirus is shredding insurers' profits right now, underlining the fact that private insurance is simply not built to handle a medical crisis. Having to cover a surge of expensive treatment — and, in some cases, having to waive co-pays — is antithetical to the premise of for-profit insurance. Saddled with these unexpected costs, private insurers' only alternative to drastically raising our premiums will be to request a massive government bailout to avoid bankruptcy.

Allowing private companies to bankroll our health care system has always been a terrible policy choice, but the horror of this approach is about to become even more evident. Hiking premiums in the midst of a devastating pandemic to make up for their losses is an act of cruelty, to be sure. But it's also the only logical act for companies whose sole purpose is to chase accrescent ("ever-growing") profits.

Instead of allowing our premiums to skyrocket or bailing out a heartless industry with public funds, thereby prolonging a profit-driven nightmare, we need to seize this watershed moment by taking the step many Americans have demanded for over a century. It's time to abolish the private insurance industry and create a single, national insurance plan in its place.

There has never been a more obvious moment to take the leap to single-payer health care. The familiar arguments against it, disingenuous in the first place, are suddenly outwardly ridiculous and easy to refute.

Joe Biden has been using his scarce media appearances to assure viewers that he still opposes Medicare for All, Bernie Sanders's popular single-payer plan that would comprehensively cover all Americans at no out-of-pocket cost. But President Biden's arguments — that Medicare for All would be too expensive, that it would disrupt people's employer-sponsored coverage, and that it would bring too large a change from the status quo — no longer carry the weight they once did. Even CNN's Anderson Cooper recently pressed Biden to explain how his health care plan would solve the problems made evident by the current pandemic.

On the question of cost, Sanders and his fellow Medicare for All advocates have long argued that single-payer health care will cost substantially less than our current system. This is backed up by virtually every major economic analysis of his plan, although these studies have long been ignored by Medicare for All's opponents in Congress and the media. But they become harder to ignore the more expensive the current system gets — and a massive hike in premiums or a major government bailout will only underscore Sanders's argument further.

As for the criticism that Medicare for All would throw people off their employer-sponsored insurance, it's a bit more difficult to defend this argument when the country is projected to possibly reach its highest ever levels of unemployment. The major flaw in tethering health care to employment has never been clearer: workers (and their dependents) are constantly at risk of losing their employer-sponsored insurance.

Now it's happening on a mass scale — millions of Americans have already lost their jobs during the pandemic, and it's only going to get worse.

Liberals have spent the last decade celebrating the fact that the Affordable Care Act lowered the number of uninsured people in the United States from 44 million to a still-astonishing 28 million. Suddenly, that modest improvement is being reversed. Because we've relied on a fragile method of coverage instead of a bulletproof approach of automatic, universal enrollment in a public plan, all of the progress made by liberals is subject to erasure by a single crisis.

Perhaps the biggest obstacle to building the public demand for Medicare for All has been the mere fact that it will bring a major disruption to the status quo. The concept of socializing one-sixth of the US economy — which is what Medicare for All entails — has been used to frighten those wary of change.

But the pandemic has already disrupted the status quo. We no longer face a choice between keeping things as they were and implementing a major change. Change is coming, no matter what, and it's our choice whether we respond to it by using public funds to prop up a broken system that constantly kills and bankrupts Americans in the name of profit, or by using those same funds to create a stable, single-payer program designed in the interest of public health.

Don't Bail Out an Industry That Shouldn't Exist

We've already tried bailouts. The Affordable Care Act (ACA) was essentially a bailout in that it heavily subsidized insurance companies in order to get them to take measures that otherwise would not be sufficiently profitable. In fact, the government continues to pump hundreds of billions of public dollars each year into the industry to protect its profits.

It's a broken approach no matter the scale. But what's coming will be massive — it will make the ACA subsidies look incredibly meager. We cannot allow such a historic bailout of an industry that should not exist in the first place.

The logical fix to the problems of our health care system has *always* been to implement a single, national insurer. Instead of profit, we need to prioritize public health and well-being. Even when we're not facing such a monumental crisis, our current system causes millions to suffer, physically and financially.

But this crisis has brought us to a unique crossroads. With our health care providers crying out for the help they need, with millions finding themselves suddenly uninsured, and with the insurance industry proving itself fundamentally incapable of protecting public health, we have the opportunity to choose a better way.

It's long past time for single-payer health care. We've been demanding it for more than a century — people have fought their entire lives and died without ever seeing it become a reality. But we've never had a moment quite like this, where the flaws and shortcomings of our long-standing multi-payer system are so abundantly clear.

So let's make our demand even clearer: instead of bailing out the industry that murders and bankrupts us and our families, let's erase the industry altogether and take health coverage into public hands through a Medicare for All, single-payer program.

https://www.desmoinesregister.com/story/opinion/columnists/2018/10/04/its-time-get-profits-out-health-care/1514500002/
(See hyperlink for full text and references.)

It's Time to Get Profits Out of Health Care
Michael Lighty, Register Opinion Contributor, 10/4/2018

Now we know the numbers on Iowa's experiment with for-profit Medicaid. Not surprisingly, costs went up faster per participant than in the pre-reform period, regardless of Gov. Kim Reynolds' spin. Private insurers are profiting at taxpayer expense.

But that's how the health care system is gamed. We pay tax subsidies to employers and individuals for our health insurance so then we can "afford" to give insurance companies 20 cents (or more) on the dollar. What do they do in return? Deny coverage, hassle over claims, charge high co-pays, and don't pay a dime until huge deductibles are met.

So Iowa's Medicaid is just another stop on the gravy train for UnitedHealth (over $12 billion in profits in two years under the ACA), and their executives. Shareholders, especially in the drug companies, make out like bandits. The price of insulin, without any formula changes, has climbed more than 500% in just a few years because Novo Nordisk and the rest can charge whatever they want and people need it to live.

Hospital corporations did very well during the prime years of the ACA. Now – after further consolidations under new care models that emphasize high-margin boutique services, concierge doctors for the wealthy, and mandates for the rest of us to get procedures done in clinics not governed by hospital safety rules – profitability is rebounding.

Since hospitals, prescription drug corporations and insurance companies set their prices without any limit, runaway health care costs overwhelm us. Why does health care in the U.S. cost so much? Because prices are high. And who pays? Taxpayers and workers. The ACA limits out-of-pocket health care costs to under 10% of income or less. But that includes only in-network costs, and the cost of insurance for an individual, not a family. Typically, large employers who generally provide the best benefits spend $18,800 on health care for each worker. But all the rising costs have been shifted to workers in the form of higher co-pays, deductibles and premiums. Taxpayers provide $342 billion per year to employers as subsidies. Meanwhile, 42% of the insured population has deferred either a doctor visit, prescription or other medical need because of cost.

The solution to these runaway costs is the power to control prices. And that requires a mind twist for some – maybe all of us – who have seen government identified first as the problem and now the enemy: Our taxes will go up, but our costs will go down.

It turns out that Medicare – a publicly financed and publicly administered health care system that guarantees health care to all Americans over 65 – spends a fraction (3-6%) on administration compared to the 12% (or more) by private insurance companies. And effectively controls costs – annual increases are consistently below overall medical inflation. Every other industrialized country spends less – on average, half as much – as does the U.S. on health care per person but have more equitable access, better outcomes, and stronger public health systems.

We can complete the American system of guaranteed health care for all by improving and expanding Medicare. People in Medicare now and in the near future should welcome healthy, younger people into an improved system that eliminates the co-pays and deductibles of Part B, and eliminates the need for expensive private drug coverage. Dental, vision and optometry will be automatically covered. All the benefits of Medicare Part C will be available, without the limits and restrictions on what doctor you can visit.

Even conservative economists acknowledge that improved Medicare for All will enable the U.S. overall to spend less on health care and get more coverage. That's why even 52% of Republicans in the latest Gallup poll support Medicare for All. Let's build on what's popular and works: a publicly governed, democratically accountable health care system that doesn't make money but makes better health outcomes.

Note to readers: Michael Lighty was the featured speaker at "Medicare for All" town hall meetings held Oct. 8-10, 2018 in Des Moines, Ames, Cedar Rapids and Grinnell. For more information, call Iowa CCI Action at 515-282-0484 or go to www.cciaction.org. He is a founding fellow of the (Bernie) Sanders Institute and has worked on health care policy for over 25 years.

https://www.fiercehealthcare.com/payer/health-insurance-ceos-took-home-a-hefty-pay-day-2018-how-does-compare-to-their-employees
(See hyperlink for full text and references.)

What the CEOs of the 8 Largest Insurers Earned in 2018
By Paige Minemyer ; 23 April 2019

UnitedHealth Group CEO David Wichmann: $18.1 million in total compensation in 2018 — 316 times the median salary of a company employee.

Centene's CEO Michael Neidorff: $26.1 million

Humana's CEO Bruce Broussard: $16.3 million

Anthem's CEO Gail Boudreaux: $14.1 million

WellCare's CEO Kenneth Burdick: $12.7 million

All told, the CEOs of UnitedHealth, Humana, Anthem, Centene, Cigna, CVS, Molina Healthcare and WellCare Health Plans collectively earned $143,504,848 in total compensation in 2018, according to the filings.

Column: Health Insurance Companies are Useless. Get Rid of Them

By Michael Hiltzik, Business Columnist ; 5 August 2019

The most perplexing aspect of our current debate over healthcare and health coverage is the notion that Americans love their health insurance companies.

The truth is that private health insurers have contributed nothing of value to the American healthcare system. Instead, they have raised costs and created an entitled class of administrators and executives who are fighting for their livelihoods, using customers' premium dollars to do so.

"Health insurers have been successful at two things: making money and getting the American public to believe they're essential," says Wendell Potter. He should know, because he spent decades as a corporate communications executive in the industry, including more than 10 years at Cigna.

The insurers' success in making themselves seem essential accounts for the notion that Americans are so pleased with their private coverage that they'll punish any politician who dares to take it away. But the American love affair with private insurance warrants close inspection.

Let's start by examining what the insurers say are their positive contributions to healthcare. They claim to promote "consumer choice," simplify "the healthcare experience for individuals and families," address "the burden of chronic disease" and harness "data and technology to drive quality, efficiency, and consumer satisfaction." (These claims all come from the website of the industry's lobbying organization, America's Health Insurance Plans: AHIP).

They've achieved none of these goals. The increasingly prevalent mode of health coverage in the group and individual markets is the narrow network, which shrinks the roster of doctors and hospitals available to enrollees without heavy surcharges. The hoops that customers and providers often must jump through to get claims paid impose costly complexity on the system, not simplicity. Programs to manage chronic diseases remain rare, and the real threat to patients with those conditions was lack of access to insurance (until the Affordable Care Act made such exclusion illegal).

Private insurers don't do nearly as well as Medicare in holding down costs, in part because the more they pay hospitals and doctors, the more they can charge in premiums and the more money flows to their bottom lines. They haven't shown notable skill in managing chronic diseases or bringing pro-consumer innovations to the table.

Insurers cite these goals when they try to get mergers approved by government antitrust regulators. Anthem and Cigna, for example, asserted in 2016 that their merger would produce nearly $2 billion in "annual synergies," thanks to improved "operational" and "network efficiencies."

The pitch has a long history. The architects of a wave of health insurance mergers in the 2000s also proclaimed a new era of efficient technology and improved customer service, but studies of prior mergers show that this nirvana seldom comes to pass. The best example may be that of Aetna's 1996 merger with U.S. Healthcare in a deal it hoped would give it access to the booming HMO market.

According to a 2004 analysis by UC Berkeley health economist James C. Robinson, the merger became a "near-death" experience for Aetna. The deal was expected to bring about "millions in enrollment and billions in revenue to pressure physicians and hospitals" to accept lower reimbursement rates, he wrote.

"The talk was all about complementarities, synergies, and economies of scale.... The reality quickly turned out to be one of incompatible product designs, operating systems, sales forces, brand images, and corporate cultures." Aetna surged from 13.7 million customers in 1996 to 21 million in 1999, but profits collapsed from a margin of nearly 14% in 1998 to a loss in 2001.

Even when they don't happen, insurance merger deals cost customers billions of dollars. That's what happened when two proposed deals — Aetna-Humana and Anthem-Cigna — broke down on a single day in 2017. The result was that Aetna owed Humana $1.8 billion and Anthem owed Cigna $1.85 billion in breakup fees — money taken out of the medical treatment economy and transferred from one set of shareholders to another.

In reality, Americans don't like their private health insurance so much as blindly tolerate it. That's because the vast majority of Americans don't have a complex interaction with the healthcare system in any given year, and most never will. As we've reported before, 1% of patients account for more than one-fifth of all medical spending and 10% account for two-thirds. Fifty percent of patients account for only 3% of all spending.

Most families face at most a series of minor ailments that can be routinely managed — childhood immunizations, a broken arm here or there, a bout of the flu. The question is what happens when someone does have a complex issue and a complex claim — they're hit by a truck or get a cancer diagnosis, for instance?

"We gamble every year that we're going to stay healthy and injury-free," Potter says. When we lose the gamble, that's when all the inadequacies of the private insurance system come to the fore. Confronted with the prospect of expensive claims, private insurers try to constrain customers' choices — limiting recovery days spent in the hospital, limiting doctors' latitude to try different therapies, demanding to be consulted before approving surgical interventions.

Indeed, the history of American healthcare reform is largely a chronicle of steps taken to protect the unserved groups from commercial health insurance practices.

When commercial health insurance became insinuated into the American healthcare system following World War II via employer plans, it quickly became clear who was left behind — "those who were retired, out of work, self-employed, or obliged to take a low-paying job without fringes," sociologist Paul Starr wrote in his magisterial 1982 book, "The Social Transformation of American Medicine."The process even left those groups worse off, Starr observed, because insurance contributed to medical inflation while insulating only those with health plans. "Government intervention was required just to address the inequities."

Insurers wouldn't cover the aged or retirees, so Medicare was born in 1965. Insurers refused to cover kidney disease patients needing dialysis, so Congress in 1973 carved out an exception allowing those patients to enroll in Medicare at any age. (So much for addressing the "burden of chronic disease.")

Individual buyers were charged much more for coverage than those buying group plans through their employers — or were barred from the marketplace entirely because of their medical conditions. The Affordable Care Act required insurers to accept all applicants and, as compensation, required all individuals to carry at least minimal coverage.

The health insurance industry's most telling contribution to the debate over healthcare reform has been "to scare people about other healthcare systems," Potter told me. As a consequence, discussions about whether or how to remove private companies from the healthcare system are chiefly political, not practical.

The Affordable Care Act allowed private insurers to continue playing a role in delivering coverage not because they were any good at it but because their wealth and size made them formidable adversaries to reform if they chose to fight it. They were sufficiently mollified to remain out of the fray, but some of the big insurers then did their best to undermine the individual insurance exchanges once they were launched in 2015.

Even as individual Americans fret over losing their private health insurance, big employers have begun to see the light. Boeing, among other big employers, is experimenting with bypassing health insurers as intermediaries with providers by contracting directly with major health systems in Southern California, Seattle and other regions where it has major plants. It would not be surprising to see the joint venture of Amazon, Berkshire Hathaway and JPMorgan Chase try a similar approach in its quest to bring down costs.

That's an ironic development, since the private insurers first entered the market precisely by offering to play the role of intermediaries for big employers. But instead of fulfilling the promise of efficiency and cost control, they became rent-seeking profiteers themselves.

There's no doubt that it will take years to wean the American healthcare system off the private insurance model. It's true that some countries with universal healthcare systems preserve roles for private insurance, including coverage for services the government chooses to leave out of its own programs or providing preferential access to specialists, at a price.

But the private insurers' central position in America's system is an anachronism dating back some 75 years. The sooner it is dispensed with, the better off — and healthier — America will be. The next time a debate moderator asks presidential candidates if they favor doing away with private insurance, let's see all the hands go up.

# # # # # #

One way to look at it: Either (1) you show your doctor your Medicare for All card & your doctor bills Medicare for All, or (2) an insurance company issues you a card annually (billing you premiums, co-pays, deductibles, etc) and pays your doctor after first pocketing $$$ for its self-styled administrative costs, CEO salary & comps, dividends to their stockholders, etc. Any questions ???

More Than A Third of U.S. Healthcare Costs Go To Bureaucracy
By Linda Carroll for Reuters ; 3 March 2020

(Reuters Health) – U.S. insurers and providers spent more than $800 billion in 2017 on administration, or nearly $2,500 per person – more than four times the per-capita administrative costs in Canada's single-payer system, a new study finds.

Over one third of all healthcare costs in the U.S. were due to insurance company overhead and provider time spent on billing, versus about 17% spent on administration in Canada, researchers reported in Annals of Internal Medicine.

Cutting U.S. administrative costs to the $550 per capita (in 2017 U.S. dollars) level in Canada could save more than $600 billion, the researchers say.

"The average American is paying more than $2,000 a year for useless bureaucracy," said lead author Dr. David Himmelstein, a distinguished professor of public health at the City University of New York at Hunter College in New York City and a lecturer at Harvard Medical School in

Boston. "That money could be spent for care if we had a 'Medicare for all program'," Himmelstein said.

To calculate the difference in administrative costs between the U.S. and Canadian systems, Himmelstein and colleagues examined Medicare filings made by hospitals and nursing homes. For physicians, the researchers used information from surveys and census data on employment and wages to estimate costs. The Canadian data came from the Canadian Institute for Health Information and an insurance trade association.

When the researchers broke down the 2017 per-capita health administration costs in both countries, they found that insurer overhead accounted for $844 in the U.S. versus $146 in Canada; hospital administration was $933 versus $196; nursing home, home care and hospice administration was $255 versus $123; and physicians' insurance-related costs were $465 versus $87.

They also found there had been a 3.2% increase in U.S. administrative costs since 1999, most of which was ascribed to the expansion of Medicare and Medicaid managed-care plans. Overhead of private Medicare Advantage plans, which now cover about a third of Medicare enrollees, is six-fold higher than traditional Medicare (12.3% versus 2%), they report. That 2% is comparable to the overhead in the Canadian system.

Why are administrative costs so high in the U.S.? It's because the insurance companies and health care providers are engaged in a tug of war, each trying in its own way to game the system, Himmelstein said. How a patient's treatment is coded can make a huge difference in the amount insurance companies pay. For example, Himmelstein said, if a patient comes in because of heart failure and the visit is coded as an acute exacerbation of the condition, the payment is significantly higher than if the visit is simply coded as heart failure.

This upcoding of patient visits has led insurance companies to require more and more paperwork backing up each diagnosis, Himmelstein said. The result is more hours that healthcare providers need to put in to deal with billing.

"(One study) looked at how many characters were included in an average physician's note in the U.S. and in other countries," Himmelstein pointed out. "Notes from U.S. physicians were four times longer to meet the bureaucratic requirements of the payment system."

The new study is "the first analysis of administrative costs in the U.S. and Canada in almost 20 years," said Dr. Albert Wu, an internist and professor of health policy and management at the Johns Hopkins School of Public Health in Baltimore. "It's an important paper."

"It's clear that health costs in the U.S. have soared," Wu said. "We're paying for an inefficient and wasteful fee-for-services system."

"Some folks estimate that the U.S. would save $628 billion if administrative costs were as low as they are in Canada," said Jamie Daw, an assistant professor of health policy and management at Columbia University's Mailman School of Public Health in New York City. "That's a staggering amount," Daw said in an email. "It's more than enough to pay for all of Medicaid spending or nearly enough to cover all out-of-pocket and prescription drug spending by Americans."

https://berniesanders.com/issues/how-does-bernie-pay-his-major-plans/
(See hyperlink for full text and references.)

How Bernie Would Pay for Medicare for All

According to a February 15, 2020 study by epidemiologists at Yale University, the Medicare for All bill that Bernie wrote would save over $450 billion in health care costs and prevent 68,000 unnecessary deaths – each and every year.

What our current system costs over the next decade:

Over the next ten years, national health expenditures are projected to total approximately **$52 trillion** if we keep our current dysfunctional system.

How much we will save:

According to the Yale study and others, Medicare for All will save approximately **$5 trillion** over that same time period.

$52 trillion - $5 trillion = **$47 trillion total**

How we pay for it:

Current federal, state and local government spending over the next ten years is projected to total about **$30 trillion.**

The revenue options Bernie has proposed total **$17.5 Trillion**

$30 trillion + $17.5 trillion = **$47.5 Trillion total**

Sources:

- **https://www.cms.gov/Research-Statistics-Data-and-Systems/Statistics-Trends-and-Reports/NationalHealthExpendData/NationalHealthAccountsPr ojected**

- **https://www.thelancet.com/journals/lancet/article/PIIS0140-6736(19)33019-3/fulltext#%20**

Since 2016, Bernie has proposed a menu of financing options that would more than pay for the Medicare for All legislation he has introduced according to the Yale study. These options include:

- Creating a 4 percent income-based premium paid by employees, exempting the first $29,000 in income for a family of four. In 2018, the typical working family paid an average of $6,015 in premiums to private health insurance companies. Under this option, a typical family of four earning $60,000, would pay a 4 percent income-based premium to fund Medicare for All on income above $29,000 – just $1,240 a year – saving that family $4,775 a year. Families of four making less than $29,000 a year would not pay this premium. *(Revenue raised: About $4 trillion over 10 years.)*

- Imposing a 7.5 percent income-based premium paid by employers, exempting the first $1 million in payroll to protect small businesses. In 2018, employers paid an average of $14,561 in private health insurance premiums for a worker with a family of four. Under this option, employers would pay a 7.5 percent payroll tax to help finance Medicare for all – just $4,500 – a savings of more than $10,000 a year. *(Revenue raised: Over $5.2 trillion over 10 years.)*

- Eliminating health tax expenditures, which would no longer be needed under Medicare for All. *(Revenue raised: About $3 trillion over 10 years.)*

- Raising the top marginal income tax rate to 52% on income over $10 million. *(Revenue raised: About $700 billion over 10 years.)*

- Replacing the cap on the state and local tax deduction with an overall dollar cap of $50,000 for a married couple on all itemized deductions. *(Revenue raised: About $400 billion over 10 years.)*

- Taxing capital gains at the same rates as income from wages and cracking down on gaming through derivatives, like-kind exchanges, and the zero tax rate on capital gains passed on through bequests. *(Revenue raised: About $2.5 trillion over 10 years.)*

- Enacting the "For the 99.8% Act", which returns the estate tax exemption to the 2009 level of $3.5 million, closes egregious loopholes, and increases rates progressively including by adding a top tax rate of 77% on estate values in excess of $1 billion. *(Revenue raised: $336 billion over 10 years.)*

- Enacting corporate tax reform including restoring the top federal corporate income tax rate to 35 percent. *(Revenue raised: $3 trillion, of which $1 trillion would be used to help finance Medicare for All and $2 trillion would be used for the Green New Deal.)*

- Using $350 billion of the amount raised from the tax on extreme wealth to help finance Medicare for All.

http://healthoverprofit.org/2020/03/16/20-top-economists-endorse-medicare-for-all-as-best-plan-to-cut-costs-save-tens-of-thousands-of-lives-each-year/   (See hyperlink for full text and references.)

20 Top Economists Endorse Medicare For All As Best Plan To Cut Costs, Save Tens of Thousands of Lives Each Year

"By eliminating insurance premiums and out-of-pocket expenses, and lowering overall healthcare costs, Medicare for All will result in enormous savings for almost all households, all except the richest households who will pay more in taxes."
By Jake Johnson for Common Dreams, 16 March 2020

Rejecting "loose talk" from corporate Democrats, the media, and insurance industry that a single-payer system would be unaffordable, twenty leading U.S. economists on Tuesday released an open letter endorsing Medicare for All as the best way to reduce soaring national healthcare costs, significantly cut expenses for most U.S. households, and save countless lives.

"We believe the available research supports the conclusion that a program of Medicare for All (M4A) could be considerably less expensive than the current system, reducing waste and profiteering inherent in the current system, and could be financed in a way to ensure significant financial savings for the vast majority of American households," reads the letter, whose signatories include Columbia University professor Jeffrey Sachs, former Labor Secretary Robert Reich, and University of Massachusetts at Amherst professor Robert Pollin.

"Most important," the economists write, "Medicare for All will reduce morbidity and save tens of thousands of lives each year."

The letter was provided to *Business Insider* by Business for Medicare for All, an advocacy group led by former insurance executive Wendell Potter, who is now a vocal supporter of single-payer healthcare.

"By eliminating insurance premiums and out-of-pocket expenses, and lowering overall healthcare costs, Medicare for All will result in enormous savings for almost all households, all except the richest households who will pay more in taxes," the letter states.

Dr. Gerald Friedman, economics professor at the University of Massachusetts at Amherst and one of the letter's signatories, told *Business Insider* that "what's really unaffordable" is not Medicare for All, but the current for-profit system in which price-gouging is rampant and the costs of private insurance plans are skyrocketing. "We spend about twice the average for affluent countries in the OECD on healthcare," Friedman said.

Read the open letter in full below:

We are economists interested in public policy and healthcare. Some of us have worked to estimate the cost of alternative healthcare programs. Others have reviewed such estimates. We believe the available research supports the conclusion that a program of Medicare for All (M4A) could be considerably less expensive than the current system, reducing waste and profiteering inherent in the current system, and could be financed in a way to ensure significant financial savings for the vast majority of American households. Of course, the details would depend on the design of the M4A system.

Compared with the current system, Medicare for All would achieve considerable savings on administration and by reducing payments to monopoly drug companies and hospital networks. Within a few years of operation, M4A could save hundreds of billions of dollars per year from these sources. Additional savings will come when a rational healthcare finance system allows needed investments in coordinated care and preventive care, as well as reductions in fraudulent billing.

Over time, global budgeting would slow the rate of future healthcare costs significantly, as has been done in Canada and other countries. Bending the cost curve could save more than $2 trillion over the next decade, and even more with a well-designed system. Costs will be predictable, enabling households and businesses to plan in a way that is impossible today.

There are added costs associated with Medicare for All. Universal coverage and increased utilization, coming from reduction or elimination of cost sharing, will add costs, but studies show that these added costs will be far less than the savings outlined above.

The need for increased public funds (replacing premiums) can be financed with some combination of payroll, income, and wealth taxes. By eliminating insurance premiums and out-of-pocket expenses, and lowering overall healthcare costs, Medicare for All will result in enormous savings for almost all households, all except the richest households who will pay more in taxes. Shifting the burden from per-person payments for premiums and cost sharing to income- and wealth-related taxation will magnify the savings for most households. The current system is particularly burdensome for middle-income working households who receive relatively little support through Medicaid or other public programs but are responsible for health insurance premiums either paid directly or by their employer as nonwage compensation. A system that cuts costs and shifts financing to income and wealth taxes will dramatically lower this burden, producing significant savings for workers and businesses.

The net financial savings will be accompanied by substantial improvements in productivity through improved health, and the elimination of "job lock" coming from the need to stay on a job to retain health coverage. Most important, Medicare for All will reduce morbidity and save tens of thousands of lives each year.

1. *James G. Kahn, Professor, Institute for Health Policy Studies, School of Medicine, University of California, San Francisco*

2. *Jeffrey Sachs, University Professor and Director, Center for Sustainable Development, Columbia University*

3. *Anders Fremstad, Assistant Professor, Economics, Colorado State University*

4. *Robert Reich, Carmel P. Friesen Professor of Public Policy, Goldman School of Public Policy, University of California, Berkeley*

5. *Robert Pollin, Distinguished University Professor of Economics and Co-Director of Political Economy Research Institute, University of Massachusetts Amherst*

6. *Leonard Rodberg, Professor Emeritus of Urban Studies, Queens College/CUNY*

7. *Emmanuel Saez, Professor of Economics, Director, Center for Equitable Growth, University of California at Berkeley*

8. *Gabriel Zucman, Associate Professor of Economics, University of California at Berkeley*

9. *Alison Galvani, Burnett and Stender Families' Professor of Epidemiology, Director of the Center for Infectious Disease Modeling and Analysis, Yale School of Public Health*

10. *Gerald Friedman, Professor of Economics, University of Massachusetts at Amherst*

11. *Katherine Moos, Assistant Professor of Economics, University of Massachusetts at Amherst*

12. *Lindy Hern, Associate Professor of Sociology, University of Hawaii at Hilo*

13. *Lawrence King, Professor of Economics, University of Massachusetts at Amherst*

14. *Michael Ash, Professor of Economics, University of Massachusetts at Amherst*

15. *Markus P. A. Schneider, Associate Professor of Economics, University of Denver*

16. *Jeff Helton, Associate Professor Health Care Management College of Professional Studies, Metropolitan State University of Denver*

17. *Mark Paul, Assistant Professor of Economics, New College of Florida*

18. *Elissa Braunstein, Professor & Chair, Department of Economics, Colorado State University*

19. *Dean Baker, Senior Economist, Center for Economic and Policy Research and Visiting Professor of Economics, University of Utah*

20. *Darrick Hamilton, Professor of Economics and Sociology and Executive Director of the Kirwan Institute for the Study of Race and Ethnicity at The Ohio State University*

https://www.msnbc.com/ali-velshi/watch/medicare-for-all-what-it-could-mean-for-u-s-health-care-system-1444442179884

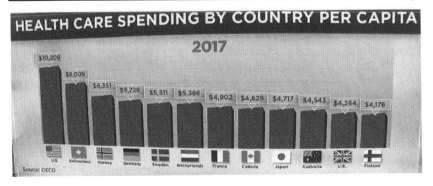

https://www.commondreams.org/newswire/2021/03/17/jayapal-introduces-medicare-all-act-2021-alongside-more-half-house-democratic
(See hyperlink for full text and references.)

Jayapal Introduces Medicare for All Act of 2021 Alongside More Than Half of House Democratic Caucus After Millions Lose Health Care During a Pandemic

Legislation guarantees health care to everyone as a human right by providing comprehensive benefits including primary care, vision, dental, prescription drugs, mental health, long-term services and supports, reproductive health care, and more with no copays, private insurance premiums, deductibles, or other cost-sharing.

WASHINGTON (March 17, 2021) - Today, U.S. Representatives Pramila Jayapal (WA-07) and Debbie Dingell (MI-12) introduced the Medicare for All Act of 2021, transformative legislation that would guarantee health care to everyone in America as a human right at a moment in which nearly 100 million people are uninsured or underinsured during a pandemic. Endorsed by 300 local, state, and national organizations and co-sponsored by more than half of the House Democratic Caucus including 14 committee chairs and key leadership Members, the landmark bill provides comprehensive benefits to all with no copays, private insurance premiums, deductibles, or other cost-sharing.

The Medicare for All Act of 2021 is being introduced in the House of Representatives one year to the day that the COVID-19 virus was first confirmed in all 50 states and the District of Columbia. This devastating public health crisis, which has taken the lives of more than 540,000 Americans, has only underscored how the country's current health care system leaves millions behind. As unemployment skyrocketed to historic levels during the pandemic, millions of additional families lost their health care and the country experienced the highest increase in the number of uninsured Americans ever recorded.

"While this devastating pandemic is shining a bright light on our broken, for-profit health care system, we were already leaving nearly half of all adults under the age of 65 uninsured or underinsured before COVID-19 hit. And we were cruelly doing so while paying more per capita for health care than any other country in the world," said Congresswoman Jayapal. "There is a solution to this health crisis — a popular one that guarantees health care to every person as a human right and finally puts people over profits and care over corporations. That solution is Medicare for All — everyone in, nobody out — and I am proud to introduce it today alongside a powerful movement across America."

"A system that prioritizes profits over patients and ties coverage to employment was no match for a global pandemic and will never meet the needs of our people," said Congresswoman Dingell. "In the wealthiest nation on earth, patients should not be launching GoFundMe pages to afford lifesaving health care for themselves or their loved ones. Medicare For All will build an inclusive health care system that won't just open the door to care for millions of our neighbors, but do it more efficiently and effectively than the one we have today. Now is not the time to shy away from these generational fights, it is the time for action."

The Medicare for All Act builds upon and expands Medicare to provide comprehensive benefits to every person in the United States. This includes primary care, vision, dental, prescription drugs, mental health, substance abuse, long-term services and supports, reproductive health care, and more. The Medicare for All Act of 2021 also includes universal coverage of long-term care with no cost-sharing for older Americans and individuals with disabilities, and prioritizes home and community-based care over institutional care. Additionally, patients have the freedom to choose the doctors, hospitals, and other providers they wish to see without worrying about whether a provider is in-network. Importantly, the legislation streamlines the health care system to negotiate drug prices and reduce exorbitant administrative waste.

This growing movement for universal, single-payer health care has robust support inside and outside of Congress. The Medicare for All Act of 2021 has several new co-sponsors including the Chair of the House Committee on Energy and Commerce, Representative Frank Pallone, Jr. (D-NJ-06) who just committed to a hearing on Medicare for All. Last Congress, the legislation had four historic hearings—the first-ever on Medicare for All—in the House Committee on Rules, the House Committee on Ways and Means, the House Committee on the Budget, and the House Committee on Energy and Commerce. Medicare for All is supported by 69 percent of registered voters including 87 percent of

Democrats, the majority of Independents, and nearly half of Republicans. Additionally, over 50 cities and towns across America have passed resolutions endorsing Medicare for All.

The Medicare for All Act of 2021 is also endorsed by 300 local, state, and national organizations that represent nurses, doctors, business owners, unions, and racial justice organizations. This includes Physicians for a National Health Program, Public Citizen, National Nurses United, Center for Popular Democracy, People's Action, Social Security Works, Labor Campaign for Single Payer, SEIU, and hundreds more.

(For a full list of endorsing organizations, see last chapter.)

"The pandemic has underscored the cruelty and irrationality of our current health care system—and the urgency of replacing it with Medicare for All. Amid the worst acute public health crisis in generations, millions lost their health insurance and health insurer profits soared," said Robert Weissman, president of Public Citizen. "Medicare for All will ensure everyone has health care coverage, including when they need it most, and will eliminate the waste and profiteering that drives ever-escalating costs. Public Citizen thanks Reps. Pramila Jayapal and Debbie Dingell, as well as the other original co-sponsors of the Medicare for All Act, for their leadership and determination in delivering health justice."

"The pandemic has highlighted in deadly detail what nurses have known for decades: Our current health care system, based on private insurance tied to employment, is a colossal failure and leaves far too many of our patients to suffer and die unnecessarily," said Bonnie Castillo, RN and executive director of National Nurses United. "We thank Rep. Pramila Jayapal and Rep. Debbie Dingell for their leadership in guaranteeing health care is a human right. While we mourn the more than 500,000 lives lost to Covid, we rededicate ourselves to the fight to ensure that everyone is provided with high-quality health care regardless of where they live, how much money they make, or their health, immigration, or employment status. Nurses will never rest until we get this done."

"Physicians have been saying it for years: We cannot give patients the care they need in a fractured and profit-driven system. For too long, doctors have watched helplessly as our patients delayed or skipped needed care—even walking out our hospital doors—because they could not afford to pay. While some are uninsured, many of these are patients enrolled in commercial insurance plans, but can't afford the thousands of dollars they must pay upfront in deductibles and copays," said Dr. Susan Rogers, President of Physicians for a National Health Program. "Medicare for All is the only plan that puts patients first: It guarantees health care for life, with free choice of hospital and provider, and no financial firewalls to stand in the way of care. It's no surprise that a majority of physicians and other health providers now support single-payer Medicare for All."

"More than any other policy, Medicare for All, would help families impacted by COVID to recover and would move to address the extreme racial disparities in health care," said Jennifer Flynn Walker, Senior Director of Advocacy and Mobilization at the Center for Popular Democracy Action. "Imagine going to the doctor without the fear of an enormous bill. Imagine losing your job, but still being able to access health care for your family. Medicare for All is a necessary policy for us to address the new normal. It is not radical. It is compassionate and sensible policy making."

"This pandemic has made it plain that our collective health and our economy depend on all of us staying healthy and safe," said People's Action Deputy Director Bree Carlson. "Our government can make this a reality by passing Medicare for All, ensuring that every one of us has access to free, high quality health care. We can and we must build a health care system strong enough to protect us all from the next health crisis."

"The costs of our current health care system remain unsustainable for too many working families, for seniors, and for employers. IFPTE applauds Rep. Jayapal, Rep. Dingell, and the cosponsors of the Medicare for All Act of 2021 for proposing a solution that will benefit all Americans by ensuring that all Americans are guaranteed high quality comprehensive health care as a right," said Paul Shearon, President of the International Federation of Professional and Technical Engineers (IFPTE). "Medicare for All would end the drag that rising health care costs have on our union members' wages and benefits, while advancing health justice and equity for all workers."

"We need to reform our national health care system now more than ever after everything we've been through this past year in battling a worldwide pandemic," said Eric Dickson, MD, President and CEO of UMass Memorial Health Care. "I believe a Medicare-for-All type of system could greatly improve health care equity in this country while ultimately reducing costs and physician burnout."

The Medicare for All Act of 2021 is co-sponsored by 14 committee chairs and several key leadership members. Co-sponsors include Alma S. Adams Ph.D., Nanette Diaz Barragán, Karen Bass, Don Beyer, Earl Blumenauer, Suzanne Bonamici, Jamaal Bowman, Brendan F. Boyle, Cori Bush, Salud Carbajal, Tony Cárdenas, André Carson, Matt Cartwright, Judy Chu, David Cicilline, Katherine Clark, Yvette D. Clarke, Emanuel Cleaver, II, Steve Cohen, Bonnie Watson Coleman, Danny K. Davis, Peter DeFazio, Diana DeGette, Mark DeSaulnier, Lloyd Doggett, Mike Doyle, Ted Deutch, Veronica Escobar, Adriano Espaillat, Teresa Leger Fernandez, Lois Frankel, Ruben Gallego, Jesús G. "Chuy" García, Jimmy Gomez, Al Green, Raúl M. Grijalva, Josh Harder, Alcee L. Hastings, Jahana Hayes, Brian Higgins, Jared Huffman, Sara Jacobs, Hakeem Jeffries, Hank Johnson, Mondaire Jones, Kaiali'i Kahele, William R. Keating, Robin L. Kelly, Ro Khanna, Daniel T. Kildee, Ann Kirkpatrick, James R. Langevin, Brenda L. Lawrence, Barbara Lee, Sheila Jackson Lee, Andy Levin, Mike Levin, Ted W. Lieu, Alan Lowenthal, Carolyn B. Maloney, James P. McGovern, Jerry McNerney, Gregory W. Meeks, Grace Meng, Jerrold Nadler, Grace F. Napolitano, Joe Neguse, Marie Newman, Eleanor Holmes Norton, Alexandria Ocasio-Cortez, Ilhan Omar, Frank Pallone Jr., Jimmy Panetta, Ed Perlmutter, Chellie Pingree, Mark Pocan, Katie Porter, Ayanna Pressley, Jamie Raskin, Lucille Roybal-Allard, Bobby L. Rush, Gregorio Kilili Camacho Sablan, Linda Sanchez, John Sarbanes, Jan Schakowsky, Adam Schiff, Robert C. "Bobby" Scott, Brad Sherman, Adam Smith, Jackie Speier, Eric Swalwell, Mark Takano, Bennie G. Thompson, Mike Thompson, Dina Titus, Rashida Tlaib, Paul Tonko, Ritchie Torres, Lori Trahan, Juan Vargas, Marc Veasey, Nydia M. Velázquez, Maxine Waters, Peter Welch, Susan Wild, Nikema Williams, Frederica Wilson, and John Yarmuth.

MEDICARE FOR ALL ACT OF 2021

The Medicare for All Act of 2021 is transformative legislation that guarantees health care to everyone in America as a human right. It does so by providing comprehensive benefits including primary care, vision, dental, prescription drugs, mental health, long-term services and supports, reproductive care, and more with no copays, private insurance premiums, deductibles, or other cost-sharing. The bill is endorsed by 300 local, state, and national organizations that represent nurses, doctors, business owners, unions, and racial justice organizations.

First 114 Co-Sponsors (% of Reps)

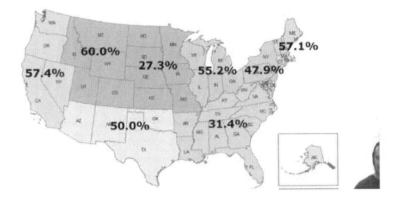

See last chapter for the full list of National, State & Local endorsing organizations.

NOTE to READER: Use hyperlinks to compare
(1) Table of Contents & (2) Full Text of H.R.1976 to S.1129

https://www.congress.gov/bill/117th-congress/house-bill/1976/text

Introduced in House (03/17/2021)

117TH CONGRESS
1ST SESSION

H. R. 1976

To establish an improved Medicare for All national health insurance program.

IN THE HOUSE OF REPRESENTATIVES

MARCH 17, 2021

Ms. JAYAPAL (for herself, Ms. ADAMS, Ms. BARRAGÁN, Ms. BASS, Mr. BEYER, Mr. BLUMENAUER, Ms. BONAMICI, Mr. BOWMAN, Mr. BRENDAN F. BOYLE of Pennsylvania, Mr. BROWN, Ms. BUSH, Mr. CARBAJAL, Mr. CÁRDENAS, Mr. CARSON, Mr. CARTWRIGHT, Ms. CHU, Mr. CICILLINE, Ms. CLARK of Massachusetts, Ms. CLARKE of New York, Mr. CLEAVER, Mr. COHEN, Mr. DEUTCH, Mr. DANNY K. DAVIS of Illinois, Mr. DEFAZIO, Ms. DEGETTE, Mr. DESAULNIER, Mrs. DINGELL, Mr. DOGGETT, Mr. MICHAEL F. DOYLE of Pennsylvania, Ms. ESCOBAR, Mr. ESPAILLAT, Ms. LOIS FRANKEL of Florida, Mr. GALLEGO, Mr. GARCÍA of Illinois, Mr. GOMEZ, Mr. GREEN of Texas, Mr. GRIJALVA, Mr. HARDER of California, Mr. HASTINGS, Mrs. HAYES, Mr. HIGGINS of New York, Mr. HUFFMAN, Ms. JACKSON LEE, Ms. JACOBS of California, Mr. JEFFRIES, Mr. JOHNSON of Georgia, Mr. JONES, Mr. KAHELE, Mr. KEATING, Ms. KELLY of Illinois, Mr. KHANNA, Mr. KILDEE, Mrs. KIRKPATRICK, Mr. LANGEVIN, Mrs. LAWRENCE, Ms. LEE of California, Ms. LEGER FERNANDEZ, Mr. LEVIN of Michigan, Mr. LEVIN of California, Mr. LIEU, Mr. LOWENTHAL, Mrs. CAROLYN B. MALONEY of New York, Mr. MCGOVERN, Mr. MCNERNEY, Mr. MEEKS, Ms. MENG, Mr. NADLER, Mrs. NAPOLITANO, Mr. NEGUSE, Ms. NEWMAN,

Ms. NORTON, Ms. OCASIO-CORTEZ, Ms. OMAR, Mr. PANETTA, Mr. PAYNE, Mr. PERLMUTTER, Ms. PINGREE, Mr. POCAN, Ms. PORTER, Ms. PRESSLEY, Mr. RASKIN, Ms. ROYBAL-ALLARD, Mr. RUSH, Mr. SABLAN, Ms. SÁNCHEZ, Mr. SARBANES, Ms. SCHAKOWSKY, Mr. SCHIFF, Mr. SCOTT of Virginia, Mr. SHERMAN, Mr. SMITH of Washington, Ms. SPEIER, Mr. SWALWELL, Mr. TAKANO, Mr. THOMPSON of Mississippi, Mr. THOMPSON of California, Ms. TITUS, Ms. TLAIB, Mr. TONKO, Mr. TORRES of New York, Mrs. TRAHAN, Mr. VARGAS, Mr. VEASEY, Ms. VELÁZQUEZ, Ms. WATERS, Mrs. WATSON COLEMAN, Mr. WELCH, Ms. WILD, Ms. WILLIAMS of Georgia, Ms. WILSON of Florida, Mr. YARMUTH, Mr. PALLONE, and Mr. PRICE of North Carolina)

introduced the following bill; which was referred to the Committee on Energy and Commerce, and in addition to the Committees on Ways and Means, Education and Labor, Rules, Oversight and Reform, and Armed Services, and the Judiciary, for a period to be subsequently determined by the Speaker, in each case for consideration of such provisions as fall within the jurisdiction of the committee concerned

A BILL

To establish an improved Medicare for All national health insurance program.

Be it enacted by the Senate and House of Representatives of the United States of America in Congress assembled,

SECTION 1. SHORT TITLE; TABLE OF CONTENTS.

(a) SHORT TITLE.—This Act may be cited as the "Medicare for All Act of 2021".

(b) TABLE OF CONTENTS.—The table of contents of this Act is as follows:

(END TABLE OF CONTENTS OF H.R. 1976)
(USE HYPERLINK TO CONTINUE READING FULL TEXT)

https://www.congress.gov/bill/117th-congress/house-bill/1976
(Summary tab)

Introduced in House (03/17/2021)
117ᵀᴴ CONGRESS
1ST SESSION

H. R. 1976

To establish an improved Medicare for All national health insurance program.

Medicare for All Act of 2021 (= Universal Healthcare!)

This bill establishes a national health insurance program that is administered by the Department of Health and Human Services (HHS).

Among other requirements, the program must (1) cover all U.S. residents; (2) provide for automatic enrollment of individuals upon birth or residency in the United States; and (3) cover items and services that are medically necessary or appropriate to maintain health or to diagnose, treat, or rehabilitate a health condition, including hospital services, prescription drugs, mental health and substance abuse treatment, dental and vision services, and long-term care.

The bill prohibits cost-sharing (e.g., deductibles, coinsurance, and copayments) and other charges for covered services. Additionally, private health insurers and employers may only offer coverage that is supplemental to, and not duplicative of, benefits provided under the program.

Health insurance exchanges and specified federal health programs terminate upon program implementation. However, the program does not affect coverage provided through the Department of Veterans Affairs or the Indian Health Service.

The bill also establishes a series of implementing provisions relating to (1) health care provider participation; (2) HHS administration; and (3) payments and costs, including the requirement that HHS negotiate prices for prescription drugs.

Individuals who are age 18 or younger, age 55 or older, or already enrolled in Medicare may enroll in the program starting one year after enactment of this bill; other individuals may buy into the program at this time. The program must be fully implemented two years after enactment.

IN THE HOUSE OF REPRESENTATIVES

MARCH 17, 2021

SPONSORS AND CO-SPONSORS AS OF MARCH 17, 2021

(IS YOUR REPRESENTATIVE INCLUDED BELOW?)

Ms. JAYAPAL (for herself, Ms. ADAMS, Ms. BARRAGÁN, Ms. BASS, Mr. BEYER, Mr. BLUMENAUER, Ms. BONAMICI, Mr. BOWMAN, Mr. BRENDAN F. BOYLE of Pennsylvania, Mr. BROWN, Ms. BUSH, Mr. CARBAJAL, Mr. CÁRDENAS, Mr. CARSON, Mr. CARTWRIGHT, Ms. CHU, Mr. CICILLINE, Ms. CLARK of Massachusetts, Ms. CLARKE of New York, Mr. CLEAVER, Mr. COHEN, Mr. DEUTCH, Mr. DANNY K. DAVIS of Illinois, Mr. DEFAZIO, Ms. DEGETTE, Mr. DESAULNIER, Mrs. DINGELL, Mr. DOGGETT, Mr. MICHAEL F. DOYLE of Pennsylvania, Ms. ESCOBAR, Mr. ESPAILLAT, Ms. LOIS FRANKEL of Florida, Mr. GALLEGO, Mr. GARCÍA of Illinois, Mr. GOMEZ, Mr. GREEN of Texas, Mr. GRIJALVA, Mr. HARDER of California, Mr. HASTINGS, Mrs. HAYES, Mr. HIGGINS of New York, Mr. HUFFMAN, Ms. JACKSON LEE, Ms. JACOBS of California, Mr. JEFFRIES, Mr. JOHNSON of Georgia, Mr. JONES, Mr. KAHELE, Mr. KEATING, Ms. KELLY of Illinois, Mr. KHANNA, Mr. KILDEE, Mrs. KIRKPATRICK, Mr. LANGEVIN, Mrs. LAWRENCE, Ms. LEE of California, Ms. LEGER FERNANDEZ, Mr. LEVIN of Michigan, Mr. LEVIN of California, Mr. LIEU, Mr. LOWENTHAL, Mrs. CAROLYN B. MALONEY of New York, Mr. MCGOVERN, Mr. MCNERNEY, Mr. MEEKS, Ms. MENG, Mr. NADLER, Mrs. NAPOLITANO, Mr. NEGUSE, Ms. NEWMAN, Ms. NORTON, Ms. OCASIO-CORTEZ, Ms. OMAR, Mr. PANETTA, Mr. PAYNE, Mr. PERLMUTTER, Ms. PINGREE, Mr. POCAN, Ms. PORTER, Ms. PRESSLEY, Mr. RASKIN, Ms. ROYBAL-ALLARD, Mr. RUSH, Mr. SABLAN, Ms. SÁNCHEZ, Mr. SARBANES, Ms. SCHAKOWSKY, Mr. SCHIFF, Mr. SCOTT of Virginia, Mr. SHERMAN, Mr. SMITH of Washington, Ms. SPEIER, Mr. SWALWELL, Mr. TAKANO, Mr. THOMPSON of Mississippi, Mr. THOMPSON of California, Ms. TITUS, Ms. TLAIB, Mr. TONKO, Mr. TORRES of New York, Mrs. TRAHAN, Mr. VARGAS, Mr. VEASEY, Ms. VELÁZQUEZ, Ms. WATERS,

Mrs. WATSON COLEMAN, Mr. WELCH, Ms. WILD, Ms. WILLIAMS of Georgia, Ms. WILSON of Florida, Mr. YARMUTH, Mr. PALLONE, and Mr. PRICE of North Carolina)

introduced the following bill; which was referred to the Committee on Energy and Commerce, and in addition to the Committees on Ways and Means, Education and Labor, Rules, Oversight and Reform, Armed Services and the Judiciary, for a period to be subsequently determined by the Speaker, in each case for consideration of such provisions as fall within the jurisdiction of the committee concerned

---

https://jayapal.house.gov/wp-content/uploads/2019/02/Medicare-for-All-Act-of-2019-Section-by-Section-Summary.pdf
(See hyperlink for full text and references.)

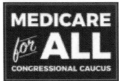

Medicare for All Act of 2019 Section-by-Section
(Last updated 2/25/19)
H.R. 1976 ("Medicare for All") BILL EXPLAINED

TITLE I—ESTABLISHMENT OF THE MEDICARE FOR ALL PROGRAM; UNIVERSAL ENTITLEMENT; ENROLLMENT

Universal coverage.

➤ Establishes the Medicare for All Program entitling all United States residents to benefits for health care services.

➤ Authorizes the HHS Secretary to determine criteria of residency.

Freedom of choice.

➤ Allows any individual entitled to benefits to obtain services from any provider qualified to participate under the Act.

Non-discrimination.

➤ Prohibits discrimination by providers or entities administering the Program on the basis of race, color, national origin, age, disability, marital status, citizenship status, primary language use, genetic conditions, previous or existing medical conditions, religion, or sex, including sex stereotyping, gender identity, sexual orientation, and pregnancy or related medical conditions (including termination of pregnancy).

➤ Requires the HHS Secretary to establish a process for adjudicating claims of discrimination.

➤ Establishes a private right of action to enforce the prohibition on discrimination.

Enrollment.

➤ Requires the Secretary to provide a mechanism for automatic enrollment at birth, time of immigration into the US, or acquisition of qualified resident status and to issue Medicare for All Program cards.

Effective date of benefits.

➤ Establishes a two-year transition period for the Medicare for All Program and makes benefits available to all eligible individuals two years after the date of enactment.

➤ Provides that individuals under 19 and 55 or older are eligible for benefits one year after the date of enactment.

Prohibition against duplicating coverage.

➤ Prohibits the sale of health insurance coverage that duplicates the benefits available under the Program.

➤ Prohibits employers from providing benefits that duplicate the benefits under the Medicare for All Program.

➤ Allows the sale of insurance and employer-sponsored benefits that provide supplemental coverage.

TITLE II—COMPREHENSIVE BENEFITS, INCLUDING PREVENTIVE BENEFITS AND BENEFITS FOR LONG-TERM CARE

Comprehensive benefits.

➢ Authorizes payment to providers for Program benefits where such items or services are medically necessary or appropriate for the individual as determined by their treating physician or other licensed health care provider with the appropriate scope of practice.

➢ Lists covered benefits including:

♣ Hospital services, including inpatient and outpatient hospital care, 24-hour-a-day emergency services and inpatient prescription drugs.

♣ Ambulatory patient services.

♣ Primary and preventive services, including chronic disease management.

♣ Prescription drugs, medical devices and biological products, including outpatient prescription drugs, medical devices, and biological products.

♣ Mental health and substance abuse treatment services, including inpatient care.

♣ Laboratory and diagnostic services.

♣ Comprehensive reproductive, maternity, and newborn care.

♣ Pediatrics.

♣ Dental, audiology, and vision services.

♣ Rehabilitative and habilitative services and devices.

♣ Dietary and nutritional therapies approved by the Secretary.

♣ Emergency services and transportation.

♣ Early and periodic screening, diagnostic, and treatment services.

♣ Transportation to receive health care services for persons with disabilities or low income individuals.

♣ Long-term care services and supports.

➢ Authorizes the Secretary to evaluate benefits and give recommendations to Congress for improvements and adjustments to the benefits package.

➤ Requires the Secretary to consult with experts to identify complementary and integrative medicine practices that are appropriate to include in the benefits package.

➤ Permits States to provide additional benefits and to provide benefits to individuals who may not be eligible for the Medicare for All Program.

No cost-sharing.

➤ Prohibits cost-sharing and balance billing for benefits provided through the Medicare for All Program.

Exclusions and limitations.

➤ Provides that Program benefits are not available to the individual unless they are medically necessary or appropriate.

➤ Authorizes the Secretary to include coverage of experimental items and services and requires the Secretary to establish an appeals process.

➤ Allows health care professionals, who by their scope of practice and licensure can exercise independent professional judgment, to override national practice guidelines if consistent with the professional's assessment of the individual, in the individual's best interest, and consistent with the individual's wishes.

Coverage of long-term care services.

➤ Entitles Program enrollees to long-term services and supports where illness, injury, or age limit their ability to perform one or more activities of daily living or similar need of assistance to perform instrumental activities of daily living.

➤ Long-term services and supports include: nursing and medical services, long-term rehabilitative and habilitative services, and services to support activities of daily living and instrumental activities of daily living whether provided in an institution, home, or community-based setting.

➤ Requires that such services be provided in the most integrative and least restrictive setting and that they maximize the recipient's autonomy as well as their civic, social, and economic participation.

➤ Requires that the Program presume that recipients of all ages and disabilities will receive long-term services and supports through home and community-based services unless the individual chooses otherwise.

➤ Requires that the Secretary develop regulations in consultation with an advisory commission that includes those who use long-term supports and services, their representatives and family caregivers; providers of such supports and services; and disability rights, academic, and labor organizations

TITLE III—PROVIDER PARTICIPATION

Provider participation and standards; whistleblower protections.

➤ Describes provisions required in the participation agreement between providers and the Program.

➤ Requires disclose to the Secretary any system or index of coding or classifying patient symptoms, diagnoses, clinical interventions, episodes, or procedures that such provider utilizes for global budget negotiations.

➤ Establishes a duty of provider ethics for participating physicians and other health care providers and prohibits hospitals and other institutional providers from limiting the ability of such professionals to advocate for medically necessary and appropriate care.

➤ Prohibits bonuses, incentive payments, or compensation based on utilization of services or the financial results of any health care provider and requires providers to disclose financial interests or relationships with other providers to the Secretary.

➤ Establishes the process for terminating a participation agreement.

➤ Establishes protections for participating providers and whistleblower protections for individuals that report potential violations of the Act.

➤ Prohibits providers or their board members from serving on the board of or receiving compensation, stock, or other financial investments in any other entity that furnishes items and services (including pharmaceuticals and medical devices) to the provider.

Qualifications for providers.

> Establishes that providers are qualified to participate in the Program if they have the requisite license from the state in which they practice and meet minimum provider standards including adequate facilities, safe staffing, and patient access.

Use of private contracts.

> Prohibits participating providers from entering into private contracts for covered services with individuals eligible for Program benefits and establishes penalties for violating this prohibition.

> Permits participating providers to enter into private contracts with individuals ineligible for benefits under the Program and with eligible individuals for non-covered services, and establishes conditions for these contracts.

> Establishes conditions under which nonparticipating providers may enter into a private contract with individuals eligible for benefits under the Program.

> Entering into a private contract with an eligible individual for covered services bars the provider from participating in the Program for one calendar year.

TITLE IV—ADMINISTRATION

Administration.

> Outlines the duties of the Secretary to include developing policies, procedures, and guidelines to ensure the timely and accessible provision of benefits under the Act.

> Lists the types of information that providers must report including and data the provider is required to report to any State or local agency and annual financial data.

> Requires the Secretary to report on the Program to Congress and regular audits by the Comptroller General.

Consultation.

> Requires the Secretary to consult with other federal agencies, Indian tribes, labor organizations representing health care workers, health care experts, etc. in the administration of the Act.

Regional administration.

➢ Requires the Secretary to establish regional offices and appoint regional directors, incorporating the existing offices of the Centers for Medicare & Medicaid Services (CMS) where possible. Also requires appointment of deputy directors to represent American Indian and Alaska Native tribes in each region.

➢ Details the duties of regional directors including performing health care needs assessments, recommending changes in provider reimbursement or payment, and establishing quality assurance mechanisms in their respective regions.

Beneficiary ombudsman.

➢ Establishes a beneficiary ombudsman to receive complaints and grievances and to provide assistance to individuals entitled to benefits under the Act.

Conduct of related health programs.

➢ Requires the Secretary to direct activities of other health-related programs to complement this Act and contribute to the health of the people.

Subtitle B — Control Over Fraud and Abuse

Application of federal sanctions to all fraud and abuse under the Medicare for All Program.

➢ Incorporates the fraud and abuse sanctions as well as limitations on referrals that already exist under Medicare or Medicaid.

TITLE V—QUALITY ASSESSMENT

Quality standards.

➢ Requires that all Program standards and quality measures be implemented and evaluated by the CMS Center for Clinical Standards and Quality in coordination with the Agency for Healthcare Research and Quality and other HHS offices.

➢ Establishes the Center's duties to include reviewing and evaluating practice guidelines, quality standards, and performance measures; creating methodology to monitor and evaluate patterns of practice for appropriate utilization; developing competency criteria to qualify independent organizations to conduct quality reviews at the regional level; and reporting findings to the Secretary.

Addressing health care disparities.

➢ Requires CMS's Center for Clinical Standards and Quality to evaluate data collection methods to ensure accurate reporting of health care disparities on the basis of race, ethnicity, gender, geography, and socioeconomic status and report the results to Congress and the Secretary.

➢ Requires the Secretary to implement effective approaches for data collection.

TITLE VI—HEALTH BUDGET; PAYMENTS; COST CONTAINMENT MEASURES

Subtitle A — Budgeting

National health budget.

➢ Requires the Secretary to establish a national health budget covering the following: operating expenditures, capital expenditures, special projects for rural or medically underserved areas, quality assessments, health professional education, administrative costs, and prevention and public health activities.

➢ Requires the Secretary to allocate funds to each regional office to carry out the Program in such region.

➢ Allocates at least 1 percent of the budget for the first five years to worker assistance programs for those displaced or affected by the implementation of the Act. Assistance programs shall include wage replacement, retirement benefits, job training, and education benefits.

➢ Requires the Secretary to establish a reserve fund to cover the costs of treating epidemics, natural disasters, and other health emergencies, and for market-shift adjustments necessary due to patient volume.

Subtitle B — Payments to Providers

Payments to institutional providers based on global budgets.

➢ Establishes that institutional providers—including hospitals, skilled nursing facilities, federally qualified health centers, home health agencies, and independent dialysis facilities—be paid a lump sum global operating budget on a quarterly basis to provide covered items and services.

➤ Requires regional directors to review institutional providers' performance on a quarterly basis and determine whether adjustments to the budget are needed.

➤ Requires regional directors to negotiate the global budget with institutional providers each fiscal year and establishes factors addressed in the negotiations including:

♣ The historical volume of services in the previous 3-year period and provider capacity.

♣ Actual expenditures based on the most recent Medicare cost report of the provider and compared to other providers within the region and to the normative payment rates established under a national comparative rate system.

♣ Projected changes in volume and type of items and services to be furnished.

♣ Employee wages, including staffing increases necessary for safe registered nurse-to-patient staffing ratios and optimal staffing of physicians and other health care professionals.

♣ Education and prevention programs.

♣ And other relevant factors and adjustments.

➤ Requires regional directors to review institutional providers' performance on a quarterly basis and determine whether adjustments to the budget are needed, including for additional funding needed for unanticipated care for individuals with complex medical needs or market-shift adjustments.

➤ Establishes that the operating expenses in the global budget must not include capital expenditures, and that funding from an institution's global budget cannot be used for capital expenditures.

➤ Requires that a system be established to enable cost comparisons among institutional providers.

Payment to individual providers through fee-for-service.

> Requires that individual providers, including individuals in medical group practices, be paid on a fee-for-service basis.

> Requires the Secretary to establish a national fee schedule that takes into account the prevailing rates under Medicare, provider expertise, and the value of the items and services furnished.

> Establishes a physician consultation review board to review quality, cost effectiveness, and fair reimbursement of services and items delivered by physicians.

> Requires a periodic audit by the Comptroller General.

Ensuring accurate valuation of services under the Medicare physician fee schedule.

> Amends the Social Security Act to include a standardized documentation and review process of the relative values of physician services to determine appropriate fee payments.

Payment prohibitions; capital expenditures; special projects.

> Prohibits providers from using payments from the Medicare for All Program for marketing expenses, increasing profit or revenue, incentive payments or bonuses based on patient utilization, compensation for labor relations consultants, or for political activity.

> Requires providers seeking capital expenditure funds to present an application to fund such capital project for review by regional directors and prohibits comingling of operations funding with capital expenditures.

> Requires regional directors seeking funding for special projects for construction, renovation, or staffing of health care facilities in rural, underserved, or shortage areas to present a budget for review to the Secretary.

Office of primary health care.

> Establishes an Office of Primary Health Care, which develops and coordinates national goals related to education of health care professionals and expanding the number of primary care practitioners.

Payments for prescription drugs and approved devices and equipment.

➢ Requires the Secretary to negotiate prices for pharmaceuticals, medical supplies, and medically necessary equipment based on factors including comparative clinical and cost effectiveness, budget impact of providing coverage, number of similarly effective drugs, and total revenues from global sales obtained by the manufacturer for such drug.

➢ Requires the Secretary, in the case of an unsuccessful negotiation at an appropriate price and price period, to authorize the use of any patent, clinical trial data, or other exclusivity with respect to such drug as the Secretary determines appropriate for purposes of manufacturing such drug for sale under the Medicare for All Program.

➢ Prohibits anticompetitive behavior by manufacturers that may interfere with issuance and implementation of a competitive license.

TITLE VII—UNIVERSAL MEDICARE TRUST FUND

Universal Medicare Trust Fund.

➢ Establishes a Universal Medicare Trust Fund in the Treasury.

➢ Requires that, during the first fiscal year benefits are available under the Medicare for All Program, amounts equal to those appropriated the preceding year to Medicare, Medicaid, and other federal health programs be deposited in the Fund. Thereafter, funds equal to the previous year (adjusted for cost savings resulting from implementation of the Medicare for All Program and for changes in the consumer price index) shall be deposited.

➢ Prohibits restrictions on the Fund related to reproductive health services.

TITLE VIII—CONFORMING AMENDMENTS TO THE EMPLOYEE RETIREMENT INCOME SECURITY ACT OF 1974

Prohibition of employee benefits duplicative of benefits under the Medicare for All Program; coordination in case of workers' compensation.

➢ Adds new sections to ERISA including a prohibition on employee benefits plans that duplicate payment for items or services that are benefits under the Medicare for All Program and a requirement that workers' compensation carriers reimburse the Medicare for All Program for costs of services furnished.

Application of continuation coverage requirements under ERISA and certain other requirements relating to group health plans.

➤ Amends ERISA's continuation of coverage requirements to apply only to plans that do not duplicate payment for items and services that are benefits under the Medicare for All Program.

Effective date of title.

➤ The effective date of Title 8 is the date on which benefits are available under the Medicare for All Program.

TITLE IX—ADDITIONAL CONFORMING AMENDMENTS

Relationship to existing Federal health programs.

➤ Maintains existing medical benefits or services under the Department of Veteran Affairs and the Indian Health Service.

➤ Requires the Secretary to provide for continuation of benefits for people who are receiving inpatient hospital services and extended care services under Medicare, Medicaid, or the Children's Health Insurance Program during the transition to the Medicare for All Program.

➤ Continues school related health programs under the Medicare for All Program.

Sunset of provisions related to the State Exchanges

➤ Sunsets the Federal and State Exchanges two years after the enactment of the Medicare for All Act of 2019.

Sunset of provisions related to pay for performance programs.

➤ Sunsets federal programs related to pay for performance payments and value-based purchasing for medical benefits or services.

TITLE X—TRANSITION

Subtitle A — Medicare for All Transition Over Two Years on and Transitional Buy-In Option

Medicare for All transition over two years.

➤ Establishes a transition period of two years for the Medicare for All Program and amends the Social Security Act to entitle individuals age 55 or older, age 18 or younger, or who are currently enrolled in Medicare to enroll and obtain benefits under the Medicare for All Program.

➤ Establishes that enrollment in the Medicare for All Program satisfies the individual mandate for health care coverage requirements under the Internal Revenue Code.

➤ Requires the Secretary to consult with beneficiary representatives, health care providers, employers, and insurance companies during the transition.

Establishment of the Medicare buy-in plan.

➤ Establishes a Medicare Transition buy-in plan during the two-year transition period that will be offered through the Federal and State Exchanges. The benefits will be the same benefits available under the Medicare for All Program.

➤ Allows those who are ineligible to enroll in Medicare for All during the two year transition, to enroll in the Medicare Transition buy-in plan.

➤ Authorizes the CMS Administrator to set premiums for the Medicare Transition buy-in plan.

➤ Requires that tax credits, premium assistance, and cost-sharing subsidies currently available under the Patient Protection and Affordable Care Act apply to Medicare Transition buy-in enrollees and makes them available to Medicare Transition buy-in enrollees who live in a Medicaid non-expansion state.

Subtitle B — Transitional Medicare Reforms

Eliminating the 24-month waiting period for Medicare coverage for individuals with disabilities.

➤ Strikes the 24-month waiting period for Medicare coverage for individuals with disabilities.

Ensuring continuity of care.

➤ Requires that the Secretary ensure continuity of care during the Medicare for All transition period for individuals enrolled in health insurance plans.

➤ Prohibits health insurers from ending coverage of enrollees during the Medicare for All transition period except for reasons expressly agreed upon under the terms of a plan.

➤ Protects people with disabilities, complex medical needs, or chronic conditions from disruptions in their care from health insurers ending coverage or imposing plan or coverage exclusions during the transition period.

TITLE XI—MISCELLANEOUS

Definitions.

Rules of Construction.

➤ Permits States and local government to expand benefits or eligibility and to set additional state provider standards if there is no reduction of benefits or access and does not limit the professional judgment of providers.

➤ Prohibits States from barring providers of reproductive services from participating in the Program for reasons other than the provider's ability to provide such services.

➤ Establishes that this shall not be construed to preempt state licensing, practice, or education laws, unless expressly preempted under the Act.

➤ Establishes that no other workplace rights under Federal or State law or collective bargaining agreement is diminished or altered by the Act

NOTE to READER: Use hyperlinks to compare
(1) Table of Contents & (2) Full Text of S.1129 to H.R.1976

https://www.congress.gov/bill/116th-congress/senate-bill/1129/text

Introduced in Senate (04/10/2019)

116TH CONGRESS
1ST SESSION

S. 1129

To establish a Medicare-for-all national health insurance program.

IN THE SENATE OF THE UNITED STATES

APRIL 10, 2019

Mr. SANDERS (for himself, Ms. BALDWIN, Mr. BLUMENTHAL, Mr. BOOKER, Mrs. GILLIBRAND, Ms. HARRIS, Mr. LEAHY, Mr. MARKEY, Mr. MERKLEY, Mr. SCHATZ, Mr. UDALL, Ms. WARREN, Mr. WHITEHOUSE, Ms. HIRONO, and Mr. HEINRICH) introduced the following bill; which was read twice and referred to the Committee on Finance

A BILL

To establish a Medicare-for-all national health insurance program.
Be it enacted by the Senate and House of Representatives
of the United States of America in Congress assembled,

SECTION 1. SHORT TITLE; TABLE OF CONTENTS.

(a) SHORT TITLE.—This Act may be cited as the "Medicare for All Act of 2019".

(b) TABLE OF CONTENTS.—The table of contents for this Act is as follows:

(END TABLE OF CONTENTS OF S.1129)

(USE HYPERLINK TO CONTINUE READING FULL TEXT)

NOTE: Senator Bernie Sanders introduced S.1129 (Medicare For All Act of 2019) in the 116th Congress (January 2019 – January 2021). It died in committee, never making it to the floor for debate. Neither Bernie nor any other senator has introduced a similar bill in the current Congress.

This is precisely why activist groups and the media need to press to turn the dual Medicare for All bills S.1129 and H.R.1976 into law – and hopefully that can be accomplished using reconciliation the next time we have majorities in both the Senate and the House of Representatives!

https://www.congress.gov/bill/116th-congress/senate-bill/1129/text
(See "SUMMARY TAB" at this hyperlink)

Summary: S.1129 — 116th Congress (2019-2020)

Note to reader: Underlined items contradict H.R.1976.

This bill establishes a national health insurance program that is administered by the Department of Health and Human Services (HHS).

Among other requirements, the program must (1) cover all U.S. residents; (2) provide for automatic enrollment of individuals upon birth or residency in the United States; and (3) cover items and services that are medically necessary or appropriate to maintain health or to diagnose, treat, or rehabilitate a health condition, including hospital services, prescription drugs, mental health and substance abuse treatment, dental and vision services, and home- and community-based long-term care.

The bill prohibits cost-sharing (e.g., deductibles, coinsurance, and copayments) and other charges for covered services, with the exception of prescription drugs. Additionally, private health insurers and employers may only offer coverage that is supplemental to, and not duplicative of, benefits provided under the program.

Health insurance exchanges and specified federal health programs terminate upon program implementation. However, the program does not affect coverage provided through the Department of Veterans Affairs or the Indian Health Service. Additionally, state Medicaid programs must cover certain institutional long-term care services.

The bill also establishes a series of implementing provisions relating to (1) health care provider participation; (2) HHS administration; and (3) payments and costs, including the requirement that HHS negotiate prices for prescription drugs and establish a formulary.

Individuals who are age 18 or younger may enroll in the program starting one year after enactment of this bill; other individuals may buy into a transitional plan or an expanded Medicare program at this time, depending on age. The bill's program must be fully implemented four years after enactment.

https://pnhp.org/news/doctors-group-welcomes-sen-sanders-medicare-for-all-bill-2/ (See hyperlink for full text and references.)

Doctors' Group Welcomes Sen. Sanders' Medicare-for-All Bill

Physician Leaders Urge Congress to Move Past Incremental Proposals towards Full Single-Payer Reform

FOR IMMEDIATE RELEASE, April 10, 2019
Contact: Clare Fauke, communications specialist,
312-782-6006, clare@pnhp.org

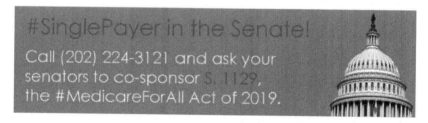

#SinglePayer in the Senate!
Call (202) 224-3121 and ask your
senators to co-sponsor S. 1129,
the #MedicareForAll Act of 2019.

WASHINGTON, D.C. — Physicians for a National Health Program (PNHP), a nonprofit research and education organization of 23,000 physicians, medical students and health professionals, welcomes the Medicare for All Act of 2019 as an important step towards the organization's goal of a single-payer national health plan. Introduced today by Sen. Bernie Sanders (I-Vt.), the bill would improve Medicare to include all medically necessary services, while expanding coverage to everyone in the U.S.

"The Affordable Care Act has taught us that merely tinkering around the edges of our broken health care system will only perpetuate its problems: skyrocketing costs, falling health outcomes, medical bankruptcy, and needless death," said Dr. Adam Gaffney, PNHP's president and a critical care physician and faculty member at Harvard Medical School. "It's time to eliminate the greed and waste of private health insurance and move to a Medicare for All system that puts patients ahead of profits."

Dr. Gaffney notes that despite the advances of the ACA, more than 28 million Americans remain uninsured, with tens of millions more under-insured. Sen. Sanders' bill would reduce the number of uninsured to zero, allowing everyone in the U.S. to visit the doctor or hospital of their choice for medically necessary care, including dental, vision, and mental health care. It would also largely eliminate patient cost-sharing, which deters many Americans from seeking needed care.

Besides expanding coverage, the Medicare for All Act would go a long way towards containing the nation's overall health care costs, which are double the per-capita spending of other industrialized nations that provide universal coverage. Without single-payer reform, U.S. annual health spending is projected to reach $5.96 trillion — 19.4 percent of GDP — by 2027.

PNHP commends the inclusion of community and home-based long-term care services in the new bill. However, PNHP also recommends several additional improvements to the Medicare for All Act that would save money and improve patient care. In particular, healthy payment strategies are needed, including global budgeting and the separation of capital and operating payments to hospitals and other institutional providers; ending "value-based" payment systems; and providing a path for the orderly conversion of investor-owned, for-profit health-care providers to not-for-profit status.

Dr. Gaffney encouraged members of Congress to move past the recent flurry of incremental proposals, such as those that claim to "strengthen" the ACA by further subsidizing the private insurance industry, or add a costly public option to our already fragmented system. "Only a true single-payer plan can provide both universal coverage and the hundreds of billions in annual savings necessary to work," added Dr. Gaffney.

"We look forward to working with Sen. Sanders to strengthen and advocate for this important bill."

OVERVIEW OF THE BILL

Based on our analysis, we find the [S. 1129] Medicare For All Act of 2019 to be a significant step forward in the fight for single payer. Taken together with Rep. Pramila Jayapal's Medicare for All Act (H.R. 1976), it would transform the U.S. health care system, making health care a human right.

Eligibility: Covers everyone residing in U.S.

Benefits: Covers medically-necessary services including primary and preventive care, mental health care, reproductive care (bans the Hyde Amendment), vision and dental care, and prescription drugs. Also provides home- and community-based long-term services and supports, which were not covered in the 2017 bill.

Patient Choice: Provides full choice of any participating doctor or hospital. Providers may not dual-practice within and outside the Medicare system.

Patient Costs: Provides first-dollar coverage without premiums, deductibles, or copays for medical services, and prohibits balance billing. Copays for some brand-name prescription drugs.

Cost Controls: Prohibits duplicate coverage. Drug prices negotiated with manufacturers.

Timeline: Provides for a four-year transition. In year one, improves Medicare by adding dental, vision, and hearing benefits and lowering out-of-pocket costs for Parts A &B; also lowers eligibility age to 55 and allows anyone to buy into the Medicare program. In year two, lowers eligibility to 45, and to 35 in year three.

HOW CAN THE BILL BE IMPROVED?

Based on decades of careful analysis and research, PNHP recommends several improvements to the Medicare for All Act that would save even more money and improve patient care:

- **Fund hospitals through global budgets, with separate funding for capital projects:** A "global budget" is a lump sum paid to hospitals and similar institutions to cover operating expenses, eliminating wasteful per-patient billing. Global budgets could *not* be used for capital projects like expansion or modernization (which would be funded separately), advertising, profit, or bonuses. Global budgeting minimizes hospitals' incentives to avoid (or seek out) particular patients or services, inflate volumes, or upcode. Funding capital projects separately, in turn, allows us to ensure that new hospitals and facilities are built where they are needed—not simply where profits are highest. They also allow us to control long term cost growth.

- **End "value-based" payment systems and other pay-for-performance schemes:** This bill continues current flawed Medicare payment methods, including alternative payment models (such as Accountable Care Organizations) established under the ACA, and the Medicare Access and CHIP Reauthorization Act of 2015 (MACRA). Studies show these payment programs fail to improve quality or reduce costs, while penalizing hospitals and doctors that care for the poorest and sickest patients. <u>PNHP recommends that Sen. Sanders end all value-based payment and pay-for-performance programs, as outlined in Section 903 of Rep. Pramila Jayapal's single-payer bill, H.R. 1976.</u>

- **Establish a national long-term care program:** This bill includes home- and community-based long-term services and supports, a laudable improvement from the 2017 bill. However, **institutional** long-term care coverage for seniors and people with disabilities will continue to be covered under state-based Medicaid plans, complete with a maintenance of effort provision. <u>PNHP recommends that Sen. Sanders include institutional long-term care in the national Medicare program, as it is in Rep. Pramila Jayapal's single-payer bill, H.R. 1976.</u>

- **Ban investor-owned health facilities:** For-profit health care facilities and agencies provide lower-quality care at higher costs than nonprofits, resulting in worse outcomes and higher costs compared to not-for-profit providers. Medicare for All should provide a path for the orderly conversion of investor-owned, for-profit health-care providers to not-for-profit status.

- **Fully cover all medications, without copayment:** Sen. Sanders' bill excludes cost-sharing for health care services. However, it does require small patient copays (up to $200 annually) on certain non-preventive prescription drugs. Research shows that copays of any kind discourage patients from seeking needed medical care, increasing sickness and long-term costs. Experience in other nations proves that they are not needed for cost control.

BUILDING MOMENTUM FOR SINGLE PAYER

See hyperlinks for a list of current Medicare For All Act co-sponsors:

S.1129 – **https://www.congress.gov/bill/116th-congress/senate-bill/1129/cosponsors**

H.R. 1976 – **https://www.congress.gov/bill/117th-congress/house-bill/1976/cosponsors**

It is important to build as much support for single payer as possible, and you can help!

1. If your senators have already co-sponsored the Medicare For All Act, call and email to thank them. Also, ask them to help improve the bill by covering institutional long-term care, establishing global budgets for hospitals, ending pay-for-performance schemes, banning investor-owned health facilities, and fully eliminating copayments.

2. If your senators have not cosponsored the Medicare For All Act, call and email to **encourage them to co-sponsor**. If you believe one or both of your senators may be skeptical, visit **pnhp.org/gop** to brush up on the conservative case for single payer.

To find your senators by state -
https://www.senate.gov/senators/senators-contact.htm.

If you have trouble locating contact information for your senators and/or your Representative, you can always call the U.S. Capitol switchboard at (202) 224-3121.

Physicians for a National Health Program (www.pnhp.org) is a nonprofit research and education organization whose 23,000 members support single-payer national health insurance.

NOTE: Senator Bernie Sanders introduced S.1129 (Medicare For All Act of 2019) in the 116th Congress (January 2019 – January 2021). It died in committee, never making it to the floor for debate. Neither Bernie nor any other senator has introduced a similar bill in the current Congress. **This is precisely why activist groups and the media need to press to turn Medicare for All from legislation into law!**

LOBBYING YOUR MEMBERS OF CONGRESS TO ENACT MEDICARE FOR ALL

John Feal and Jon Stewart – in the 2021 documentary "**No Responders Left Behind**" – give advocates of the "Medicare for All" movement a powerful and inspiring example of how to organize supporters and lobby members of Congress to turn legislative bills into law. This documentary is "must viewing" for advocacy groups who want to strategize to transform our current costly, fragmented and dysfunctional system of health insurance into Universal Health Care for every US citizen and resident.

# # #

Congressman Andy Kim (D) represents New Jersey's third district of approximately 900 square miles from just east of Philadelphia to the Jersey shore with just under 736,000 constituents.

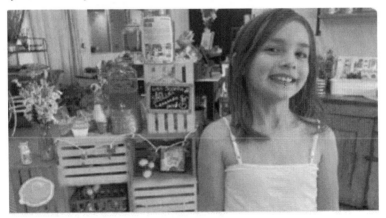

 cbs42.com   'I hope I make it': 7-year-old Alabama girl selling lemonade to fund her... Liza Scott, an Alabama 7-year-old, is selling lemonade to help pay for brain surgeries she desperately needs.

Congressman Kim <u>did not</u> sign on as a co-sponsor to H.R.1976 (Medicare for All) in March of 2021. WHY NOT?

Yet in June of 2021 – just a few months later – he proposed to add to the complexity, cost and inefficiency of our dysfunctional current health "care" system by introducing H.R.3512 "Healthcare for our Troops". H.R.3512 is to ensure TRICARE Reserve Select coverage at no cost for over 800,000 members of the Reserves and National Guard (including roughly 130,000 who don't have private health insurance).

There are 31 million uninsured Americans in this country – and rather than co-sponsor H.R.1976 "Medicare For All", Congressman Kim seems to be pandering to a small specific group of citizens by promoting a "bipartisan" bill that covers fewer than 1 million Americans.

We're not asking Congressman Kim to abandon his bill for our troops. But we ARE asking him to become (without delay) a co-sponsor of H.R.1976 "Medicare For All" – a bill that will completely cover the health needs of the 800,000 troops his bill targets while also completely covering all Americans.

A coalition of progressive organizations within New Jersey's First Congressional District (next door to Congressman Kim's Third District) have made "Medicare for All" (H.R.1976) an immediate priority and are calling on Representative Donald Norcross to sign the legislation as a co-sponsor. "Medicare For All is the only choice. People over profits" – says Pastor Amir Khan of New Beginnings, who works in conjunction with Sue Altman, Executive Director of the NJ Working Families Alliance and Mario De Santis, lead organizer with Our Revolution Gloucester County, NJ. Congressman Kim needs to hear from them – and all in NJ-03 who would benefit from "Medicare for All"!

This is a model for activists across The United States to join forces to put pressure on their members of Congress to pass "Medicare for All" (S.1129 & H.R.1976) in both the Senate and The House of Representatives.

https://www.insidernj.com/press-release/coalition-local-progressive-groups-call-rep-norcross-support-medicare/
(See hyperlink for full text and references.)

Coalition of Local Progressive Groups Call on Rep. Norcross to Support Medicare for All
Insidernj.com ; May 4, 2021

Cherry Hill, NJ – On March 17, 2021, Representatives Pramila Jayapal and Debbie Dingell introduced the Medicare for All Act of 2021 (H.R. 1976). For many suffering families across the country, the timeliness of this bill could not be more urgent.

Understanding this urgency, a coalition of progressive organizations within New Jersey's first congressional district have made this issue an immediate priority and are calling on Representative Donald Norcross to sign the legislation as a co-sponsor. "Medicare For All is the only choice. People over profits" – says Pastor Amir Khan of New Beginnings.

"At few moments in history have we collectively understood the gravity and importance of a well functioning, universal healthcare system. We cannot afford to let profiteers keep control of our healthcare any longer. This is a heavily Democratic district. If Rep. Norcross isn't going to lead on this issue, the left will find it easy to unify to challenge him in the years to come," said Sue Altman of the NJ Working Families Alliance.

Mario De Santis, lead organizer with Our Revolution Gloucester County added, "Well before the pandemic, our for-profit healthcare system was characterized by GoFundMe campaigns, medical bankruptcies, and deaths due to rationing medicine and avoiding care due to costs; COVID-19 has only exacerbated these injustices. Any reform that does not permanently guarantee healthcare as a human right is inadequate."

If passed, the legislation would expand the existing Medicare system and provide comprehensive healthcare coverage and services including primary care, hospital and outpatient care, dental, vision, audiology, women's reproductive health services, maternity and newborn care, long-term services and supports, prescription drugs, mental health, substance abuse treatment, laboratory and diagnostic services, and ambulatory services. Patients would maintain the freedom to choose the doctors, hospitals, and other providers they prefer, and the legislation would eliminate insurance premiums, co-pays, and deductibles—no out-of-pocket costs.

Academics suggest that this bill would save 68,000 American lives and save $300-450 billion annually – savings largely due to the reduction in administrative costs and the negotiating power of a Medicare for All system.

Representative Donald Norcross understands the failure of a for-profit healthcare system. On March 17, 2021, he celebrated the bill's introduction on social media: "The United States is the richest country in the world, but millions of Americans still can't afford health care. #MedicareForAll will change that – it's time for a bold change."

Donald Norcross is right; Medicare for All will change that, and, as <u>he did in 2018 with the Expanded & Improved Medicare for All Act, he can support this reform by signing onto the Medicare for All Act of 2021 (H.R. 1976) as a co-sponsor.</u>

<u>https://www.manchin.senate.gov/newsroom/in-the-news/check-up-reveals-major-problems-the-health-of-west-virginia-truly-in-crisis-exponent-telegram</u> (See hyperlink for full text and references.)

Check-Up Reveals Major Problems: The Health of West Virginia Truly in Crisis
18 June 2017 @ manchin.senate.gov

It might be easy to lose sight of this amid a state with a plethora of other problems, but West Virginia has a crisis in health.

Gov. Jim Justice ran his 2016 campaign by rallying West Virginians around a common disillusionment with a penchant for finishing last in measures of national success.

And though West Virginia isn't in last place, many would likely find it disconcerting to know the state ranks 48th in mortality rate, according to a study by the Institute for Health Metrics and Evaluation (IHME).

Various researchers with IHME, an independent population health research organization based out of the University of Washington, used death registration data in order to compile mortality rates for every county in America since 1980. The picture it paints of West Virginia is not a pretty one.

In 2014, the state had a mortality rate of nearly 997 deaths per 100,000 people (the flat rate used nationwide by the study), or roughly 1 percent of the population. For comparison, neighboring Ohio has a rate of about 868, and Virginia 783.

Consultation with the U.S. Centers for Disease Control and Prevention (CDC) gives a similarly stark view of the problems. According to Jeff

Lancashire, a public affairs officer and the acting associate director for communications science with the CDC's National Center for Health Statistics, the mortality rate in 2015 for West Virginia was 943.4 deaths per 100,000 — more than 200 higher than the national rate of 733.1.

The data is alarming and, according to Dr. Lindsay Allen, an incoming assistant professor of health economics at WVU's School of Public Health, the IHME study cannot be explained away by pointing to a large elderly population in West Virginia. "The study in question took age into account, so we can be reasonably sure that the mortality rates stated can be mostly explained by health status," she said. "Health problems in the area can be passed down through generations in ways that aren't necessarily biological. Parental characteristics such as education, income level and insurance status all impact the health of children."

Conventional wisdom would state that most businesses require a healthy populace in order to function at optimal levels. A dearth of that resource is likely a significant contributing factor, then, to the State's economic struggles. "One thing for certain is businesses won't locate here if they can't find the workers they need, and that means drug-free, healthy and trained," said Dr. John Deskins, director of the Bureau of Business and Economic Research at WVU. "It serves as a major barrier to growing the economy, and it puts a major strain on government."

The impact of the health crisis shows in a survey of the state's population trends. According to the 2017-2021 West Virginia Economic Outlook prepared by Deskins' Bureau, 40 of the state's 55 counties saw population decline between 2014 and 2015, even as the United States continues to show consistent and rapid growth.

"And who is going to leave for new jobs?" Deskins asked rhetorically. "The people who have the best education, better health outcomes, who are younger."

Conversely, U.S. Senator Joe Manchin, D-W.Va., said that fixing the economy is key to improving the health situation in West Virginia, noting the importance of keeping youth in the state. "Not only do we need to help people fight addiction so they can rebuild their lives and help rebuild our communities, but we need to bring meaningful job opportunities back to our state," he said. "For decades, our state has faced a decreasing aging population, and we must find ways to keep

West Virginians here and to attract young people to our state to raise families and grow communities." "Why is West Virginia the second poorest state in the country? It goes hand-in-hand with the fact that we have the smallest share of our population in the labor force."

There isn't simply one ailment causing the health issues faced in West Virginia, Lancashire said, but there are a few key contributors. "A few specific causes of death are certainly contributing to high mortality rates in West Virginia," Lancashire said. "For example, cancer is the leading cause of death in West Virginia. In 2015, the mortality rate from cancer in West Virginia was 190.4 deaths per 100,000, significantly higher than the national cancer mortality rate of 158.5."

Regarding cancer, Lancashire noted that lung cancer, in particular, is a problem in West Virginia, especially in the southern portion of the state, well-known for its mining tradition. That might be a significant factor, Allen said. "In the study by Dwyer-Lindgren et al. (the iHME study), the authors found that more people died from chronic respiratory disease in southwestern West Virginia than almost anywhere else in the country," she said. "This is likely due to higher exposure to coal dust in these areas, where there is a lot of coal production. Previous studies have found a direct link between coal dust exposure and chronic respiratory diseases."

And cancer isn't the only problem Lancashire listed. "Also, drug overdose deaths have become a major problem nationally over the last several years, but particularly in certain states, including West Virginia," he said. "In 2015, the mortality rate from drug overdoses in West Virginia was 41.5 deaths per 100,000, significantly higher than the national drug overdose mortality rate of 16.3."

Manchin drew attention to the fact that, as would be expected, West Virginia is also "the most addicted state." "In order to begin combating this problem we need to dramatically increase funding for substance abuse treatment," he said. "That is why I introduced my LifeBOAT bill to require pharma companies to pay a 1 cent fee per milligram to fund substance abuse treatment."

On top of that bill, which congressional records show was last referred to the Senate Committee on Finance and which was co-sponsored by 10 Democrats and one independent, Manchin said a plethora of other action needs to occur. That includes improvement of drug abuse education, improvement of state prescribing practices and the protection of Medicaid funding in the state. "Of the 175,000 West Virginians who have gained health insurance coverage through the Medicaid expansion, 50,000 of them were diagnosed with a substance abuse treatment disorder in 2016," Manchin said. "The state received $112 million in federal funding through the Medicaid expansion to provide services and treatment to those individuals. We desperately need to maintain funding for treatment, not cut it."

More than half a decade has passed since the Affordable Care Act passed under the pen of President Obama in 2010. The act appears to have gained popularity as of late, with a majority of Americans approving of the ACA in most polls taken in 2017.

Allen concurred with Manchin in noting the impact of ACA on Medicaid expansion, calling a future in which the ACA is repealed "unclear" for those who received coverage from the expansion.

Other issues, such as a decrease in government subsidies for care and the likelihood that healthier individuals might not buy care without an individual mandate could serve to drive up premiums and impact affordability for the less affluent, Allen said.

"Rural counties tend to have lower median incomes, and a primary aim of the ACA was making health insurance coverage possible for those who previously could not afford it," she said.

Manchin commented that "we cannot repeal the Affordable Care Act unless we have human legislation to replace it with." "West Virginians would suffer if the House repeal plan was passed today," he said. "In fact, one estimate shows that the House Republican bill would kick more than 120,000 West Virginians off of their health insurance. It would also reduce federal funding through Medicaid for seniors who need nursing home care, students who get health services through their schools, and — as I mentioned before — significantly reduce funding for substance abuse treatment."

Manchin also said that those he has spoken with in rural hospitals fear they might be forced to close their doors if large numbers of their patients lose insurance as some predict.

(Note to readers: It sounds like Senator Joe Manchin – who says "we cannot repeal the Affordable Care Act unless we have human legislation to replace it with" - should be in favor of "Medicare for All" when it is next introduced in the U.S. Senate.)

Also about West Virginia: An excerpt from the article "To Understand Life Expectancy Fall, Start in West Virginia" by Mike Stobbe (apnews.com, 18 December 2018): "We want to give people hope that we can be knocked off the unhealthiest list" of states, said Kayla Wright, director of an organization called Try This West Virginia (https://trythiswv.com/).

https://www.riseupwv.org/medicareforall
(See hyperlink for full text and references.)

RISE UP WEST VIRGINIA
www.facebook.com/RiseUpWV

Healthcare is a human right. Yet too many West Virginians cannot get the care they need.

Meanwhile, CEOs in the healthcare and pharmaceutical industries are among the highest paid in the country. The largest six health insurance corporations earned $6 billion in profits in the second quarter of 2017, up 29% from the prior year. We pay more for healthcare than any other developed country, but we have among the worst health outcomes. We need a healthcare system that works for all of us.

That's why - even as we advocate against repeal of the Affordable Care Act and cuts to Medicaid - we are pushing for a "Medicare for All" universal healthcare system that would cover everyone.

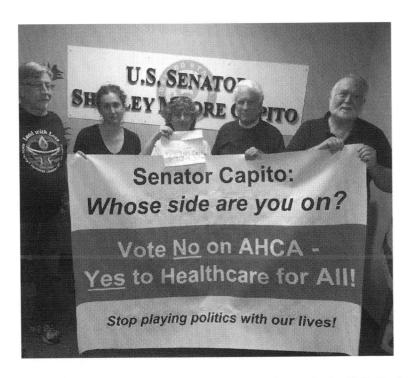

To locate your Senators and/or your Representative, call the U.S. Capitol switchboard at (202) 224-3121. Or find your senators by state at: **https://www.senate.gov/senators/senators-contact.htm**

SPREADING THE WORD on MEDICARE FOR ALL

President Biden has spoken of improving The Affordable Care Act. Does the ACA make provisions for 21-year-old orphans who can't be on their parents' health insurance? How do we improve on a program that has a 40-year-old non-smoking individual being forced annually to decide between premiums of $436 per month for the lowest-cost silver plan and $328 per month for a bronze plan through "The ACA Marketplace"?

You have a body and that should have nothing to do with silver or bronze! You need healthcare – comprehensive health care – no matter what life throws your way! It shouldn't matter that you live in New York City or in Tombstone, Arizona. Nor should it matter your age, employment, income, military status or ethnicity.

Two cable hosts – Ali Velshi and Lawrence O'Donnell – have taken a clear stand in favor of Medicare For All. They and other commentators need to give this critically important issue the full attention it deserves.

THE TIME IS NOW for frequent in-depth on-air interviews of the many M4All advocates, experts and organization leaders mentioned in this book.

In closing, we provide as comprehensive a list of advocates and organizations as we can – and we look forward to their names, organizations and outreach becoming familiar (with the help of the media) to voters all across our country:

> Dr. Susan Rogers, President of PNHP (Physicians for a National Health Program)

> Bonnie Castillo, Executive Director and Co-Presidents Deborah Burger, Zenei Triunfo-Cortez and Jean Ross, National Nurses United

> Benjamin Day, Executive Director of Healthcare-NOW!

> Rhiannon Duryea, National Coordinator of the Labor Campaign for Single-Payer Health Care

> Sue Saltmarsh, Founder DUH (Demand Universal Healthcare!) and PEP (https://www.peopleenergizingpolitics.org/)

> Dr. Margaret Flowers, H.O.P.E. (Health Over Profit for Everyone)

> Dr. Wendell Potter, Creator of Tarbell.org: https://tarbell.org/what-is-tarbell/ - "a global source for objective news in Healthcare, Culture, Environment, Aerospace and Defense."

> Bishop William Barber: Founder, Repairers of The Breach and Co-Chair, Poor People's Campaign

> Single Payer Action: **https://www.singlepayeraction.org/**

http://healthoverprofit.org/join-as-an-organization/

Member Organizations of
HOPE: Health Over Profit for Everyone

Backbone Campaign - CODEPINK - Colleges Organizing for Medical Access of Connecticut (COMA-CT) - Demand Universal Healthcare (DUH) - Eastern Panhandle Single Payer Action Network - Healthcare For All Hawaii - Health Care for All-Los Angeles Chapter - Healthcare for All Texas - Healthcare for All, Y'all! - Healthcare is a Human Right Maryland - Indivisible Omaha - Indivisible Montgomery County - Medicare for All Michigan - Medicare for All, NJ - Medicare for All, Northern IL - People For a New Society - People's Health Movement USA - Popular Resistance - Santa Clara County Single Payer Health Care Coalition - Single Payer Action - United for Single Payer - Women's Health Institute

https://www.ncm4a.org/member_organizations

Member Organizations of
The North Carolina Medicare for All Coalition

Action NC - AMEXCAN - Apoyo NC - Asheville DSA - Black Workers for Justice - Carolina Peace Center - Center for Justice and Reconciliation (NC NAACP) - Charlotte DSA - The Coalition for Health Care of NC - Down Home - Duke SNAHP - Durham For All - Emancipate NC - Fayetteville PACT - Health Care for All Western NC - Health Care for All NC - Health Care for All UNC - Health Care Justice UNCC - Health Care Justice NC - Health Care for All Y'all - League of Women Voters of the Piedmont Triad - Muslims for Social Justice - Muslim Women For - NARAL Pro Choice NC - National Nurses United - NC Alliance for Retired Americans - NC Citizens For Public Health -

NC Council of Churches - NC Green Party - NC NAACP - NC Raise Up/Fight for $15 - NC Poor People's Campaign - NC Public Service Workers Union, UE Local 150 - Planned Parenthood South Atlantic - Red Oak United Methodist - Southern Anti Racism Network (SARN) - Southern Workers Assembly - Triangle DSA - Winston Salem DSA - Women's International League for Peace and Freedom of the Triangle (WILPF).

Organizations Endorsing H.R. 1976 as of 17 March 2021
https://www.commondreams.org/newswire/2021/03/17/jayapal-introduces-medicare-all-act-2021-alongside-more-half-house-democratic (orgs endorsing 1976)

National Organizations endorsing H.R.1976

AF3IRM - AIDS Healthcare Foundation - American Medical Student Association - American Muslim Health Professionals - American Postal Workers Union - Asian Pacific American Labor Alliance - AFL-CIO - Association of Flight Attendants - CWA - Bayard Rustin Liberation Initiative - Be A Hero - Blue Future - Brotherhood of Maintenance of Way Employees - Business Leaders for Health Care Transformation - Businesses for a Livable Climate - CASA - Catch Fire Movement - CatholicNetwork.US - Center for Health and Democracy - Center for LGBTQ Economic Advancement & Research (CLEAR) - Center for Popular Democracy Action - Color Of Change - Debs-Jones-Douglass Institute - Democracy for America - Democratic Socialists of America – DUH (Demand Universal Healthcare) - Earth Action, Inc. - Equality Federation - Faith in Healthcare For All - GreenFaith - Healthcare-NOW - Indivisible - International Alliance of Theatrical Stage Employees (IATSE) - International - Federation of Professional and Technical Engineers (IFPTE) - Justice Democrats - Labor Campaign for Single Payer - MoveOn - MPower Change - Muslim Delegates and Allies - NAACP - National Council of Churches of Christ in the USA - National Domestic Workers Alliance - National Center for Lesbian Rights - National Education Association, National Educators United (NEU) - National Health Care for the Homeless Council - National Immigration Law Center - National Korean American Service & Education Consortium (NAKASEC) - National Nurses United - National Organization for Women - National Union of Healthcare Workers - NETWORK Lobby for Catholic Social Justice - One Fair Wage - Opioid

Network - Center for Popular Democracy Action - Other98 - Our Revolution - P.A.I.N. (Prescription Addiction Intervention Now) - Partners for Dignity & Rights - People's Action - Pharmacists for Single Payer - Physicians for a National Health Program - Positive Women's Network-USA - Progressive Democrats of America - Progressives for Democracy in America - Public Citizen - RAICES - RapidShift Network - SEIU - Social Security Works - Sunrise Movement - The Committee of Interns and Residents - SEIU - The Zero Hour with RJ Eskow - UltraViolet Action - Union for Reform Judaism - United Electrical, Radio & Machine Workers of America (UE) - United Mine Workers of America - United We Dream - Utility Workers Union of America - Voto Latino - Women's March.

State Organizations endorsing H.R.1976

Action NC - AF3IRM Hawai'i - Alaskans Take A Stand - Arizona Educators United (AEU) - Arizona People's Party - Arizona Progressive People's Alliance - Arkansas Community Organization - Arkansas Community Organizations - Arizona Working Families Party - AZ Medicare for All Updated March 17, 2021 Coalition - Call to Action Colorado - Campaign for NY Health - CASA - Citizen Action of Wisconsin - Colorado Businesses for a Livable Climate - Colorado Foundation for Universal Health Care - Columbia Legal Services - Communities United - DelACA (Delaware Alliance for Community Advancement) - Democratic Progressive Caucus of Florida - FreedomBLOC - Health Care for All Minnesota - Health Care for All Oregon - Health Care for All Oregon-Action - Health Care for All Pennsylvania - Healthcare is a Human Right Maryland - Hometown Action - HOPE in the Midwest - Health Over Profit for Everyone - Indivisible California Statewide - Indivisible Colorado Action Network - Indivisible Illinois - Indivisible Tennessee - Iowa Citizens for Community Improvement - Land Stewardship Project - Maine AFL-CIO - Mainers for Accountable Leadership - Make the Road Nevada - Make the Road New York - Maryland Progressive Healthcare Coalition - Massachusetts Nurses Association - Mass-Care: the Massachusetts Campaign for Single-Payer Health Care - Michigan United - Minnesota Indivisible Alliance - Minnesota Nurses Association - Montana Human Rights Network - NAKASEC Virginia - New Hampshire Youth Movement - NJ State Industrial Union Council - New Jersey Working

Families Alliance - New York State Nurses Association - NJ State Industrial Union Council - Not Me Us, FL - Ohio Organizing Collaborative - OLÉ (Organizers in the Land of Enchantment) - One Fair Wage Arizona, OneAmerica - Our Revolution Washington Berniecrats Coalition - Our Future WV - Our Revolution Maryland - Our Revolution New Jersey - Our Revolution Ohio - Our Revolution Oregon - Our Revolution Texas - Our Revolution Virginia - PDA California - PDA Colorado - PDA Nebraska - PDA NJ - PDA Oregon - PDA South Carolina - Phoenix Democratic Socialists of America - Physicians for a National Health Program, Maryland Chapter - Physicians for a National Health Program, Minnesota (PNHP-MN) - Progressive Democrats of America, Arizona Chapter - Progressive Democrats of America, Massachusetts - Progressive Democrats of America, Central New Mexico - Progressive Democrats of America, Central New Mexico Chapter - Progressive Democrats of America, Florida Chapter - Progressive Democrats of America, Maryland - Progressive Democrats of America, Virginia - Progressive Democrats of Colorado Initiative of CDP - Progressive Democrats of Guam - Progressive Democrats of Hawaii - Rights & Democracy (NH + VT) - River Valley Organizing - South Carolina AFL-CIO - SPAN Ohio - Stand Up Alaska - Step Up Louisiana - Sustainable Energy & Economy Network - TakeAction Minnesota - Texas Organizing Project – Whole Washington - WV Citizen Action Group - Vermont State Labor Council, AFL-CIO.

Local Organizations endorsing H.R.1976

Action for a Better Tomorrow - Sauk Valley - AF3IRM NY/NJ - AF3IRM SF Bay Area - Arvadans for Progressive Action - Asian Counseling and Referral Service - Asian American Health Research Group (AAPIHRG) - AWAKE Palm Beach County - Bend the Arc: Champaign-Urbana - Broward For Progress, Broward PDA - Bus For Progress - Butte County Health Care Coalition - Cape May County Indivisible - Cobb Progressive Democrats of America, CobbPDA - Cuyahoga County Progressive Caucus - Democracy for Monroe County - Democratic Progressive Caucus of Tampa Bay - Democratic Socialists of America, Los Angeles - Democrats of Hemet-San Jacinto - Denver PDA - DFA Palm Beach County - Essex Rising - Freeport Indivisible - Fremont County Indivisible of Colorado - Goshen Indivisible - Green Mountain Labor Council, AFL-CIO - HANA Center Health Updated

March 17, 2021 - Care is a Human Right - Maryland, Frederick County - Health Care Justice--NC - Healthcare is an Act of Love - Indivisible 121 - Indivisible Brookfield - Indivisible Cayuga - Indivisible Chicago-South Side - Indivisible DuPage - Indivisible Evansville - Indivisible GA 04 - Indivisible Grapevine Area - Indivisible in Anchorage - Indivisible Indiana District 2 - Indivisible Indiana 8th District - Indivisible Northwestern University - Indivisible Printers Row - Indivisible Rochester - Indivisible San Francisco - Indivisible Shawnee - Indivisible South Bay Los Angeles - Indivisible South Suburban Chicago - Indivisible West Suburban Action League - Indivisible Western Springs and Surrounding Communities – Indivisible WIL Crystal Lake - Jane Addams Senior Caucus - Jefferson County Progressives - LA Poor People's Campaign - LD24 Democrats - Lehigh Valley Medicare for All - Los Amigos of Orange County CA - Metro DC Democratic Socialists of America - Michiana Medicare4all - Monmouth County Democratic Progressive Caucus - Muncie Resists - Northridge Indivisible - NYC Democratic Socialists of America - Ocean County Progressives - Orange County Equality Coalition - Our Revolution, Gloucester County, New Jersey - Our Revolution Central Willamette - Our Revolution Colorado Springs & CD 5 - Our Revolution Essex County - Our Revolution Howard County - Our Revolution MD Anne Arundel - Our Revolution Metro Denver - Our Revolution Monmouth County NJ - Our Revolution Mountain Colorado - Our Revolution Northern Virginia (ORNOVA) - Our Revolution Portland - Our Revolution Prince William - Our Revolution South Central Virginia - Our Revolution Trenton Mercer - Our Revolution/ Progressive Democrats of America Antelope Valley - OurRev305 - PDA CD-24 - The People's Progressive Caucus of Miami-Dade - PDA Central Florida - PDA Oakland Chapter - PDA Orange Co CA Chapter - PDA Rockdale County - PDA San Francisco Chapter - PDA South Orange County - PDA-Chapter Leader-Central Texas - PDA-Riverside - PDA-San Fernando Valley Chapter - Phoenix Democratic Socialists of America - Phoenix Workers Alliance - Prince George's County Peace & Justice Coalition - Progressive Democrats of America (PDA) - East Valley Arizona - Progressive Democrats of America Calumet Region - Progressive Democrats of America of North Central Texas - Progressive Democrats of America - Palm Beach County Chapter - Progressive Democrats of America: Tucson Chapter - Progressive Democrats of the Santa Monica Mountains - Progressives for

Democracy in America Central Florida - Rio Grande Indivisible - Rise Up WV - San Antonio PDA - San Gabriel Valley Progressives - San Luis Obispo County Democratic Party - San Mateo County Democracy for America - SEIU 888 - Sierra County Indivisible - Social Justice Indivisible - South Bay SNaHP - South Hampton Roads for Bernie - SPACEs in Action - Sumter Speaks - Sunrise Movement Tempe - UNITE HERE Local 11 - Uptown Progressive Action - Western Front Indivisible - Woori Center.

https://www.commondreams.org/news/2021/07/24/medicare-all-advocates-take-streets-over-50-us-cities
(See hyperlink for full text and references.)

Medicare for All Advocates Take to the Streets of Over 50 US Cities

By Jessica Corbett, Staff Writer, Common Dreams ; 25 July 2021

Just days before the 56th anniversary of Medicare being signed into law, advocates for creating a public, universal health insurance program in the United States to replace the largely private, for-profit system held marches in more than 50 cities across the country on Saturday.

The day of action was organized by a coalition of over 100 groups, from Mainers for Accountable Leadership, the Chicago Teachers Union, and Sunrise Movement Seattle to various arms of Democratic Socialists of America, Physicians for a National Health Program (PNHP), and Our Revolution.

"Our movement was founded from a place of compassion and love," the coalition's website explains (see m4m4all.org). "We came together out of frustration with the lack of action from the powers that be."

"Many of us have our own personal stories as to why we are in this fight," the coalition continues. "All of us know that healthcare is a right, not a privilege. It is a basic freedom. How can we have life, liberty, and the pursuit of happiness when we live in constant fear of illness, bankruptcy, or homelessness because of the outrageous for-profit healthcare system?"

Highlighting that "universal healthcare isn't radical," the coalition points to more than 30 other countries that have it — from Australia, Canada, Germany, and Iceland, to Japan, Kuwait, South Korea, and the United Kingdom.

"Like most Americans, when the Covid pandemic shut down our country, we thought this was it — America would finally catch up to the rest of the developed world and have a healthcare system that is free at the point of service," says a petition from the coalition. "As we all know, this did not happen... yet!"

UNIVERSAL HEALTHCARE ISN'T RADICAL

☑ Australia
☑ Austria
☑ Bahrain
☑ Belgium
☑ Brunei
☑ Canada
☑ Cyprus
☑ Denmark
☑ Finland
☑ France
☑ Germany

☑ Greece
☑ Hong Kong
☑ Iceland
☑ Ireland
☑ Israel
☑ Italy
☑ Japan
☑ Kuwait
☑ Luxembourg
☑ Netherlands
☑ New Zealand

☑ Norway
☑ Portugal
☑ Singapore
☑ Slovenia
☑ South Korea
☑ Spain
☑ Sweden
☑ Switzerland
☑ U.A.E.
☑ United Kingdom
⊗ United States

30-SECOND M4A CONVERSATIONS: You Can Advocate for Universal Healthcare Anywhere, Anytime! https://www.ncm4a.org/30_second_m4a_conversations

https://www.ncm4a.org/m4a2021

N.C. OFFICIALS AND BIDEN ADMINISTRATION:
PEOPLE ARE DYING WITHOUT MEDICARE FOR ALL! PASS THE BILL!

Dear President Joseph Biden, Vice-President Kamala Harris, the Health and Human Services Secretary Xavier Becerra, Senator Richard Burr, Senator Thom Tillis, Rep. G.K. Butterfield, Rep. Elect Deborah Ross, Rep. Greg Murphy, Rep. David Price, Rep. Virginia Foxx, Rep. Elect Kathy Manning, Rep. David Rouzer, Rep. Richard Hudson, Rep. Dan Bishop, Rep. Patrick McHenry, Rep. Elect Madison Cawthorn, Rep. Alma Adams, and Rep. Ted Budd -

People are continuing to get sick, die, and face financial ruin from COVID-19 raging out of control. Our jobs and insurance plans are not secure, if we have them. We must, as a country, find policy solutions that address our interconnected problems, and we believe that starts by passing Improved Medicare For All. Therefore we are urging the entire N.C. Congressional delegation as well as the Biden administration to support the passage and implementation of the H.R. 1976 - The Medicare For All Act of 2021 - and then its Senate companion bill when it is re-introduced.

We must admit that even before COVID-19, our country was facing a healthcare crisis. We continue to spend almost double what other industrialized countries spend per capita on healthcare, and yet more than 87 million of our people are either uninsured or underinsured, meaning they can't afford to use the insurance they have.

In addition, our nation's health outcomes in areas like life expectancy and maternal and infant mortality rates continue to be among the worst in the developed world. The Affordable Care Act and our employer-based healthcare system have failed us during this public health crisis and no amount of tweaking will make this profit-driven system cover everyone and control costs. A public option will just be another layer in our costly, inefficient multi-payer system.

This pandemic has produced immense economic strain, a climbing death toll, and rapid loss of employer-based insurance (for those fortunate to have it). Within this unjust system, Black, Latinx, Indigenous, and other marginalized people are forced to bear the harshest impacts. Dying of COVID-19 at higher rates, people of color also account for 54 percent of North Carolina's uninsured while making up only 37 percent of the population. Furthermore, an estimated 257,000 North Carolinians lost their health insurance and jobs during the first six months of the COVID-19 pandemic, increasing our state's uninsured rate to 20 percent for people under age 65, one of the highest uninsured rates in the nation.

This "crossroads" moment demands we imagine a new future where healthcare is a human right for all of us - youth, seniors, low-wage workers, disabled individuals, justice-system involved folk, domestic violence and sexual assault survivors, veterans, the LGBTQIA community, the undocumented community, people who need reproductive health services, and more. We must join together in an intersectional movement that shines light on the interconnected injustices we face and builds power to overcome them. We must reject platitudes and half-measures as we work to achieve true health justice and equity with a universal, single-payer healthcare system that eliminates financial barriers to seeking care.

Improved Medicare for All not only means freedom from the financial stress of medical bills, it also means a country that is safer, healthier and more productive because every person is covered. Moreover, a single-payer, universal health-care system is estimated to lead to a 13 percent savings in national healthcare expenditure, equivalent to more than **$450 billion annually**, according to a recent study by Yale University. Additionally, researchers estimated that ensuring healthcare access for all Americans with a universal system would save more than **68,000 lives** each year compared with the status quo.

Not only is a universal, single-payer system the right and most economically feasible policy, it's also clearly more popular among Americans than the current system. According to a November 2020 Fox News poll, 72 percent of voters favor a universal, government-administered health care plan. A CNN exit poll of N.C. voters in the 2020 Democratic primary found majority support for replacing private insurance with a "government" plan. Overall, Republicans and

Democrats have tended to favor Medicare For All with consistency.

The COVID-19 pandemic has made the need for a healthcare system that values people over profits more urgent than ever before. Therefore, we the undersigned urge the Biden administration to support passage of Medicare For All. We urge the entire N.C. Congressional delegation to sign on as co-sponsors of the new bills - H.R. 1976 in the House and the companion bill when introduced in the Senate, so the U.S. may join the rest of the developed world in making healthcare a human right and not a privilege.

Sincerely,

The North Carolina Medicare for All Coalition

and

Bipartisan Americans across our great country, President Biden!

YES, PEOPLE ARE DYING WITHOUT MEDICARE FOR ALL!

PASS THE BILL!

AND PUT A "MEDICARE FOR ALL" CARD IN EVERY WALLET.

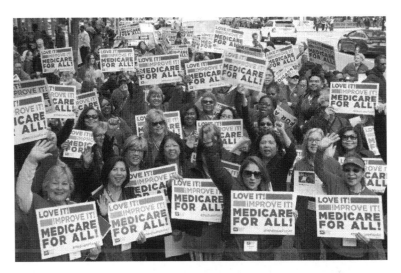

Become a Citizen Co-Sponsor by posting to
#MedicareForAll & https://medicare4all.org/

 MEDICARE FOR ALL!

BIBLIOGRAPHY

DEDICATION

- https://www.peopleenergizingpolitics.org/
- https://youtu.be/BoiarllLjD4

FOREWORD

- https://catalog.upenn.edu/courses/hcin/

CHAPTER 1: Now Is The Time

- https://pnhp.org/news/two-thirds-of-voters-support-providing-medicare-to-every-american/
- https://www.defense.gov/Explore/Spotlight/FY2021-Defense-Budget/
- https://www.fiercehealthcare.com/payer/unitedhealth-s-wichmann-to-earn-2-years-salary-bonuses-post-retirement
- https://www.congress.gov/bill/116th-congress/senate-bill/1129/text
- https://www.congress.gov/bill/117th-congress/house-bill/1976/text

CHAPTER 2: True Bipartisanship

- https://www.washingtonpost.com/opinions/2021/02/10/why-dont-republicans-get-challenged-bipartisanship/
- https://www.politifact.com/article/2021/feb/08/what-you-need-know-about-budget-reconciliation-pro/
- https://www.rasmussenreports.com/public_content/politics/mood_of_america/rate_congress_april13
- https://www.newsweek.com/69-percent-americans-want-medicare-all-including-46-percent-republicans-new-poll-says-1500187
- https://www.politico.com/interactives/2019/how-to-fix-politics-in-america/gridlock/

CHAPTER 3: Personal Stories

- https://www.cdc.gov/wtc/about.html
- https://nymag.com/intelligencer/2019/06/how-lawmakers-protected-and-failed-9-11-first-responders.html
- https://www.cc.com/video/i58xmo/the-daily-show-with-jon-stewart-worst-responders
- https://abcn.ws/2y1suRx
- https://www.youtube.com/watch?v=zmYiW_xMTKc
- https://www.youtube.com/watch?v=_uYpDC3SRpM
- https://www.youtube.com/watch?v=LdbROxCyEx8
- https://www.youtube.com/watch?v=ICnUJl0t0Xw
- https://en.wikipedia.org/wiki/James_Zadroga_9/11_Health_and_Compensation_Act
- https://fealgoodfoundation.com/
- https://www.vice.com/en/article/xgq5jw/surprise-medical-bill-stories-and-private-health-care-insurance
- https://pnhp.org/news/health-care-horror-stories/
- http://www.moderntimesbeer.com/blog/medicare-all-yesterday

CHAPTER 4: A Republican for Single Payer

- http://www.healthcareforalltexas.org/I_Am_A_Republican_Can_We_Talk_About_A_Single_Payer_System.pdf
- https://www.icd10data.com/

CHAPTER 5: Rural Hospitals Are Failing

- http://healthoverprofit.org/2020/03/16/453-rural-hospitals-are-failing-medicare-for-all-would-save-them/

CHAPTER 6: Our Current System

- https://www.kff.org/health-reform/issue-brief/no-surprises-act-implementation-what-to-expect-in-2022/

CHAPTER 7: The Uninsured

- https://www.kff.org/uninsured/report/the-uninsured-and-the-aca-a-primer-key-facts-about-health-insurance-and-the-uninsured-amidst-changes-to-the-affordable-care-act/

- https://www.kff.org/medicaid/issue-brief/the-coverage-gap-uninsured-poor-adults-in-states-that-do-not-expand-medicaid/

CHAPTER 8: Undocumented Immigrants

- https://www.kff.org/racial-equity-and-health-policy/fact-sheet/health-coverage-of-immigrants/

- https://www.healthcare.gov/immigrants/lawfully-present-immigrants/

- https://www.cbsnews.com/news/does-medicare-for-all-cover-undocumented-immigrants-depends-on-who-you-ask/ (hyperlink only w/o article)

CHAPTER 9: The Affordable Care Act

- https://en.wikipedia.org/wiki/Affordable_Care_Act

- https://xpostfactoid.blogspot.com/2016/05/

- https://www.healthinsurance.org/blog/a-post-aca-subsidy-that-already-exists/

CHAPTER 10: The ACA Improved by Biden March 2021

- https://www.yahoo.com/now/obamacare-gets-a-makeover-192140275.html

CHAPTER 11: Medicaid

- https://www.macpac.gov/medicaid-101/

- https://www.healthcare.gov/medicaid-chip/eligibility/

- http://www.medicaid.gov

- https://www.kff.org/medicaid/issue-brief/status-of-state-medicaid-expansion-decisions-interactive-map/

- https://www.nj.com/coronavirus/2020/05/this-troubled-nursing-home-has-most-deaths-in-nj-but-there-were-problems-long-before-deadly-outbreak.html

CHAPTER 12: Children's Health Insurance Program (CHIP)

- https://www.kff.org/other/state-indicator/chip-program-name-and-type/?currenttimeframe=0&sortModel=%7B%22colId%22:%22Location%22,%22sort%22:%22asc%22%7D

- https://en.wikipedia.org/wiki/Children%27s_Health_Insurance_Program

- https://www.healthcare.gov/medicaid-chip/childrens-health-insurance-program/

CHAPTER 13: Indian Health System

- https://en.wikipedia.org/wiki/Indian_Health_Service

CHAPTER 14: World Trade Center Health Program

- https://www.cdc.gov/wtc/about.html

- https://www.cdc.gov/wtc/programvideos.html

- https://fealgoodfoundation.com/updates/

- https://fealgoodfoundation.com/

- www.fox6now.com/news/there-needs-to-be-a-better-system-in-place-wisconsin-9-11-responder-left-waiting-for-treatment

- https://wisconsintechnologycouncil.com/logistics-health-story-is-bright-spot-for-wisconsin/

CHAPTER 15: FEHB Program for Federal Employees

- https://en.wikipedia.org/wiki/Federal_Employees_Health_Benefits_Program

CHAPTER 16: Military & TRICARE Health Systems

- https://www.health.mil/About-MHS

- https://logisticshealth.com/our-company.aspx

- https://en.wikipedia.org/wiki/Tricare

- https://en.wikipedia.org/wiki/Veterans_Health_Administration

CHAPTER 17: VA Health Administration

- https://en.wikipedia.org/wiki/Veterans_Health_Administration

CHAPTER 18: Healthcare For Our Troops Act

- https://kim.house.gov/media/press-releases/reps-kim-and-kelly-introduce-bill-expand-no-fee-healthcare-reserve-and-national

CHAPTER 19: Employment-Based Health Insurance

- https://stanmed.stanford.edu/2017spring/how-health-insurance-changed-from-protecting-patients-to-seeking-profit.html

- https://www.commonwealthfund.org/publications/newsletter-article/us-workers-employment-based-health-insurance-continues-decline

- https://thehill.com/opinion/healthcare/499907-its-time-to-say-goodbye-to-employment-based-health-insurance

- https://www.businessinsider.com/most-americans-employer-based-plans-healthcare-medicare-for-all-2019-8

CHAPTER 20: Original Medicare Parts A & B and Hospice

- www.medicare.gov/coverage

- https://en.wikipedia.org/wiki/Medicare_(United_States)

- https://www.medicare.gov/what-medicare-covers/your-medicare-coverage-choices/how-original-medicare-works

- https://www.medicare.gov/your-medicare-costs/part-a-costs

- https://www.medicareresources.org/basic-medicare-information/what-is-medicare/

- https://www.bcbs.com/medicare/original-medicare?utm_medium=sem&utm_campaign=nmac_sem&utm_sour ce=google_ad&gclid=EAIaIQobChMIubiJvbmD8AIVvOy1Ch3TFQ 2MEAAYASAAEgK2pfD_BwE

- https://www.medicare.gov/what-medicare-covers/what-part-a-covers/how-hospice-works

- https://www.medicare.gov/Pubs/pdf/02154-medicare-hospice-benefits.pdf

CHAPTER 21: MEDIGAP

- https://www.medigapplanners.com/medicare-supplements/medicare-supplement-vs-medicare-advantage/

- https://www.aarp.org/health/medicare-insurance/info-2017/choosing-right-medigap-plan

- https://en.wikipedia.org/wiki/Medigap

CHAPTER 22: Medicare Advantage Part C

- https://www.policygenius.com/medicare/medicare-part-c-plans/

- **https://www.policygenius.com/about**

- https://www.healthline.com/health/medicare/what-are-the-advantages-and-disadvantages-of-medicare-advantage-plans#disadvantages

CHAPTER 23: Medicare Dual-Eligible Plans

- https://eligibility.com/medicare/programs/dual-eligible-definition-qualifications

- https://www.medicaidplanningassistance.org/dual-eligibility-medicare-medicaid/

- https://en.wikipedia.org/wiki/Medicare_dual_eligible

CHAPTER 24: Medicare Special Needs Plans

- https://en.wikipedia.org/wiki/Special_needs_plan

- https://www.cms.gov/Medicare/Health-Plans/SpecialNeedsPlans

- https://www.medicare.gov/sign-up-change-plans/types-of-medicare-health-plans/special-needs-plans-snp

- https://www.medicare.gov/sign-up-change-plans/types-of-medicare-health-plans/how-medicare-special-needs-plans-snps-work

- https://www.cms.gov/Medicare/Health-Plans/SpecialNeedsPlans/I-SNPs

- https://www.macpac.gov/subtopic/medicare-advantage-dual-eligible-special-needs-plans-aligned-with-medicaid-managed-long-term-services-and-supports/

- https://www.macpac.gov/about-macpac/

- https://www.state.nj.us/humanservices/dmahs/clients/d_snp.html

- https://bmchealthservres.biomedcentral.com/articles/10.1186/s12913 -021-06228-3   Cite this article: https://bmchealthservres.biomedcentral.com/articles/10.1186/s12913 -021-06228-3#citeas

CHAPTER 25: Medicare DSNP Food Card

- https://www.uhccommunityplan.com/dual-eligible/benefits/healthy-food-benefit

- https://populationhealth.humana.com/food-card-added-for-70000-members/

CHAPTER 26: Medicare Prescription Part D

- https://www.kff.org/medicare/fact-sheet/an-overview-of-the-medicare-part-d-prescription-drug-benefit/#:~:text=In%202020%2C%2046%20million%20of,enrolled %20in%20Part%20D%20plans.

- https://en.wikipedia.org/wiki/Medicare_Part_D

- https://www.seniorliving.org/prescription-discount-cards/best/

- https://en.wikipedia.org/wiki/GoodRx

- https://www.drugchannels.net/2020/08/how-goodrx-profits-from-our-broken.html

- https://clark.com/health-health-care/singlecare-vs-goodrx-which-is-cheaper/

CHAPTER 27: How Medicare is Paid For

- https://en.wikipedia.org/wiki/Medicare_(United_States)

- https://www.medicare.gov/about-us/how-is-medicare-funded

- https://www.medicare.gov/drug-coverage-part-d/costs-for-medicare-drug-coverage/monthly-premium-for-drug-plans

- https://www.taxpolicycenter.org/briefing-book/what-medicare-trust-fund-and-how-it-financed

- https://www.policygenius.com/medicare/how-is-medicare-funded/
- https://www.medicalnewstoday.com/articles/how-is-medicare-advantage-funded

CHAPTER 28: Medical Savings Accounts: HSA-FSA

- https://en.wikipedia.org/wiki/Health_savings_account
- https://en.wikipedia.org/wiki/Flexible_spending_account

CHAPTER 29: Auto Medical Coverage

- https://www.allstate.com/tr/car-insurance/medical-payments-coverage.aspx

CHAPTER 30: COBRA

- https://www.dol.gov/general/topic/health-plans/cobra
- https://www.dol.gov/sites/dolgov/files/EBSA/about-ebsa/our-activities/resource-center/faqs/cobra-continuation-health-coverage-consumer.pdf

CHAPTER 31: The Downside of Medicare Advantage

- https://www.singlepayeraction.org/2021/03/09/kay-tillow-on-the-downside-of-medicare-advantage-and-the-upside-of-single-payer/
- https://publicintegrity.org/health/why-medicare-advantage-costs-taxpayers-billions-more-than-it-should/
- https://www.fiercehealthcare.com/payer/big-name-payers-earned-35-7-billion-2019-here-s-one-common-thread-their-reports

CHAPTER 32: The Public Option is Bad Policy

- https://www.thenation.com/article/archive/insurance-health-care-medicare/

CHAPTER 33: Kamala Harris' Public Option is Bad Policy

- https://www.thenation.com/article/archive/insurance-health-care-medicare/

CHAPTER 34: Neera Tanden vs True Medicare for All

- https://www.commonwealthclub.org/events/archive/video/citizens-guide-medicare-all

- https://pnhp.org/news/caps-medicare-extra-for-all-what-it-really-is/

- https://pnhp.org/news-category/quote-of-the-day/

- https://www.healthcare-now.org/about/regarding-hcan/

CHAPTER 35: Liz Fowler is Back!

- https://www.counterpunch.org/2021/06/07/liz-fowler-is-back-and-shes-writing-us-health-policy-again/

CHAPTER 36: Our Elected Officials

- https://student.pnhp.org/category/blog/

- Published in The Lens: https://thelensnola.org/2019/04/18/rep-richmond-should-co-sponsor-the-medicare-for-all-act/

CHAPTER 37: Lobbyist: Partnership for America's Health Care Future

- https://theintercept.com/2018/11/20/medicare-for-all-healthcare-industry/

- https://www.politico.com/news/2020/02/26/anti-medicare-for-all-south-carolina-117771

CHAPTER 38: Lobbyist: AHIP

- https://www.ahip.org/ahip-submits-statement-for-congressional-hearing-on-medicare-for-all-legislation/

- https://thehill.com/policy/healthcare/458252-head-of-health-insurance-lobby-responds-to-sanders-we-disclose-all-of-our

CHAPTER 39: RICO: Racketeer Influenced and Corrupt Organizations

- http://www.fbi.gov/elpaso/press-releases/2010/ep090210.htm

- https://www.justice.gov/usao-wdtx/pr/four-sentenced-connection-el-paso-corruption-investigation

- https://www.fiercehealthcare.com/regulatory/health-insurer-lobbying-single-payer-democrats-campaign-contributions

- https://www.theglobalist.com/republican-tax-bill-trump-corruption/

- http://www.differencebetween.net/miscellaneous/politics/difference-between-lobbying-and-bribing/

- https://www.opensecrets.org/federal-lobbying/top-spenders?cycle=2021

CHAPTER 40: History of Single Payer: HC-NOW

- https://www.healthcare-now.org/legislation/national-timeline/

CHAPTER 41: History of Single Payer: PNHP

- https://pnhp.org/a-brief-history-universal-health-care-efforts-in-the-us/

CHAPTER 42: The Congressional Progressive Caucus

- https://progressives.house.gov/caucus-members/

- https://progressivecaucusactionfund.org/issues/healthcare

- https://progressives.house.gov/universal-health-care

- https://static1.squarespace.com/static/53cab2c3e4b0207d2957d0d2/t/605b72e1d6fc1a50a52c01d0/1616605921216/House+Support+for+Medicare+for+All+Growing.pdf

CHAPTER 43: Organizations Promoting Medicare For All

- www.healthcare-now.org

- https://www.laborcampaign.org/resources

- https://pnhp.org/

- https://student.pnhp.org/about/

- https://www.nationalnursesunited.org/

- https://www.facebook.com/groups/858099384918591/

- https://www.facebook.com/groups/182119008587323

- http://healthoverprofit.org/

- tarbell.org

- https://networklobby.org/issues/healthcare/

- https://www.americanswhotellthetruth.org/portraits/dr-rev-william-barber-ii

- https://en.wikipedia.org/wiki/Poor_People%27s_Campaign:_A_Nati onal_Call_for_a_Moral_Revival

- https://wholewashington.org/

CHAPTER 44: Songs & Documentaries

- https://www.youtube.com/watch?v=UQfzAdBhObk

- https://www.youtube.com/watch?v=NsgHm-ZMYvQ

- https://wicklinefamilyandfriends.bandcamp.com/track/medicare-for-all-single-payer-2

- https://www.youtube.com/watch?v=_XWgw3Ea4WU

- http://www.escapefiremovie.com/trailer

- https://www.youtube.com/watch?v=KS-olhBvEkc

- https://www.youtube.com/watch?v=W6c3yhBGGMU

- https://fixithealthcare.com/watch-the-movie/big-money-agenda/

- https://www.youtube.com/watch?v=olRR_wNTd9A&t=237s

- https://www.youtube.com/watch?v=pyC4grL-Uag

- https://www.youtube.com/watch?v=jCVmY1iOJQs

- https://www.commonwealthclub.org/events/archive/video/citizens-guide-medicare-all

- https://www.youtube.com/watch?v=hQV4SZic0lE

- https://www.youtube.com/watch?v=IyGYXEKRQ7c

- https://www.youtube.com/watch?v=1DLHLHpeA-E

- https://www.youtube.com/watch?v=dvP1IaI8m44

- https://www.youtube.com/watch?v=PuqYC-1abVM

- https://vimeo.com/314654894

- https://www.laborcampaign.org/resources

- https://edvideoplus.net/the-healthcare-movie/
- www.nowisthetimemovie.com
- https://www.youtube.com/watch?v=SMiZ1co0S0M
- https://www.youtube.com/channel/UCzAyfuoKs0kc_3fiUQd2PXQ/ videos
- https://www.youtube.com/watch?v=hObcysTDEcE
- https://www.youtube.com/watch?v=YtHYMokr940
- https://www.facebook.com/groups/182119008587323

CHAPTER 45: Books on Medicare For All

- https://www.abebooks.com/first-edition/Case-Medicare-Paperback-Gerald-Friedman-Polity/30558616408/bd
- https://www.forewordreviews.com/reviews/medicare-for-all/
- https://pnhp.org/news/timothy-faust-health-justice-now-a-must-read/
- https://www.youtube.com/watch?v=x0ikEx-qXtg
- http://www.ezekielemanuel.com/
- https://fivebooks.com/best-books/austin-frakt-healthcare-reform/

CHAPTER 46: True Universal Healthcare Fact Sheet

- https://www.congress.gov/bill/116th-congress/senate-bill/1129/text
- https://www.congress.gov/bill/117th-congress/house-bill/1976/text
- https://www.facebook.com/groups/858099384918591/
- www.peopleenergizingpolitics.org/
- https://spanwv.org/
- https://www.nbcnews.com/politics/2020-election/if-roe-v-wade-struck-down-would-sanders-medicare-all-n1024566
- https://www.youtube.com/watch?v=hQV4SZic0lE

CHAPTER 47: PNHP Compares Medicare for All_2021

- https://pnhp.org/system/assets/uploads/2021/03/HouseBill2021_Chart.pdf

CHAPTER 48: Socialized vs Universal

https://www.facebook.com/groups/858099384918591/

CHAPTER 49: Public Health

- https://www.commondreams.org/views/2021/03/20/all-health-public-health?utm

CHAPTER 50: Job Growth with Medicare for All

- https://www.epi.org/publication/medicare-for-all-would-help-the-labor-market/

- https://youtu.be/FEzGZOGuDOA

CHAPTER 51: The Congressional Budget Office (CBO)

- https://www.cbo.gov/system/files/2020-12/56811-Single-Payer.pdf

- https://www.healthaffairs.org/do/10.1377/hblog20210210.190243/full/

- https://pnhp.org/news/congressional-budget-office-scores-medicare-for-all-universal-coverage-for-less-spending/

- https://www.vox.com/policy-and-politics/2019/3/8/18251707/medicare-for-all-bill-senate-filibuster-budget-reconciliation-byrd-rule

- https://www.cbo.gov/publication/56898

CHAPTER 52: Medicare for All Cost Studies

- https://khn.org/news/does-medicare-for-all-cost-more-than-the-entire-budget-biden-says-so-but-numbers-say-no/

- https://www.pnhpnymetro.org/medicare_for_all

- http://www.pnhp.org/publications/nejmadmin.pdf

- https://www.theguardian.com/commentisfree/2019/oct/25/medicare-for-all-taxes-saez-zucman

- https://taxjusticenow.org/#/

- https://www.thelancet.com/journals/lancet/article/PIIS0140-6736(19)33019-3/fulltext

- https://www.salon.com/2020/02/22/multiple-studies-show-medicare-for-all-would-be-cheaper-than-public-option-pushed-by-moderates/

- https://www.acpjournals.org/doi/10.7326/M19-2818

- https://journals.plos.org/plosmedicine/article?id=10.1371/journal.pmed.1003013

- https://www.thenation.com/article/archive/insurance-health-care-medicare/

- https://thehill.com/blogs/congress-blog/healthcare/484301-22-studies-agree-medicare-for-all-saves-money

- https://justcareusa.org/

- https://journals.plos.org/plosmedicine/article?id=10.1371/journal.pmed.1003013

- https://jacobinmag.com/2020/04/coronavirus-medicare-for-all-m4a-single-payer-health-insurance

- https://www.desmoinesregister.com/story/opinion/columnists/2018/10/04/its-time-get-profits-out-health-care/1514500002/

- https://www.fiercehealthcare.com/payer/health-insurance-ceos-took-home-a-hefty-pay-day-2018-how-does-compare-to-their-employees

- https://www.latimes.com/business/story/2019-08-05/health-insurance-useless

- http://healthoverprofit.org/2020/03/03/more-than-a-third-of-u-s-healthcare-costs-go-to-bureaucracy/

- https://berniesanders.com/issues/how-does-bernie-pay-his-major-plans

- https://www.cms.gov/Research-Statistics-Data-and-Systems/Statistics-Trends-and-Reports/NationalHealthExpendData/NationalHealthAccountsProjected

- https://www.thelancet.com/journals/lancet/article/PIIS0140-6736(19)33019-3/fulltext#%20

- http://healthoverprofit.org/2020/03/16/20-top-economists-endorse-medicare-for-all-as-best-plan-to-cut-costs-save-tens-of-thousands-of-lives-each-year/

- https://www.msnbc.com/ali-velshi/watch/medicare-for-all-what-it-could-mean-for-u-s-health-care-system-1444442179884

CHAPTER 52: Cost Studies links in plos.org article

- https://www.mercatus.org/system/files/blahous-costs-medicare-mercatus-working-paper-v1_1.pdf

- https://www.cbo.gov/publication/16595

- https://www.healthcare-now.org/wp-content/uploads/2017/08/Maryland-Friedman-2013.pdf

- https://www.healthcare-now.org/single-payer-studies/gerald-friedman-2013/

- https://www.healthcare-now.org/wp-content/uploads/2017/08/Pennsylvania-Friedman-2013.pdf

- http://www.infoshare.org/main/Economic_Analysis_New_York_Health_Act_-_GFriedman_-_April_2015.pdf

- https://www.gao.gov/products/T-HRD-91-35

- https://jamanetwork.com/journals/jama/article-abstract/385948

- https://hcr.vermont.gov/sites/hcr/files/FINAL_REPORT_Hsiao_Final_Report_17_February%202011_3.pdf

- https://www.healthcare-now.org/wp-content/uploads/2017/08/Maryland-Lewin-Group-2000.pdf

- https://www.healthcare-now.org/wp-content/uploads/2017/08/California-Lewin-2002.pdf

- https://www.healthcare-now.org/single-payer-studies/minnesota-lewin-group-2012/

- https://www.rand.org/pubs/rgs_dissertations/RGSD375.html

- https://www.rand.org/pubs/research_reports/RR2424.html

- https://www.peri.umass.edu/publication/item/996-economic-analysis-of-the-healthy-california-single-payer-health-care-proposal-sb-562

- https://www.peri.umass.edu/publication/item/1127-economic-analysis-of-medicare-for-all

- https://www.bu.edu/sph/files/2012/07/UHC-1-Nov-00-FINAL.pdf

- https://www.rand.org/pubs/research_reports/RR1662.html

CHAPTER 53: HR 1976 Rolled Out March 17, 2021 for 117th Congress

https://www.commondreams.org/newswire/2021/03/17/jayapal-introduces-medicare-all-act-2021-alongside-more-half-house-democratic

CHAPTER 54: HR Bill 1976 Table of Contents_Pramila Jayapal

- https://www.congress.gov/bill/117th-congress/house-bill/1976/text

CHAPTER 55: HR Bill 1976 Explained

- https://www.congress.gov/bill/117th-congress/house-bill/1976

- https://jayapal.house.gov/wp-content/uploads/2019/02/Medicare-for-All-Act-of-2019-Section-by-Section-Summary.pdf

CHAPTER 56: Senate Bill 1129 Table of Contents_Bernie Sanders

- https://www.congress.gov/bill/116th-congress/senate-bill/1129/text

CHAPTER 57: Senate Bill 1129 Explained

- https://www.congress.gov/bill/116th-congress/senate-bill/1129/text

CHAPTER 58: PNHP on S1129 & HR 1976

- https://pnhp.org/news/doctors-group-welcomes-sen-sanders-medicare-for-all-bill-2/

- https://www.congress.gov/bill/116th-congress/senate-bill/1129/cosponsors

- https://www.congress.gov/bill/117th-congress/house-bill/1976/cosponsors

- https://www.senate.gov/senators/senators-contact.htm.

- www.pnhp.org

CHAPTER 59: Lobbying Your Members of Congress

- https://www.insidernj.com/press-release/coalition-local-progressive-groups-call-rep-norcross-support-medicare/

- https://www.manchin.senate.gov/newsroom/in-the-news/check-up-reveals-major-problems-the-health-of-west-virginia-truly-in-crisis-exponent-telegram

- https://trythiswv.com/

- https://www.riseupwv.org/medicareforall

- https://www.senate.gov/senators/senators-contact.htm

CHAPTER 60: Get Involved

- https://www.peopleenergizingpolitics.org/

- https://tarbell.org/what-is-tarbell/

- https://www.singlepayeraction.org/

- http://healthoverprofit.org/join-as-an-organization/

- https://www.ncm4a.org/member_organizations

- https://www.commondreams.org/newswire/2021/03/17/jayapal-introduces-medicare-all-act-2021-alongside-more-half-house-democratic (orgs endorsing 1976)

- https://www.commondreams.org/news/2021/07/24/medicare-all-advocates-take-streets-over-50-us-cities

- https://www.ncm4a.org/30_second_m4a_conversations

- https://www.ncm4a.org/m4a2021

- #MedicareForAll & https://medicare4all.org/

Made in the USA
Columbia, SC
29 May 2022